INTRODUCTION TO NUTRITION

Pantelis Protopapas

ALLIED HEALTH PRESS

Introduction to Nutrition

Author: **Pantelis Protopapas**

Allied Health Press
4164 Lakeshore Road
Burlington ON L7L 1A4
Canada
www.alliedhealthpress.com
Email: orders@arclereducation.com

ISBN: 978-1-77956-255-5

ABOUT THE AUTHOR

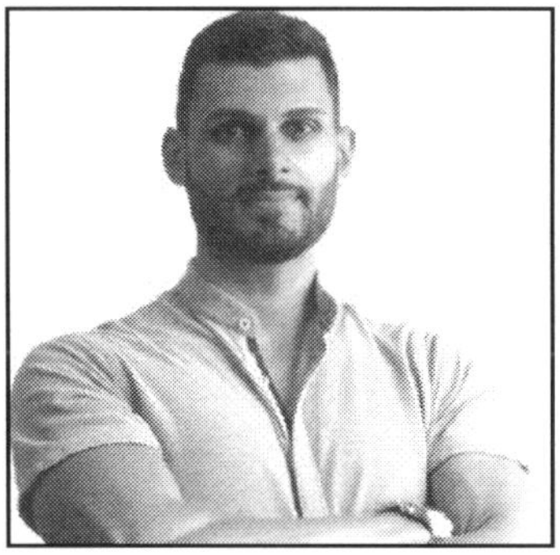

Pantelis Protopapas has acquired his Bachelor's degree in Food Science & Nutrition (with Honours) from Coventry University, England in 2017. After obtaining a Master's degree in Clinical Dietetics from the University of Nicosia in 2021, he has been working as a Clinical Dietitian - Nutritionist ever since, focusing on prevention and treatment of various conditions & illnesses through dietary intervention and nutritional education.

Word Roots, Prefixes, and Suffixes by Chapter

Chapter 1 Introduction to Nutrition

nutri: (food) nourish, nourishment, nutrient, nutrition
Phage: To eat
Derm-: Skin
-ose: Simple sugar
-in: Protein

Chapter 2 Tools of Nutrition

Troph: Food, nutrition, nourish
Vore: One who eats
im-: imbibe (drink in, take in)
-ose: Simple sugar
-in: Protein

Chapter 3 Energy

Stoma: Mouth
aqua-: water
corp-, corpor-, corpu-: body
dyn-: be able; power; energy
-cracy: rule; strength

Chapter 4 Macronutrients

Sacchar-: Monosaccharide (simple sugar)
Di-: Disaccharide (two sugar molecules)
Lip-: Lipid (fat)
-ose: Glucose, Fructose
-ase: Enzymes

Chapter 5 Micronutrients

Vita-: Vitamin (essential for life)
Micro-: Micronutrient (a nutrient needed in small amounts)
Macro-: Macronutrient (a nutrient needed in large amounts)
myo-: Muscle
Anti-: Antioxidant (a substance that inhibits oxidation)
-oid: Carotenoid (a class of pigments found in plants)
-ate: (salt or ester of an acid)

Chapter 6 Water and Electrolytes

calc/i: calcium
caud/o: tail, toward the lower part of the body
ichthy/o: fish
Electro-: electrolyte
Hypo-: Indicates a lower amount
estuar-: the sea
fum-: smoke

Chapter 7 Nutrients Important for Metabolism and Blood Function

Phago: Eat, Feed
Gyn: Woman
-cyte: Cell
-emia: Blood condition
lact-: Milk
-ol: Alcohol
-ine: Amino acid

Chapter 8 Medical Nutrition Therapy and Evidence-Based Nutrition Care

Somat/o-, Somatico-: Body; Bodily
Pharmaco-: Drug; Medicine
Oxy-: Sharp; Acute; Oxygen
Crani/o-: Brain
Gastr-: Stomach
carcin-: cancer
-tuss-, -tussi-: cough

Chapter 9 Nutrition Counseling and Documentation

Diabet: related to diabetes (e.g., diabetic, diabetes)
glyco -: Glycometabolism
anti-: against (e.g., antioxidant, antibiotic)
- lysis: Glycolysis
-trophy: nourishment or development (e.g., hypertrophy, atrophy)

Table of Contents

LIST OF FIGURES

LIST OF TABLES

PREFACE

Nutrition occupies a pivotal role in the foundation of health and the overarching process of human development. It is an essential determinant of well-being, profoundly influencing an individual's health trajectory from the earliest stages of life into old age. The relationship between nutrition and health is reciprocal and dynamic; optimal nutrition not only supports physical and cognitive development but also fortifies the immune system, enhances maternal health outcomes, sharpens mental faculties, and significantly reduces the likelihood of encountering a myriad of chronic conditions, including but not limited to diabetes, cardiovascular diseases, and various metabolic disorders.

A well-balanced and nutritious diet serves as the cornerstone for sustaining a healthy pregnancy, mitigating the risk of chronic health issues, and maintaining an ideal body weight. The quality and composition of the food consumed play a crucial role in determining an individual's nutritional status. Diets rich in essential nutrients support the body's needs, promoting growth, vitality, and the prevention of diseases. Conversely, a diet deficient in these vital components, or one that excessively includes processed, sugary, fatty, and overly salted foods, can lead to malnutrition. This state of nutritional imbalance encompasses both spectrums of malnutrition: undernutrition, which includes micronutrient deficiencies, and overnutrition, characterized by overweight and obesity. Both conditions pose significant health risks and are increasingly prevalent in the contemporary world, reflecting the complexities of modern dietary patterns and food systems.

For the human body to operate at its optimum, to grow and develop correctly, and to maintain robust health, a sufficient intake of both macronutrients (such as proteins, carbohydrates, fats, and water) and micronutrients (including vitamins and minerals) is imperative. Macronutrients provide the energy necessary for the body's fundamental functions and activities, whereas micronutrients, required in smaller quantities, are crucial for the processes that sustain life, including metabolic pathways, immune function, and cell and tissue repair.

The adverse effects of consuming processed and unhealthy foods are manifold; such dietary habits can deplete the body's energy levels, impede proper functioning, and contribute to the development of chronic diseases. In stark contrast, a diet that prioritizes fresh, whole, and natural foods can significantly enhance health outcomes. Foods in their natural state are more likely to provide a balanced spectrum of the nutrients the body needs to generate energy, support metabolic activity, prevent micronutrient deficiencies, guard against chronic illnesses, and overall promote a state of health and well-being.

Understanding the critical importance of these seven fundamental types of nutrients—proteins, carbohydrates, fats, vitamins, minerals, fiber, and water—is essential for anyone looking to maintain or improve their health. While the body requires larger quantities of macronutrients for energy and basic functions, micronutrients, despite being needed in smaller amounts, are equally vital for maintaining health and preventing diseases. The balance between these nutrient groups forms the backbone of nutritional science and underscores the importance of a well-rounded and nutritious diet in achieving and maintaining optimal health throughout the lifespan.

This book is aimed to provide a comprehensive foundation in the principles of nutrition, exploring the essential nutrients required for optimal health, the physiological processes influenced by nutrition, and the impact of dietary choices on overall well-being. This book is designed to elucidate the complex science of nutrition, making it accessible and engaging for readers who are beginning their journey into the study of nutrition, as well as for those seeking to deepen their understanding of how dietary habits influence physical and mental health.

Intended for students in introductory nutrition courses, health enthusiasts, and individuals aiming to make informed decisions about their diet and lifestyle, this book serves as both an educational tool and a practical guide. It addresses the current nutritional challenges and controversies, providing evidence-based recommendations and insights into emerging research trends. By bridging the gap between scientific theory and everyday practice, this book empowers its readers to apply nutritional knowledge in personal health management and advocacy for healthier communities. Through clear explanations, real-world examples, and practical tips, it aims to inspire a lifelong commitment to nutritional well-being among its diverse audience.

Chapter 1

INTRODUCTION TO NUTRITION

Contents

Unit Introduction

The study of nutrition focuses on how food and drink affect our bodies, especially in relation to the vital nutrients that are needed to maintain human health. It examines the physiological and biochemical mechanisms of feeding as well as the ways in which nutrients are transformed into bodily tissues or used as energy in food. These nutrients—which provide our bodies with energy—are categorized as follows: water, minerals, proteins, fats, carbohydrates, and fiber. A healthy diet consists of eating the correct foods in the right amounts with the right combinations of nutrients. Examining the diseases that can arise from malnutrition and the part food plays in the development of chronic disease is an important aspect of the study of nutrition.

Orientation and Directional Terms

Term	Definition	Illustration
Diet	Diet is the sum of food consumed by a person or other organism. The word diet often implies the use of specific intake of nutrition for health or weight-management reasons (with the two often being related).	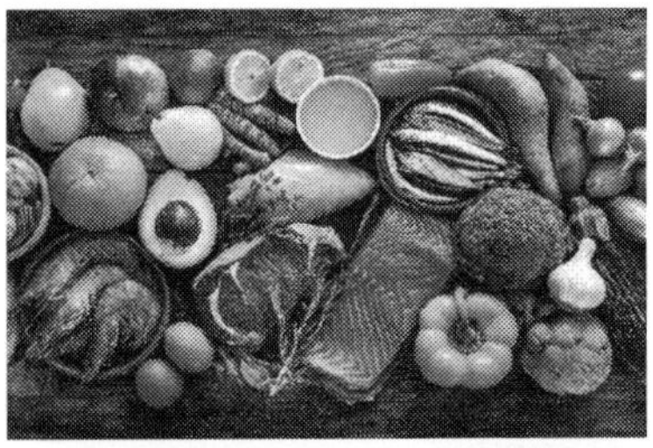
Protein Energy Malnutrition (PEM)	Protein–energy malnutrition (PEM) is a form of malnutrition that is defined as a range of pathological conditions arising from coincident lack of dietary protein and/or energy (calories) in varying proportions.	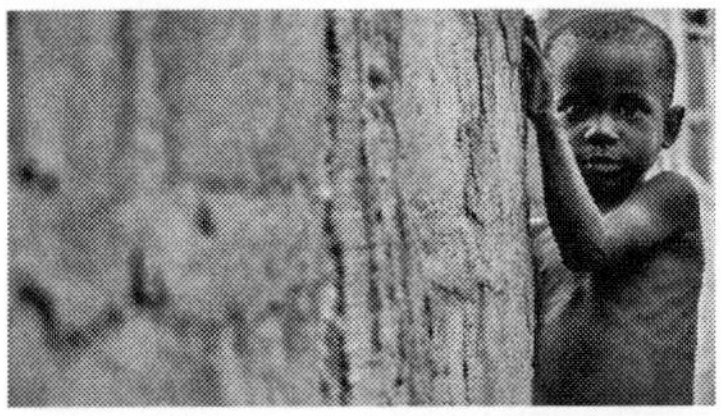
Cookie	A cookie is a baked or cooked food that is typically small, flat and sweet. It usually contains flour, sugar and some type of oil or fat.	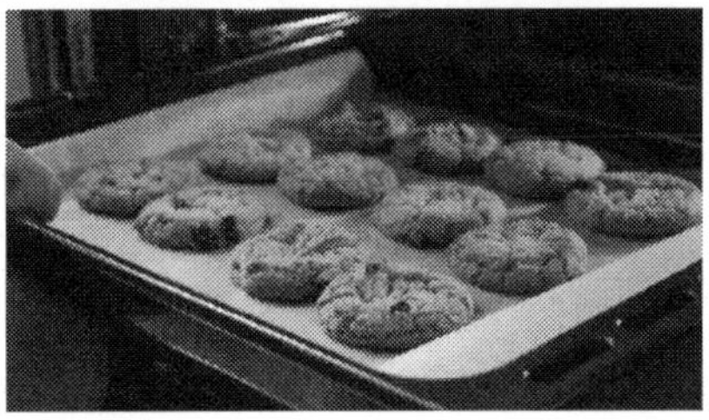
Fat-free Mass	Fat-free mass, also known as lean body mass, refers to all of your body components except fat. It includes your body's water, bone, organs and muscle content.	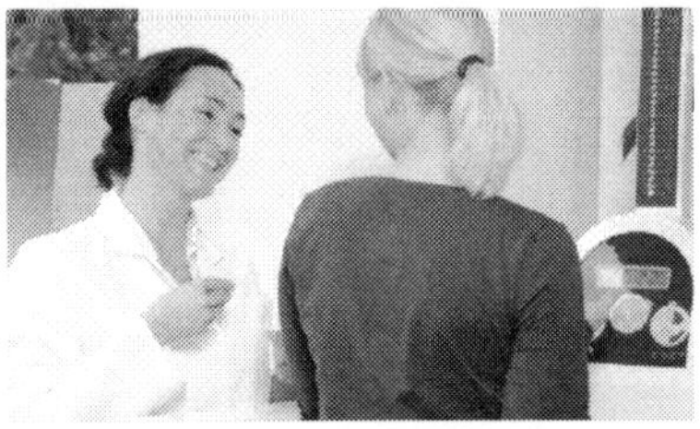
Body Mass Index	Body mass index is a value derived from the mass and height of a person. The BMI is defined as the body mass divided by the square of the body height, and is universally expressed in units of kg/m^2, resulting from mass in kilograms and height in meters.	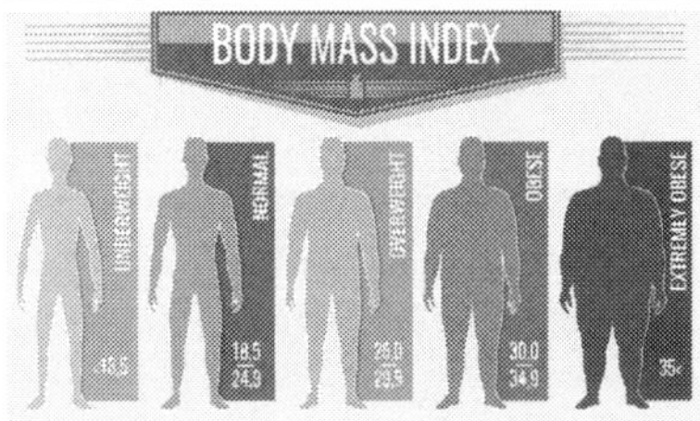

1.1. Concept of Nutrition

The processes by which a plant or animal absorbs and makes use of food materials are referred to as nutrition. Protein, carbohydrates, fats, vitamins, minerals, and electrolytes are examples of essential nutrients. Typically, 15% comes from protein and 85% comes from fat and carbs during daily energy use. Humans primarily obtain nutrition by placing food in our mouths, chewing it, and then swallowing it. Age and the condition of the body, such as physical activity and the presence of diseases, determine the necessary amounts of essential nutrients. (eg., cancers of the prostate, breast, or weakened bones osteoporosis), drugs, pregnancy, and nursing. For health and well-being, as well as for growth and development, nutrition is crucial. Maintaining a healthy diet helps extend life and improve quality of life by warding off illness in the future. Your health as it relates to what you eat is known as your nutritional status. The evaluation of nutritional status can be done in a number of ways, such as anthropometric (i.e. measurement of the physical body), food consumption, and biochemical measurement (Figure 1.1).

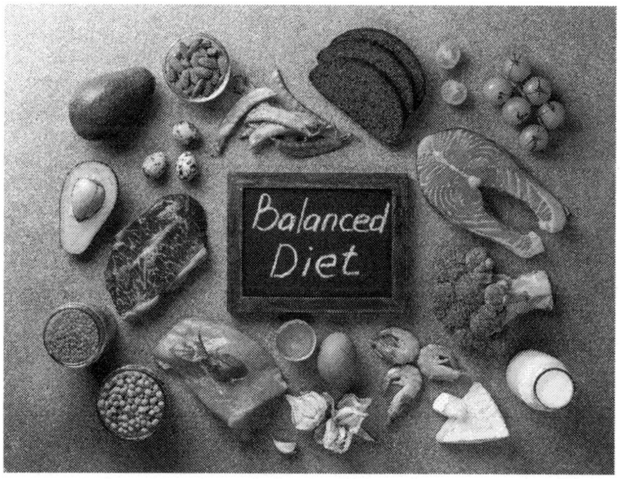

Figure 1.1. *A balanced diet.*

Source: https://cdn.prod.website-files.com/5ca5fe687e34be0992df1fbe/611bdef355c6b7d4f6e9b659_balanced-diet-concept-VX8E3ZW-min.jpg.

The science of nutrition exists. Nutrition is a relatively new science when it comes to some other fields, like chemistry, which has been studied for thousands of years. Nutrients like carbs are the focus of many nutritional facts. The nourishing ingredients in food, known as nutrients, give us energy and aid in the development and upkeep of our bodies. Nutrients also support the body's optimal health by controlling bodily functions like digestion and heart rate. Researchers studying nutrition examine the relationship between health and disease and nutrients and other ingredients in food. We are inundated with news reports almost every day suggesting that certain foods, like fat, are bad for us and can potentially cause or worsen conditions like heart disease and some types of cancer. Scholars scrutinize the correlations between nutrients and illnesses, in addition to the methods through which you make food selections and the equilibrium of foods and nutrients in your diet. The science of nutrition examines the effects of nutrients and other ingredients in food on the body, particularly about health and illness. Nutrition also looks at the motivations behind your food preferences and diet choices. The word "diet" has multiple definitions. Without a doubt, everyone who has attempted to lose weight has gone on a diet. In this context, diet refers to a weight-loss diet and is generally associated with negative connotations. However, a broader definition of diet is the kinds of foods and drinks you typically consume.

1.1.1. History of Nutrition

The development of nutrition careers and centuries of scientific discovery are revealed by the history of the study of food as medicine. Contrary to popular belief, people have been studying the very real connection between food and health for far longer. Modern science and the most recent findings in biology, medicine, and health provide information on today's field of nutrition and diet.

1.1.1.1. Food and the History of Healing Through Nutrition

In 400 B.C., the Greek physician Hippocrates, the "Father of Medicine," said, "Let thy food be thy medicine and thy medicine be thy food." Hippocrates realized that food impacts a person's health, body, and mind to help prevent illness as well as maintain wellness. In Hippocrates' Greece, as well as across pre-modern Europe and Asia since ancient times, foods were used to affect health. For instance, the juice of liver was squeezed on the eye to treat eye diseases, connected to Vitamin A deficiency. Garlic was used to cure athlete's foot, and eating ginger was thought to stimulate the metabolism. In 1747, a British Navy physician, Dr. James Lind, saw that sailors were developing scurvy, a deadly bleeding disorder, on long voyages. He observed that they ate only nonperishable foods such as bread and meat. Lind's experiment fed one group of sailors salt water, one group vinegar, and one group limes. Those given limes didn't develop scurvy. And although Vitamin C was not discovered until the 1930s, this experiment changed the way physicians thought about food, creating a market for nutrition careers.

1.1.1.2. Scientific Developments in Nutrition

The advances in science and medicine during the Enlightenment and into the Victorian era grew rapidly. The "Father of Nutrition and Chemistry," Antoine Lavoisier, made the discovery of metabolism in 1770. Metabolism is the process by which food and oxygen are converted by the body into heat and water, which produces energy. Additionally, the elements that make up food—carbon, nitrogen, hydrogen, and oxygen—were isolated in the early 1800s and were later linked to health.

Justus Liebig of Germany conducted research on the chemical makeup of foods, specifically proteins, fats, and carbohydrates. This work paved the way for vitamin research in the early 20th century. The word "vitamins" was first used to describe vital components of the diet in 1912 by Polish physician Casimir Funk. The words "vital" and "amine," which refer to vitamins because they are necessary for life, are the origins of the term "vitamin," which was formerly thought to be an amine—a compound derived from ammonia.

In 1912, E.V. McCollum, a United States Department of Agriculture researcher at the University of Wisconsin, began using rats instead of humans in his experiments rather than cows and sheep. He found the first fat-soluble vitamin, Vitamin A, and discovered that rats were healthier when they were fed butter rather than lard, as butter contains more Vitamin A. Other diseases were linked to vitamin deficiencies, such as beri-beri, resulting from a lack of Vitamin B, and rickets, brought on by a lack of Vitamin D.

1.1.1.3. The Growth of the Health Products Industry

Numerous vitamins were identified and isolated in the early 1900s, leading to the idea of using vitamins to improve health. The first vitamin supplements were introduced in the 1930s, sparking the creation of a new industry centered around scientifically-backed health products. The Dietary and Supplement Health and Education Act, passed by Congress in October 1994, established guidelines on the information that can be provided about nutritional supplements without needing FDA approval, highlighting the influence of this industry.

When the importance of a healthy diet for overall health started to be recognized in the late 19th century, dietitians and nutritionists began to work in hospitals. In order to monitor and enhance the health of World War I veterans, the Public Health Service in the United States started adding dietitians to PHS Hospital staffs in 1919. Over time, the PHS expanded its involvement in the country's healthcare system and even ventured into the private sector.

Nutrition careers and dietitian jobs gained popularity as nutrition and dietitian programs became more common. Dietitians are members of the American Dietetic Association and can only use the title "dietitian" after completing a national registration exam and meeting stringent requirements regarding their training, work history, and education. Many but not all states in the US protect and designate the title "nutritionist." Although there is some overlap, nutritionists and dietitians typically work in private practice, education, and research, with the former serving in hospitals, schools, and prisons. The fields of nutrition and alternative medicine have experienced unparalleled growth and expansion as our awareness of the impact of nutrition on our health has grown. There are now more career options than ever, thanks to this ongoing demand, which has also fueled the growth of the nutrition industry. A great way to learn more about this fascinating field with a long and illustrious history is through online nutrition programs and distance learning at colleges.

1.1.2. What Is Food?

Anything we eat that provides nourishment for our bodies is referred to as "food." Liquids, semi-solids, and solids are all included. Thus, two important features for any item to be called food are:

1. It should be worth eating; that is, it should be 'edible.'
2. It must nourish the body.

Have you ever wondered why food is considered a basic necessity?

1.1.2.1. Functions of Food

There are basically three important functions of food:

1. **Social Function:** Eating and food have important social connotations. Any food sharing implies acceptance by the community. Food plays a crucial role in celebrations everywhere in the world. In addition to having special significance and meaning in the religious context, food is also celebrated with feasts and delicacies on special occasions like birthdays, marriages, and the birth of a child.
2. **Psychological Function:** Everybody has emotional needs, including the need for love, affection, and security. One means of meeting these needs is through food. When your mother makes your favorite meal, for instance, you get a sense that she loves and cares for you. Food is also frequently offered as a reward. Do you remember offering someone a chocolate because they had been kind to you? In a similar vein, some foods—like khichri and bland foods—become linked to illness. Since being ill is an unpleasant experience, even the food that is served to you while you're sick may make you feel bad.
3. **Physiological Function:** Three physiological roles are fulfilled by food, that supply energy, help to build muscle, control bodily functions, and guard against illness.
   i. **Food Provides Energy:** For everyone to work, they need energy. It takes energy to work outside or inside the home,

study, eat, and walk. The food you eat provides you with this energy. Even when at rest, you still require energy. What is the reason behind this? Various bodily organs are constantly in operation. For instance, the heart continuously pumps blood, the stomach breaks down food, the lungs take in oxygen, and so on. Food supplies the energy that each of these organs requires to perform its specific job.

ii. **Food Helps in Bodybuilding:** Our body is already composed of thousands of tiny cells; have you ever wondered how a small child grows into an adult? New cells are added to the growth of the body. For new cells to form, food is required. Injuries also cause cells to die or become damaged. Food aids in the formation of new cells, which are necessary for cell repair.

iii. **Food Regulates Body Processes and Provides Protection Against Diseases:** The term "regulatory functions" describes how food affects how the body operates. For instance, our body temperature is kept at 37°C, or 98.6°F. In a similar vein, the heartbeat is kept constant at 72 beats per minute. The body excretes waste materials on a regular basis. If not, the body becomes ill with a condition called constipation, which can cause more issues. Your diet affects every single one of these processes. Our food provides us with the energy to combat disease-causing microorganisms.

1.1.3. Inter-Relationship of Food, Nutrition, and Health

Food is a primary area of interest in the scientific field of nutrition. The study of what happens to food after it enters the mouth is the most basic definition of nutrition. A more formal definition of nutrition is the study of the mechanisms through which a living thing obtains and makes use of the substances required for bodily component growth, renewal, and maintenance. Every food has certain necessary ingredients that serve vital purposes for our bodies. We refer to these vital components that come from our diet as nutrients. These nutrients support healthy growth and organ protection, two processes that are essential to maintaining bodily functions. A person's health is influenced by the kinds and amounts of food they eat. A person needs a healthy diet to grow and develop normally as well as to stay healthy throughout their life. A person runs the risk of their body not developing normally if they don't eat the right foods. There's a possibility that an illness could develop or that some of the body's organs will begin to fail. Inadequate diet can also have a negative impact on social and mental health.

1.1.4. Importance of Good Nutrition

Eating well improves your life expectancy and lowers the risk of illness. It gives you the calories and nutrients your body requires to function at its best and to feel well.

Calories, or more accurately, kilocalories, are units of heat that are used to quantify the energy that the body uses and receives from food. Everything you do, including working out, playing sports, doing your homework, and chatting with friends, is powered by this energy. The ingredients in food, known as nutrients, are what your body needs to develop, heal, and provide energy. Eating a balanced diet will give your body the nutrients it needs to function at its best and look your best.

1.1.4.1. Influences Your Food Choices

Taste, of course, is a major factor in food selection, but have you ever wondered why you make the choices you do?

If a food doesn't taste good, you probably won't eat it even if you know it's healthy.

Understanding the distinction between your psychological need for food—known as appetite—and your physical need for food will help you better understand your eating habits. Making the distinction between the two will enable you to choose foods that are healthier.

1.1.4.1.1. Hunger and Appetite

A natural physical drive that keeps you from starving, hunger is an unlearned, inborn reaction. The walls of your stomach constrict when it is empty, stimulating nerve endings. The body's need for food is communicated to the brain by the nerves. The stomach's walls expand during eating, and the nerve endings stop being stimulated. Your physical hunger has been satiated. People eat for purposes other than satisfying their bodily needs. When you eat something "just to be sociable" or in reaction to a familiar feeling, like the smell of freshly baked bread, you are not eating out of hunger, but rather out of appetite. Rather than being a necessity, appetite is the desire to eat. Your emotions and various environmental factors are among the many factors that influence the eating habits and food choices, regardless of whether you are eating out of hunger or appetite (Figure 1.2).

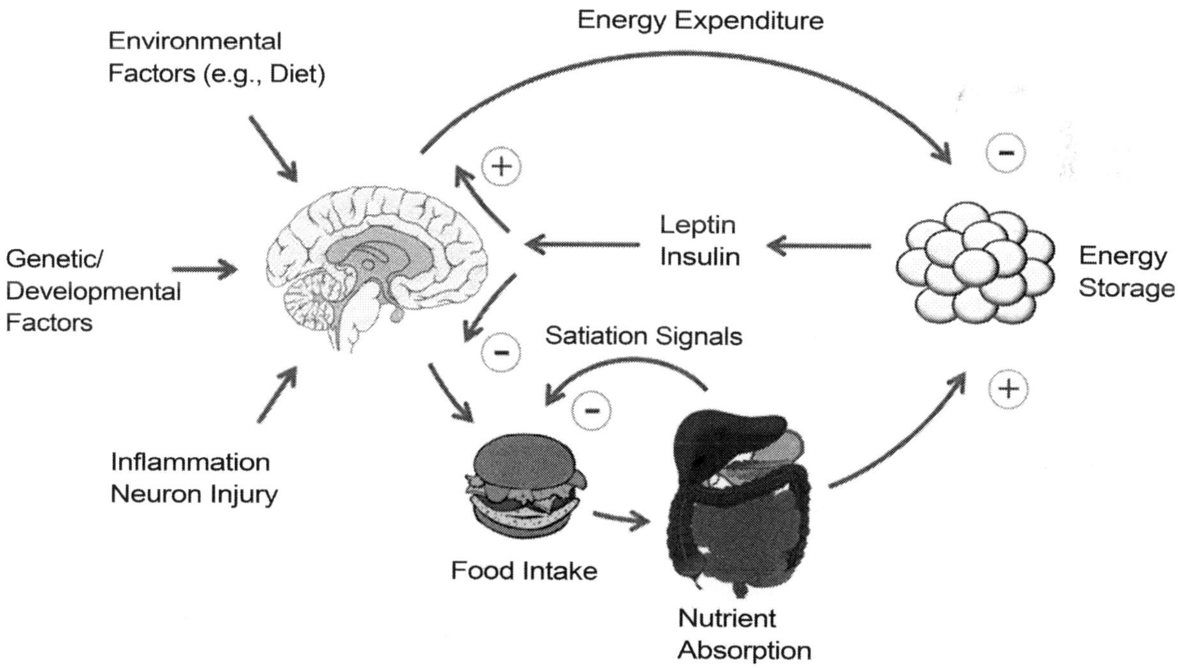

Figure 1.2. *Weight loss, nutrition, and hunger.*

Source: https://www.dietvsdisease.org/weight-loss-tips-hypothyroidism/.

1.1.4.1.2. Food and Emotions

Eating can be used as a coping mechanism. Using food to relieve tension or boredom or to reward yourself when you've achieved a goal can lead to overeating and unhealthy weight gain.

For instance, do you tend to eat more or less when you feel stressed, frustrated, or depressed? Do you sometimes snack just because you are bored? However, you run the risk of not consuming enough of the nutrients your body needs if you stop eating when you are angry. You can break such patterns and change your eating habits by recognizing the times when your emotions are influencing the foods you choose to eat.

1.1.4.2. Food and Your Environment

A number of environmental factors influence food choices:

1. **Family, Friends, and Peers:** Growing up, when meals were planned by adults, shaped a lot of your eating habits. Now that you have grown up eating a certain food, you might prefer it. You may be persuaded to try new foods by friends and peers.
2. **Cultural and Ethnic Background:** Your food choices may reflect your cultural heritage or ethnic background. For example, corn, beans, and tortillas might be common foods in many Mexican-American households.
3. **Convenience and Cost:** For some people, the cost and convenience of food may be the most important factors. For instance, time-pressed families might depend on easily prepared foods, like meals that can be microwaved.
4. **Advertising:** Every year, marketers spend millions of dollars trying to sway your eating choices. Making educated food decisions also entails closely examining the health messages propagated by food advertising in the media. Then you will decide what to eat instead of advertising.

1.1.5. Nutrition Throughout the Life Span

Good nutrition is important for health at all stages of life, but it is especially important during adolescence, which is one of the fastest growth periods in a human life. Eating a healthy diet gives you the nutrients you need for development and growth, energy for sports and other activities, mental clarity, and the best possible appearance and feeling. Obesity, type 2 diabetes, and unhealthy weight gain can all be avoided with a balanced, healthful diet. Making good dietary decisions now also reduces your chance of growing older and developing several serious illnesses. Heart disease, stroke, some malignancies, and osteoporosis are among these ailments.

1.1.6. Role of Nutrition in Maintaining Health

The role of nutrition in maintaining health is paramount, serving as a cornerstone of overall well-being and vitality. A balanced diet provides essential nutrients—such as vitamins, minerals, carbohydrates, proteins, and fats—that are vital for supporting various bodily functions. Adequate nutrition supports optimal growth and development, enhances immune function, and helps prevent chronic diseases such as obesity, diabetes, cardiovascular diseases, and certain cancers. Nutrients play specific roles in the body, from providing energy for daily activities to supporting cellular repair and maintenance. Moreover, dietary habits influence mental health and cognitive function, with deficiencies in certain nutrients linked to mood disorders and impaired cognitive performance. Beyond individual health, nutrition also has broader societal implications, affecting productivity, healthcare costs, and the overall quality of life. Therefore, promoting access to nutritious foods and fostering healthy eating habits are essential strategies for promoting public health and well-being. Education on nutrition, coupled with initiatives to improve food accessibility and affordability, can empower individuals to make informed dietary choices, ultimately contributing to the prevention of disease and the promotion of optimal health throughout the lifespan.

1.2. Nutrients

The nutrients in food are essential for the human body's normal growth and functioning. They can be categorized into six groups: carbohydrates, proteins, fats, vitamins, minerals, and water. Each of these nutrients plays a distinct role in supporting your body's health and well-being. Collectively, they are crucial for maintaining overall health and wellness (Figure 1.3).

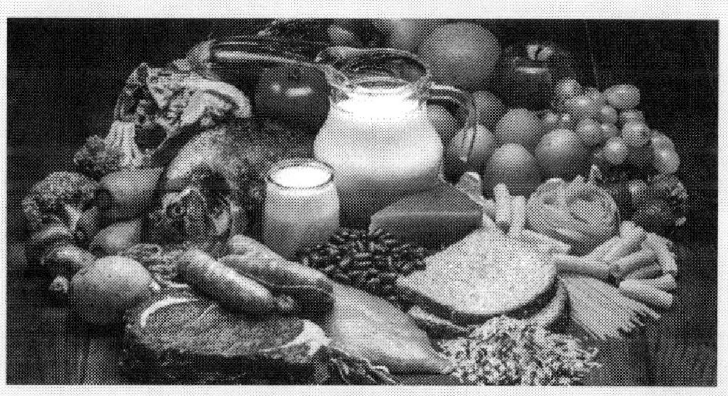

Figure 1.3. *Importance of nutrients in our body.*

Source: https://www.healthandfood.com.au/wp-content/uploads/2020/02/nutrients.jpg.

Seldom do foods contain a single nutrient. Most food sources offer a variety of nutrients. For instance, while bread is commonly associated with carbohydrates, it also contains significant amounts of several vitamins and minerals. Food is not just about nutrients. Foods can include colorings, flavorings, caffeine, phytochemicals—minute compounds found in plants that have biological activity and potential health benefits—and other ingredients.

Carbohydrates, lipids, and protein are called energy-yielding nutrients because they can be burned as fuel to provide energy for the body. They provide kilo calories (kcal) as follows:

- **Carbohydrates:** 4 kcal per gram;
- **Lipids:** 9 kcal per gram;
- **Protein:** 4 kcal per gram.

(A gram is a unit of weight in the metric system; there are about 28 g in 1 ounce.) Vitamins, minerals, and water do not provide energy or calories.

Micronutrients are defined as vitamins and minerals that the body requires in minute amounts (micro means small). On the other hand, the body requires high concentrations of fats, proteins, and carbohydrates; these are referred to as macronutrients because the word "macro" means large. Analyzing the classes of nutrients from a chemical perspective is another way to group them. Any compound that contains carbon is referred to as organic in chemistry. A compound is referred to as inorganic if it is carbon-free. Vitamins, proteins, lipids, and carbohydrates are all organic. Both water and minerals are inorganic.

1. **Carbohydrates:** The body uses a broad class of nutrients called carbohydrates, which includes sugars, starches, and fibers, as its main source of energy. The most commonly known refined forms of sugar are table sugar and high-fructose corn syrup, which are found in soft drinks, candies, jams, jellies, cakes, pies, cookies, and other

sweetened foods. Moreover, milk and fruits naturally contain sugar (even though milk does not taste sweet). Breads, pastas, potatoes, beans, and breakfast cereals all contain starch. Starch and sugar are both significant sources of energy for the body. Fiber is eliminated from the body because it cannot be digested or broken down by the body. As a result, it doesn't give the body energy. The body benefits greatly from fiber in many ways, one of which is improved digestive tract health. Legumes (dried beans and peas), fruits, vegetables, whole-grain foods like whole-wheat bread and cereal, nuts, and seeds are good sources of fiber.

2. **Lipids:** Triglycerides and cholesterol are examples of fatty substances that belong to the class of lipids. They are soluble in fat rather than water and give cells a rich source of energy and structure. The most well-known types of lipids are fats and oils, which can be found in salad dressings, butter, margarine, and vegetable oils. Fatty streaks in meat, the fat beneath chicken skin, milk and cheese (apart from fat-free milk and its derivatives), baked goods like cakes, fried foods, nuts, and a lot of processed foods like canned soups and frozen dinners are other sources of lipids. Most pasta, breads, cereals, fruits, and vegetables are low in fat or contain none at all. The primary lipid form is triglycerides. They give the body energy and a means of storing it as fat. The majority of the calories we consume come from fats or carbohydrates. Protein accounts for only 15% of total calories. This is not to say that protein is any less significant. Protein, on the other hand, serves as the primary structural element in every cell in the body. It is composed of building blocks known as amino acids, which are special because they contain nitrogen.

In addition to being a crucial component of cells, protein can be burned to produce energy and regulate bodily functions (though the body prefers to burn fats and carbohydrates so protein can be used to build new cells). Foods derived from animals, such as beef, pork, chicken, fish, eggs, milk, and cheese, are high in protein. Smaller amounts of protein can be found in plant-based foods like grains, beans, and vegetables. Protein is found in very small amounts in fruits. Around 13 distinct vitamins can be found in food. Organic, non-caloric nutrients, vitamins can be found in a wide range of foods. In tiny amounts, they are necessary for the maintenance of the body, control of bodily functions, and facilitation of growth and reproduction. Vitamins serve as aids to the body rather than being burned to produce energy. They support the bodily functions that maintain your health.

3. **Minerals:** The body needs minerals, but only in trace amounts—they don't give us energy. Similar to vitamins, they function as allies in the body and are present in a wide range of meals. Certain minerals, like calcium and phosphorus, are used in the development of teeth and bones, giving the body structure. Minerals are inorganic and unbreakable, unlike vitamins. Just a few people have the ability to endure for months without any

deficiencies in energy. In terms of necessity for life, experts rank water second only to oxygen. Water makes up slightly more than half of the body weight and is essential to all physiological functions. It provides the environment for the body's numerous chemical reactions, supports circulation, facilitates digestion and absorption, and lubricates joints.

Water is a key component of blood, helping to transport nutrients to cells and waste to the kidneys for removal. As the saying goes, "You are what you eat," meaning that the nutrients you consume can be found in your body. Water is the most abundant nutrient, making up about 60% of body weight. Protein makes up about 15%, fat 20 to 25%, and carbohydrates only 0.5%. The rest of body weight consists of minerals like calcium in bones and trace amounts of vitamins. Most nutrients are essential, including carbohydrates, vitamins, minerals, water, some lipids, and parts of protein.

4. **Fiber:** Whole grains, vegetables, and fruits that have tough, stringy sections contain fiber, an indigestible complex carbohydrate. Fiber helps move waste through the digestive system and thereby helps prevent intestinal problems like constipation, even though it cannot be digested and used as energy. By lowering the chance of heart disease, eating adequate fiber throughout your life may improve your health. Certain forms of fiber have also been demonstrated to lower blood glucose levels, which aids in the management of diabetes. Consume 20 to 35 g of fiber daily to stay healthy. Good sources of dietary fiber include fruits and vegetables with edible skins as well as whole-grain products like brown rice, oatmeal, and bran cereals.
5. **Proteins:** Amino acid chains are the building blocks of proteins. Around 19 of the 20 different amino acids that make up proteins can be produced by your body. The nine amino acids that your body is unable to produce are known as essential amino acids, and you must obtain them through diet.

1.2.1. Computation of Nutrient Requirements

Many different nutrients are necessary for humans to live a healthy and active life. Only a diet that is well-balanced can provide the necessary nutrients for the various physiological groups.

Dietary components must be carefully chosen to supply all the nutrients needed by humans in the right amounts for their various physiological functions.

Individual nutrient requirements differ greatly from dietary allowances for populations or groups. The former is based on the person's age, weight, and metabolic and physiological state. The latter must also account for individual differences within the group, diet quality, the impact of processing and cooking, and the bioavailability of the nutrients in the food.

A desirable body composition and a high potential for both physical and mental work are the goals of good nutrition. To maintain a desired body weight, energy intake and expenditure must be balanced. Age, sex, weight, and levels of physical and metabolic activity all affect how much energy is used. Weight gain occurs when energy intake surpasses energy expenditure. Weight loss occurs when energy intake is less than energy used.

1.2.2. Nutrient Density

In terms of the calories and nutrients they contain, not all foods are created equal. Certain foods—like milk—contribute a significant amount of calcium to your diet, particularly when weighed against other drinks—like soft drinks. A standard 12-ounce can of cola contains a whopping 40 g (roughly 10 teaspoons) of sugar, zero vitamins, and almost no minerals. When comparing calories, you will discover that skim milk has fewer calories than cola (97 kcal per cup), even though it contains many vitamins and minerals. As a result, we can state that milk is more "nutrient-dense" than cola, i.e., it has more nutrients per kilocalorie.

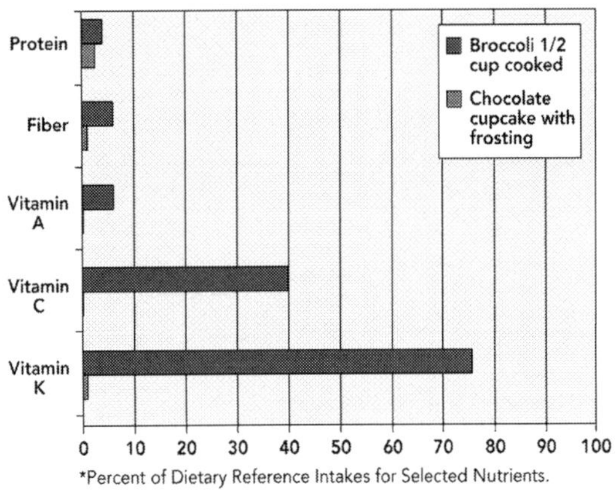

Figure 1.4. *Nutrition density comparison.*

Source: https://slideplayer.com/slide/12900894/.

A food's nutrient density is determined by counting its nutrients and dividing that total by its calorie content. Stated differently, nutrient density represents the amount of nutrients present in each kilocalorie of food. As Figure 1.4 shows, broccoli offers many nutrients for its few calories. Broccoli is considered to have a high nutrient density because it is high in nutrients relative to its caloric value. Vegetables and fruits are examples of nutrient-dense foods. In comparison, a cupcake contains many more calories and fewer nutrients. By now, you no doubt recognize that some foods, such as candy bars, have a low nutrient density, meaning that they are low in nutrients and high in calories. These foods are called empty-calorie foods because the calories they provide are "empty" (that is, they deliver few nutrients).

1.2.3. Characteristics of a Nutritious Diet

A nutritious diet has four characteristics. It is:

1. Adequate;
2. Balanced;
3. Moderate;
4. Varied.

Nutrients must be present in your diet in moderation. Here's where moderate and adequate diets come into play. A moderate diet steers clear of consuming excessive amounts of calories or more of one food group than is advised, while an adequate diet gives you the necessary amount of calories, fiber, and essential nutrients to keep you healthy. For instance, eating too many calories can result in obesity.

The idea of moderation enables you to select sensible serving sizes for any food item and to occasionally treat yourself to high-fat, high-calorie foods like French fries and fine ice cream. Eating enough of the right nutrients in moderation may seem easy, but research indicates that most adult Americans struggle with this. Choosing foods that are high in nutrients is one of the best strategies to solve this issue. As previously mentioned, foods high in nutrients have a high nutrient content relative to their calorie content. A balanced diet is necessary. Consuming a balanced diet entails consuming fewer servings of nutrient-poor foods like cakes, cookies, and chips and more servings of nutrient-dense foods like whole grains, fruits, and vegetables.

For instance, if you consume a lot of soft drinks, you may be consuming too much sugar and insufficient amounts of calcium, a mineral that is present in milk. Children should be especially concerned about this since their bones are growing and they are more likely than ever to be obese. An unbalanced diet is the norm in America. We consume excessive amounts of soda and overindulge in fried and fatty foods. We also consume far too few whole grains, fruits, and vegetables at the same time. Additionally, a balanced diet is probably sufficient and moderate. Finally, to ensure that you are getting all the nutrients you need, you should eat a varied diet, or a wide variety of foods. A varied diet is important because it increases the likelihood that you will get the essential nutrients in the right amounts. If you picture everything you eat for a week piled into a grocery cart, how much variety is in that cart from week to week? Do you eat the same bread, the same brand of cereal, the same types of fresh fruit, and so on, every week? Do you constantly eat favorite foods? Do you try new foods?

1.3. Body Composition

The percentage of fat and fat-free mass in the body is referred to as body composition. A lower percentage of body fat and a higher percentage of fat-free mass are characteristics of a healthy body composition. One way to gauge your level of fitness and health is to take your body composition.

Your body is composed of two types of mass: body fat and fat-free mass.

- Body fat is fat that is located within the body. Body fat can be in muscle tissue, under skin or around organs. Some fat is necessary for overall health. It helps protect internal organs, provides energy and regulates important body hormones.
- Fat-free mass includes bone, water, muscle, and tissues. Fat-free mass is also important for the body to function properly.

A comparison of your body's fat and fat-free mass is called body composition. Body fat percent, or the proportion of body fat, is typically discussed in relation to body composition. Fat-free mass (FFM) is the percentage of your body that is not fat. Your percentage of body fat is within a normal range if your body composition is good. Compared to people with poor body composition, you typically feel better, move more freely, and are healthier. People with a healthy body composition usually have bodies that look more fit and trim. If you can improve your body composition you can improve your quality of life and overall wellness.

- If you are overweight or obese, you have an excessive amount of body fat. Your body fat percent is too high. Your body composition is unhealthy.
- Your body may feel more sluggish and it may not function as well with excess body fat.
- Weighing yourself on a regular bathroom scale does not truly assess your body composition, because a regular scale cannot tell the difference between how much of your total weight is comprised of water, fat, or muscle.
- To know if your body composition is healthy, you should get an estimate of your body fat percent.

1.3.1. Method for Body Composition Assessment

Body composition has been estimated using a variety of methods. The only way to accurately determine the amount of fat in the body would be to dissect and chemically analyze bodily tissues, which is not possible with any of the existing methods. The methods commonly employed for estimating (%BF) are predicated on the correlation between (%BF) and other measurable variables, like skinfold thicknesses or underwater weight. These indirect methods can be used to estimate (%BF) because the measured value and body composition have a predictable relationship.

1.3.1.1. Anthropometric Methods: Body Mass Index

The body mass index (BMI), also known as the Quetelet index, is a commonly used clinical measure of a person's appropriate weight. BMI: weight (kg)/ height (m^2). BMI is a quick and simple way to Figure out if your weight is suitable for your height. The accepted method for interpreting the height-weight relationship is currently BMI, though height-weight charts were used in the past for this purpose as well. A problem with BMI testing for athletes with high lean mass is that it does not distinguish between fat and fat-free weight. For instance, a 6 feet 2 inch football linebacker. (1.9 m) and weighs 220 lb (100 kg), he may actually have a very low (%BF), but according to BMI standards (BMI = 28.3 kgm^{-2}), he is overweight. Conversely, an inactive individual of comparable height and weight is most likely carrying extra adipose tissue. Notwithstanding its limitations, elevated BMI is clearly associated with adverse health outcomes for the majority of adults. The recommended range for BMI is 18.5 to 24.9 kg/m^{-2}. A BMI of 25 to 29.9 kg m^{-2} is categorized as overweight, and a BMI of 30 kg m^{-2} or greater is categorized as obese. BMI can be helpful in screening situations where estimating body fat is unfeasible or impractical in order to give people feedback regarding the appropriateness of their weight. It is significant to remember that age and gender-specific BMI guidelines apply to children. Obese children are those who are 95th percentile or higher for their age and sex. To find the recommended BMI for children, refer to the CDC growth charts.

1.3.1.2. Girth Measurements

A number of girth measurements, such as limb and body circumferences, are used to characterize the proportions of the body or to estimate body composition. Measurements of circumference offer accurate and timely information. They can be used to track changes in body size and shape during weight loss, and they are occasionally included in equations to predict body composition. Their main drawback is their lack of information regarding the body's fat and fat-free components. For instance, a bodybuilder's thigh may be larger than an obese person's but still have less fat on it. A list of several commonly measured girths follows:

- **Waist:** Narrowest part of the torso between the xiphoid process and the umbilicus.
- **Abdomen:** Circumference of the torso at the level of the umbilicus.
- **Hips:** Maximal circumference of the buttocks above the gluteal fold.
- **Thigh:** Largest circumference of the right thigh below the gluteal fold.

The waist-hip ratio (WHR) is a common way to measure abdominal obesity based on girth measurements. A WHR above 0.95 in young men or 0.86 in young women is linked to health risks, while a WHR above 1.03 in men and above 0.9 in women aged 60–69 is associated with disease risk. Waist circumference (WC) alone can also indicate disease risk, with a WC above 102 cm (40 in.) in men or 88 cm (35 in.) in women significantly increasing the risk of obesity-related diseases.

When assessing girths, use the following procedures to standardize the measurements:

- Make sure the measuring tape is horizontal when measuring trunk circumference and is perpendicular to the long axis of the limb when measuring limbs. Use either a mirror or an assistant to help ensure that the tape is placed properly.
- Apply constant pressure to the tape without pinching the skin. Use a tape measure fitted with a handle that indicates the amount of tension exerted.
- When measuring limbs, measure on the right side of the body. Alternatively, measure on both sides and record the values for both right and left.
- Ensure that the person stands erect, relaxed, and with feet together.
- When measuring girths of the trunk, take the measurement after the person exhales and before the next breath begins.

1.3.1.3. Skinfold Measurements

One of the tests used most frequently to estimate (%BF) is skinfold thickness measurement. This quick, non-invasive, low-cost technique can estimate (%BF) with a reasonable degree of accuracy. The difference between the value measured with underwater weighing and the value obtained by skinfold measurement is usually within 3.5%. The foundation of skinfold measurement is the idea that an individual's increased skinfold thickness is directly proportional to their increased body weight as they gain adipose tissue. Fitness professionals should become proficient in skinfold measurement due to its widespread use. Finding the skinfold site, pinching the skinfold away from the underlying tissue, using the caliper to measure, and selecting the appropriate equation are all necessary for accurately determining skinfold thickness.

1.3.1.3.1. Locating the Skinfold Site

Finding the skinfold measurement site precisely is essential. Find the location of the measurement site and mark it with a washable marker to improve measurement accuracy, especially for the novice technician.

This makes it more likely that the calipers will be positioned correctly each time the skinfold is measured (Figure 1.5).

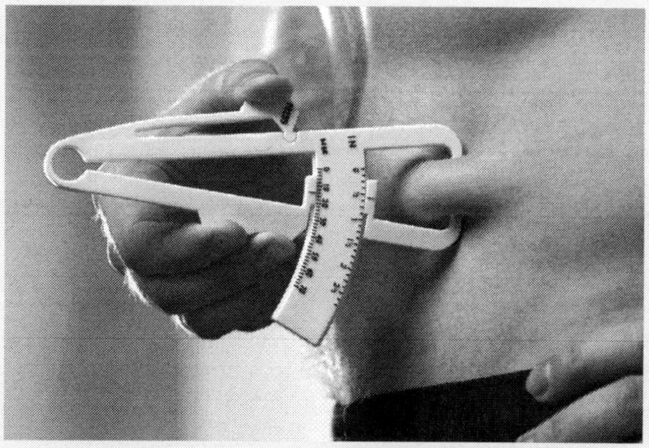

Figure 1.5. *Body composition and anthropometric measurement.*

Source: https://eadn-wc04-11125113.nxedge.io/wp-content/uploads/2022/10/Body-Composition-and-Anthropometric-Measurement-14601.jpg.

All skinfold measurements should be taken on the right side of the body unless otherwise specified. Measuring skinfolds immediately after exercise should be avoided because exercise can shift fluid volume, leading to inaccurate results (Table 1.1).

Table 1.1. *The Estimation of Body Density Using 4 Skinfold Sites*

Age (Years)	Equations for Men	Equations for Women
< 17	D = 1.1533 – (0.0643 * L)	D = 1.1369 – (0.0598 * L)
17–19	D = 1.1620 – (0.0630 * L)	D = 1.1549 – (0.0678 * L)
20–29	D = 1.1631 – (0.0632 * L)	D = 1.1599 – (0.0717 * L)
30–39	D = 1.1422 – (0.0544 * L)	D = 1.1423 – (0.0632 * L)
40–49	D = 1.1620 – (0.0700 * L)	D = 1.1333 – (0.0612 * L)
> 50	D = 1.1715 – (0.0779 * L)	D = 1.1339 – (0.0645 * L)

Source: https://www.measurement-toolkit.org/anthropometry/objective-methods/simple-measures-skinfolds.

1.3.1.3.2. Pinching the Skinfold

The tester pinches and lifts the skinfold away from the underlying muscle, gently but firmly, after determining the proper location for the skinfold measurement. The following are guidelines for measuring skinfolds correctly:

1. Place the fingers perpendicular to the skinfold approximately 1 cm from the site to be measured.
2. Gently yet firmly pinch the skinfold between the thumb and the first two fingers and lift away from the underlying tissues. Place the jaws of the caliper perpendicular to the skinfold at the measurement site. The jaws of the caliper should be halfway between the bottoms and top of the fold. Maintain the pinch while taking the measurement.
3. Read the measurement on the caliper 1 to 2 sec after the jaws contact the skin.
4. Wait at least 15 sec before taking a subsequent measurement. To allow time for the fold to return to normal, take one measurement at each site and then repeat measurements. If the second measurement varies by more than 1 to 2 mm, repeat the measurement a third time.

Assessing the skinfolds of obese people can be challenging, if not impossible. If the caliper's jaws won't open far enough to measure the skinfold, find another way to determine your body's composition.

1.3.1.3.3. Measuring with the Caliper

A skinfold caliper is used to measure skinfold thickness. The accuracy and cost of the many commercially available calipers differ. Although other calipers can also be used effectively, large and Harpenden calipers are the most commonly used in research settings due to their accuracy and dependability. It goes without saying that inaccurate skinfold measurements by the calipers will skew the estimate of body fat. Use calipers for your measurements that closely resemble the ones that were used to create the equation you are using.

1.3.1.3.4. Choosing the Proper Equation

The majority of skinfold equations, which are really meant to estimate body density, were created with underwater weighing as the standard method. The body density of numerous subjects was determined (usually by hydrostatic weighing) in order to create skinfold equations. Regression analysis was then used to compare the results with skinfold thickness. Using this statistical method, an equation representing the relationship between skinfolds and body density is developed. An estimation of the client's body density is obtained by entering their skinfold measurements (as well as occasionally additional data, like age) into these formulas. The body density is then translated into (%BF) using a model equation with two compartments, like the Siri equation. Skinfold equations that are both population-specific and generalized have been created. When estimating body composition in groups of people with significant age, fitness, and body composition variations, generalized equations are used. These equations have the benefit of being able to estimate body composition for the majority of people; however, when testing individuals who differ from those used to develop the equations, the equations become less accurate. Additionally, these formulas are less reliable for individuals who fall on either end of the fat spectrum. Body composition in a specific subgroup of the population, like female runners, is predicted by population-specific equations. Using population-specific equations has the benefit of generally having higher accuracy when testing individuals who match the physical characteristics of the subgroup of interest.

1.3.1.4. Densitometry

An object's density is determined by dividing its weight by its volume (density = weight ÷ volume). Hydrostatic weighing and air displacement plethysmography are two popular methods used to estimate body composition based on densitometry. These methods are based on the idea that the body's different tissues have distinct but uniform densities. Compared to either muscle or bone, fat tissue has a far lower density. With each of these methods, the entire body volume is evaluated, and body density is then computed.

Body density needs to be computed and then converted to (%BF). This conversion is carried out using a two-compartment model. All body tissues are categorized as either fat or fat-free in a two-compartment model.

The Siri equation is a frequently utilized formula for this process, which is (%BF) = (495 ÷ Db) – 450. In this model, the body's fat-free area is made up of all tissues with the exception of lipids, and its density is set at 1.1 kg L^{-1}. The density of fat is assumed to be 0.9 kg L^{-1}. According to some estimates, the inherent error of this method in young Caucasian adults ranges from 2% to 2.8%, depending on variations in bone density or hydration. Individual differences in fat density are rare, but there are circumstances where the assumed 1.1 kg L^{-1} is not reflected in the density of the fat-free body. The assumption that the fat-free body density is equal to 1.1 kg L^{-1} is invalid, for instance, if an individual's bone density differs from the standard used by Siri.

1.3.1.5. Hydrostatic Weighing

One of the most popular methods for determining body composition in research settings is hydrostatic (underwater) weighing, which is also frequently employed as the standard technique for determining (%BF).

A criterion method offers the benchmark by which alternative approaches are evaluated. The participant in this procedure is submerged in a warm water tank, and as technicians record the body mass, they fully exhale. The (%BF) is computed using the body mass on land and the body mass while submerged. The Archimedes principle, which states that a submerged object is buoyed up by a force equal to the volume of water it displaces, is the foundation of hydrostatic weighing.

1.3.2. Compositional Changes During Life Cycle

The correlation between rising obesity rates and chronic illnesses like diabetes and hypertension is a persistent source of concern. Body mass index (BMI) is a common measure of overweight or obesity, but few people are aware of their true body composition. Lean body mass (LBM) or fat-free mass (FFM) and fat mass (FM) are two components of body composition. Adipose tissue and necessary fats that support healthy body function combine to form fat mass. For instance, lipid, or fat, is present in all of the body's cell membranes and covers all nerves, acting as an insulator.

LBM is made up of water, electrolytes, bone, and muscle or protein. Additionally, fat mass provides calories during periods of growth, illness, pregnancy, and lactation. On the other hand, LBM stands for the body's metabolism and the area that uses energy. From early childhood through adolescence and adulthood, FM and LBM change. A stable body composition period spans the 20s to mid-60s, and by the time an individual reaches 70 or 80 years old, age-related changes in LBM have occurred.

During the first four months of life, body fat is a vital source of energy for the infant's continued growth and development. Up until late adolescence, fat mass and LBM increase during childhood and puberty. Girls typically mature one and a half years earlier than boys during the pubertal growth spurt; the biggest increase in height happens around age 8.6 years for girls vs. 10.4 years for males. Peak weight velocity follows height velocity at approximately 12 points 3 years for girls and 13 points 8 years for boys.

Men and women have reached adult body composition by their mid-20s, with a mature skeleton, stable LBM, and FM. Men have less FM as a percentage of body weight because they have higher LBM than women. The midlife years are spent upholding these ideals. The mean proportion of fat and LBM in adult males and females. But as people get older (mid-60s to mid-80s), there is a noticeable shift from LBM to more FM. Although there are changes in overall metabolism due to declining hormones like growth hormone, estrogen, and testosterone—all of which lead to lower LBM, reduced metabolism, and greater FM—this shift may also be attributed to changes in diet, exercise, and other lifestyle factors. Older people should concentrate on diets that include lean protein, complex carbohydrates like whole grains, fruits, and vegetables, as well as moderate physical activity most days of the week, in order to counteract these natural aging processes and stabilize LBM.

Since exercise benefits both muscle and bone, maintaining adequate physical activity—both aerobic and resistance training—helps to maintain LBM and bone health. Dairy products are a great source of high-quality protein and other essential nutrients, such as calcium, for healthy bones.

These nutrients are particularly important for growing adolescents to help them develop the maximum amount of bone density possible, and for older people to maintain their bone density. Dairy products might also be a more cost-effective option for seniors with low incomes who want high-quality protein. Throughout infancy, childhood, and adolescence, there are rapid changes in body composition; the biggest changes in height, weight, LBM, and FM happen in the early stages of adolescence. Maintaining a stable body composition during middle age and beyond can be achieved through proper diet and consistent exercise. Sustaining a healthy diet and exercise regimen are critical for fulfilling requirements for body composition and general well-being throughout life.

1.4. Nutritional Status

Nutrient status refers to an individual's state of health that is impacted by their intake and utilization of nutrients. You are aware that maintaining our health and well-being requires a balanced diet. We are in a state of good nutrition when our bodies get all nutrients they need in the right amounts to meet their requirements. Our nutritional status is normal. On the other hand, an imbalanced state of the body arises when the nutrients in the diet are either insufficient or improperly used. If this keeps happening for a while, it could become a serious issue that could even be fatal. An unbalanced state arises in the body when there is an excess or deficiency of one or more nutrients, as well as when our bodies utilize those nutrients improperly. Malnutrition is the term for this state. Two categories of malnutrition exist. Under-nutrition is the state of health that arises from a person's lack of one or more nutrients. On the other hand, over-nutrition occurs when there is an excessive nutrient intake.

Therefore, under-nutrition and over-nutrition are both included in the definition of malnutrition. You have probably seen people gain weight or become obese when they consume foods high in energy at quantities greater than what their bodies need. Overeating is the cause of this. Being obese is dangerous since it can result in major health issues. But under-nutrition is more prevalent in our environment. Actually, "under nutrition" has come to be synonymous with malnutrition.

1.4.1. Assessment of Nutritional Status

You may be wondering how to find out how nourished you or your friends are at this point. Nutritional assessment is the process of determining a person's or a group's nutritional status. You can find out the nutritional status of both yourself and other people in a few easy ways.

These procedures are:

1. By measuring physical growth;
2. By determining dietary intake;
3. By recognizing nutritional deficiency diseases.

1.4.1.1. Physical Growth

You are aware that early childhood is the time when growth is fastest. As a result, children under the age of five are particularly vulnerable to malnutrition. Weight and height measurements can be used to assess growth. A child needs to be a certain weight and height at a given age.

Stated differently, a child's height and body weight may serve as markers of their nutritional status. Standard weights and heights that a child should reach at a given age are established. How can you determine if a child is overweight or underweight? If the child's height and/or weight fall short of the reference, we can declare that the child is malnourished and that their growth is retarded.

1.4.1.2. Dietary Intake

It is the second evaluation technique. You will keep in mind that each of us needs a balanced diet to stay healthy. All the food consumed during the previous 24 hours must be documented in order to evaluate the nutritional status.

The food intake is tracked using household measurements. It is possible to adjust the quantity of portions (servings) to suit different physiological groups. The comparison allows one to determine if a person is following a normal or advised diet. The quantity consumed makes it evident whether or not a person has a normal nutritional status.

Let us know the method of determining your nutritional status:

- Note down whatever food items are eaten on one particular day along with the amounts of raw food items, in grams (g).
- Now group the food items into different food groups and find out the respective total amounts.
- Lastly, compare the differences in amounts of each food group with the recommended dietary intakes for the age and sex.

A normal nutritional status will result from dietary intakes that are comparable to the recommended dietary intakes. Any individual's nutritional status can be evaluated by calculating their dietary intakes in a comparable manner and comparing them to the intakes advised for their age and gender. After 6 to 12 months of lactation, diet should be gradually resumed as before. Older women: cut down on cereals and millets to two, fruit to one.

Identifying Nutritional Deficiency Diseases: You can also determine a person's nutritional status by looking for the telltale signs and symptoms of different nutritional deficiencies. A person with poor nutritional status will have one or more deficiencies. As you have already read, nutritional imbalance occurs when the body does not properly utilize the nutrients in the diet or when they are consumed at levels below what is needed. The body experiences a "nutritional deficiency" as a result. For instance, vitamin A is necessary for normal night vision. Your body will become vitamin A deficient if your diet is inadequate in this nutrient. It will interfere with your eyes' ability to function normally. For instance, you will not be able to see in the dark (night blindness), and your eyes may become hazy or muddy. Comparing the child with protein and energy malnutrition to the other children of the same age who get enough energy and protein from their diets, you will also notice that the child with this condition is shorter and thinner. These anatomical variations point to a disease caused by a nutritional deficit. These are usually specific and are, therefore, helpful in recognizing different deficiency diseases in and around you.

1.4.2. Nutritional Deficiency Diseases

Deficiency diseases result from the body not having enough of one or more nutrients. A person with this deficiency is weak and susceptible to infection. The different deficiencies are as follow:

1.4.2.1. Protein Energy Malnutrition (PEM)

PEM is one of the main issues with nutrition in our nation. While it can strike at any age, young children are the ones who are most affected.

It results due to:

- lack of energy and proteins;
- lack of proteins alone in the diet.

One may wonder how energy and protein deficiencies are related, and the truth is that energy deficiency can lead to protein deficiency. Carbs and fats provide energy to the body. The body cannot meet its energy needs if these are not included in the diet in sufficient amounts. The body then uses proteins as a source of energy, which leads to a protein shortage and PEM.

Low energy (carbohydrates and fats) intake
↓ leads to
Deficiency of energy in the body
↓ leads to
Use of proteins for giving energy because the avilability of carbo hydrates is low
↓ leads to
Deficiency of proteins in the body

Protein energy malnutrition is of two types:

- Marasmus; and
- Kwashiorkor.

Both marasmus and kwashiorkor exhibit growth retardation and a reduction in muscle mass. Yes, you are correct; could you explain why? These kids' diets are low in energy-dense foods and proteins, which are what give them energy.

1.4.2.2. Vitamin A Deficiency

Vitamin A deficiency is caused by a diet low in vitamin A.

- **Signs and Symptoms:**
    - Eye changes begin with night blindness, that is, inability to see when it is dark. If it is not treated, it leads to complete blindness.
    - Drying of the white portion of the eye.
    - Increased rate of infections especially of the respiratory system.

1.4.2.3. Anemia

Low levels of hemoglobin in the blood are referred to as anemia. The red pigment in blood called hemoglobin aids in the movement of oxygen throughout the body. A diet low in iron causes a decrease in hemoglobin levels. Put another way, an iron deficiency leads to anemia. A diet deficient in folic acid and vitamin B_{12} can also result in anemia.

- **Signs and Symptoms:**
- General body weakness. The person complains of tiredness and breathlessness.
- Loss of appetite.
- Paleness of tongue, white portion of eye and nail beds.
- Feeling of being pricked with pins and needles on the fingers and toes.
- Brittle and spoon shaped nails.
- The capacity of a person to work decreases considerably.

1.4.2.4. Iodine Deficiency

A crucial part of the hormone thyroxine is iodine. The majority of metabolic functions of the body are regulated by this hormone. The most common symptoms of iodine deficiency in adults are goiter and cretinism in young children. A maternal and paternal iodine deficiency during pregnancy is detrimental. It is important to keep in mind, though, that iodine deficiency disorders (IDD) can cause other issues as well.

- **Signs and Symptoms:**

In Adults:

- The neck becomes swollen. This is called goiter;
- The person may become fat;
- The person feels tired and is unable to work properly;
- Skin changes may also occur.

In Young Children:

- Growth retardation;
- Mental retardation;
- Speech and hearing defects;
- Disorders of nerves and muscles causing inability to control movements of limbs.

1.4.3. National Nutrition Programs

Diseases caused by nutritional deficiencies are very common in our nation. As you are aware, these illnesses have detrimental impacts on people's survival and general health. It is important for you to know that these illnesses can be prevented with minimal care. Several National Nutrition Programs have been introduced in our nation in an effort to control this situation. These initiatives benefit vulnerable populations nutritionally. It's true that young children, adolescents, pregnant women, and nursing mothers are the groups most vulnerable to deficiencies.

By knowing the services provided, you can benefit yourself as well as others from these nutrition programmes.

- Integrated Child Development Services (ICDS) Scheme.
- Mid Day Meal Programme (MDMP).
- National Control Programme for Prevention of Nutritional Blindness due to Vitamin A deficiency.
- National Nutritional Anaemia Control Programme (NNACP).
- National Iodine Deficiency Disorder Control Programme (NIDDCP).

1.4.3.1. Integrated Child Development Services (ICDS) Scheme

Today's youth will shape tomorrow; they will develop into healthy adults if we give them the care they need. Consider the possibility that children who do not eat enough will not be healthy. A child who is ill will not be motivated to learn. Similarly, giving a child extra food will not help if they have diarrhea; instead, it will not improve their nutritional status. As a result, it is critical to offer education, healthcare, and nutrition as a comprehensive package. This is the rationale behind the introduction of the ICDS program in our nation. Its success can be attributed to the inclusion of all the necessary elements for children's growth and development.

ICDS package provides:

1. **Health:**
   - Immunization;
   - Health check-ups;
   - Referral services;
   - Treatment of minor illnesses.
2. **Nutrition:**
   - Supplementary feeding;
   - Growth monitoring and promotion;
   - Nutrition and Health Education.
3. **Convergence:** Of other supportive services, such as safe drinking water, environmental sanitation, women's empowerment programs, non-formal preschool education, and adult literacy.

Anganwadis are the names of the centers where the ICDS program offers services. The Child Health Centers (CHC) offer the medical services.

Have you ever visited a Community Health Center (CHC; formerly known as a Primary Health Centre, or PHC) in your community? If so, you must have noticed that CHCs offer referral services in addition to standard health services like immunizations, health examinations, and treatment of minor illnesses. A person is referred to a larger hospital for medical treatment if they have "a serious health problem," according to referral services.

- **Beneficiaries:**
  - Children below 6 years of age;
  - Adolescent girls between 11 and 18 years;
  - Pregnant women and lactating mothers;
  - All women between 15 and 45 years.

1.4.3.2. Mid-Day Meal Program (MDMP)

The primary goal of the MDM program is to give primary school students, ages 6 to 11, supplemental meals. Thus, attendance at school is guaranteed.

- **National Control Program for Prevention of Nutritional Blindness Due to Vitamin A deficiency:** The goal of this program is to stop vitamin A deficiency-related blindness.

The services provided under this programme include:

i. Promoting consumption of vitamin A rich foods;

ii. Providing massive doses of vitamin A orally to children between 6 months to 5 years of age.

Beneficiaries:

- Children between 6 months to 5 years of age;
- Pregnant women and lactating mothers;
- All women between 15 and 45 years.

- **National Nutritional Anemia Control Program (NNACP):** The goal of this program is to dramatically lower the incidence and prevalence of anemia in young children and women.

The services provided through this program are:

- Promotion of regular consumption of foods rich in iron
- Providing iron and folic acid supplements
- Treatment of severe anemic cases.

Beneficiaries:

- Children between 6 months to 5 years of age
- Pregnant women and lactating mothers
- All women between 15 and 45 years

- **National Iodine Deficiency Disorder Control Program (NIDDCP):** This program's objective is to reduce the incidence of iodine deficiency disorder (IDD) in our nation by making iodine available in common salt (iodized salt).

The services provided are:

- To assess the extent of the problem;
- To arrange for production/ supply of iodized salt;
- To take quality control measures to ensure supply of standard quality of iodized salt to the consumer. The government is ensuring that all the salt that is produced in our country is iodized before it reaches the consumer. Steps are also taken to make the people aware about the consumption of iodized salt.

1.5. Body Fluids

Water is necessary for life, and staying hydrated is critical for both optimal physical and mental health. Water makes up the majority of the human body.

The percentage of water in the body decreases with age, going from roughly 75% in babies to 60% in adults. Even in cold climates, we can survive for only a few days without water, but we can live for up to 50 days without food.

People generally drink enough water, but for specific population groups, like the elderly, or while exercising, fluid intake might become critical. Water balance is achieved in the body by ensuring that the amount of water consumed in food and drink (and generated by metabolism) equals the amount of water excreted. The consumption side is regulated by behavioral mechanisms, including thirst and salt cravings. While almost a liter of water per day is lost through the skin, lungs, and feces, the kidneys are the major site of regulated excretion of water.

1.5.1. Body Water Compartments

The various organs and tissues that make up the body contain water. These countless fluids can be combined to form larger groups that can be the subject of physiologically relevant discussion.

These collections are referred to as "compartments."" The major division is into intracellular fluid (ICF: about 23 L) and extracellular fluid (ECF: about 19 L) based on which side of the cell membrane the fluid lies.

1.5.1.1. Intracellular Fluid

The ICF is composed of at least 10^{14} separate tiny cellular packages. The concept of a single united "compartment" called intracellular fluid is clearly artificial. The ICF compartment is really a "virtual compartment" considered as the sum of this huge number of discontinuous small collections. Intracellular though not united physically, the collections have extremely important unifying similarities which make the ICF concept of practical usefulness in physiology. In particular, similarities of location, composition and behavior (Figure 1.6):

- **Location:** The distinction between ICF and ECF is clear and is easy to understand: they are separated by the cell membranes.
- **Composition:** ICFs are high in potassium and magnesium and low in sodium and chloride ions.
- **Behavior:** ICF behave similarly to tonicity changes in the ECF.

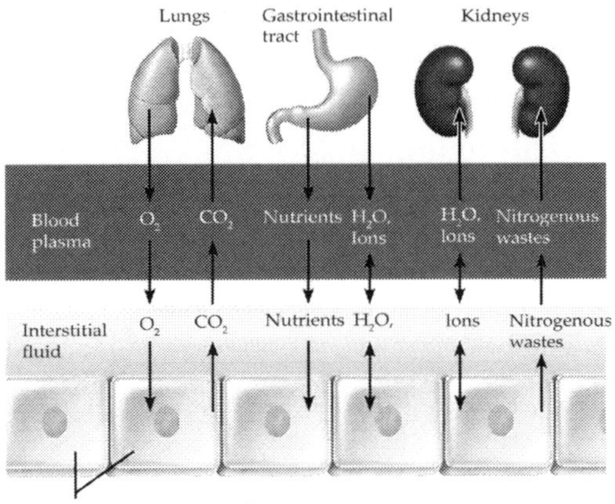

Figure 1.6. *Exchange of gases, nutrients, water, and wastes between the three fluid compartments of the body.*

Source: https://fi.pinterest.com/pin/234327986842880625/.

It is convenient to discuss an idealized ICF as though it were a single real entity due to its physiological usefulness. By using this convention, predictions about the outcomes of different interventions can be made, and these predictions are, within certain bounds, physiologically meaningful.

1.5.1.2. Extracellular Fluid (ECF)

The ECF is subject to a similar defense. The ECF is split up into multiple smaller sections, (for example. interstitial fluid (ISF), transcellular fluid (TCF), bone and dense connective tissue fluid, and plasma). These compartments can be identified by their distinct kinetic characteristics and locations. It can be said that the compositional similarity of the ECF is somewhat opposite to that of the ICF (i.e. concentrated in sodium and chloride and deficient in potassium and magnesium.

1.5.1.2.1. Interstitial Fluid

All the fluid fragments found in the spaces between all bodily tissues are collectively referred to as ISF. Furthermore, this fluid is "virtual" (i.e., despite existing in numerous discrete small pieces, it is discussed as if it were a single, homogeneous fluid pool. The intravascular compartment and the ICF are connected by the ISF, which envelops every cell in the body. The ISF is a conduit for chemicals, waste, nutrients, and oxygen. ISF shares compositional traits with ECF, but it differs from plasma in that it typically has a lower protein concentration. It is thought that lymph is a component of the ISF. Excess ISF and protein are returned to the bloodstream by the lymphatic system. Comparatively speaking to other ISF components, lymph is easier to obtain for analysis.

1.5.1.2.2. Plasma

The only significant fluid compartment that is a true fluid collection in one place is plasma. Its significantly higher protein content and high bulk flow (transport function) set it apart from ISF. Plasma is referred to as the "interstitial fluid of the blood" because blood contains suspended red and white blood cells. The blood volume fluid compartment is intriguing because it is a composite compartment that includes red cell water and ECF (plasma).

1.5.1.2.3. The Fluid of Bone and Dense Connective Tissue

About 15% of the body's total water content is found in the fluid found in bone and dense connective tissue, making it an important fluid. Since this fluid is only very slowly mobilized, its significance is diminished when analyzing the outcomes of acute fluid interventions.

1.5.1.2.4. Transcellular Fluid

TCF is a tiny compartment that is representative of all bodily fluids produced by cell transport processes. It is enclosed in spaces lined with epithelium. It consists of joint fluid, aqueous humor, bladder urine, CSF, and GIT fluids. Because of the specialized tasks involved, it is significant. GIT fluids can involve very large fluid fluxes. The different TCFs have quite different electrolyte compositions, with typical values or ranges for certain fluids. The total body water is separated into compartments, and although most of these fluid compartments do not exist as discrete real fluid collections, this approach can provide valuable physiological insight and a certain amount of clinical predictability.

1.5.1.3. Functional ECF

Although present in significant quantities, the water in bone, dense connective tissue, and TCFs mobilize considerably more slowly than the other constituents of the extracellular matrix. The functional ECF is composed of the remaining components. ICF to ECF is a ratio of 55:45. The ratio of ICF to functional ECF is 55:27.5, or 2:1, and the functional ECF is more significant when considering the effects of acute fluid interventions.

1.6. Nutrition Problems and Their Solutions

An impacted appetite can result in weight gain or loss following surgery, medication, or illness. Several nutritional issues may have the following potential fixes.

1. **Decreased Appetite:** One of the most problematic nutrition issues you can have is appetite loss, or decreased hunger. Despite being a widespread issue, its origin is unknown. Certain medications have the potential to increase your appetite. Consult your physician if taking such medications would be beneficial for you.

   Solutions:

- Eat smaller meals and snacks more frequently. Eating six or seven or eight times a day might be more easily tolerated than eating the same amount of food in three meals.
- Talk to your doctor. Sometimes, poor appetite is due to depression, which can be treated. Your appetite is likely to improve after depression is treated.
- Avoid non-nutritious beverages such as black coffee and tea.
- Try to eat more protein and fat and less simple sugars.
- Walk or participate in light activities to stimulate your appetite.

2. **Meal Guidelines:**
   - Drink beverages after a meal instead of before or during a meal so you do not feel as full.
   - Plan meals to include your favorite foods.
   - Try eating the high-calorie foods in your meal first.
   - Use your imagination to increase the variety of food you're eating.
3. **Snack Guidelines:**
   - Don't waste your energy eating foods that provide little or no nutritional value (such as potato chips, candy bars, colas, and other snack foods).
   - Choose high-protein and high-calorie snacks.
4. **Dining Guidelines:**
   - Make food preparation an easy task. Choose foods that are easy to prepare and eat.
   - Make eating a pleasurable experience, not a chore.
   - Liven up your meals by using colorful place settings.
   - Play background music during meals.
   - Eat with others. Invite a guest to share your meal or go out to dinner.
   - Use colorful garnishes such as parsley and red or yellow peppers to make food look more appealing and appetizing.
5. **Weight Loss:** The following advice will help you maintain a healthy weight if your doctor says you have lost too much weight.
   - Drink milk or try one of the "high-calorie recipes" listed below instead of drinking low-calorie beverages.
   - Ask your doctor or dietitian about nutritional supplements. Sometimes, supplements in the form of snacks, drinks (such as Ensure or Boost), or vitamins might be prescribed to eat between meals. These supplements help you increase your calories and get the right amount of nutrients every day. *Note*: Do not use supplements in place of your meals.
   - Avoid low-fat or low-calorie products unless you have been given other dietary guidelines. Use whole milk, whole milk cheese, and yogurt.
   - Use the "Calorie Boosters" listed below to add calories to your favorite foods.

6. **High-Calorie Snacks:**
   - Ice cream;
   - Cookies;
   - Pudding;
   - Cheese;
   - Granola bars;
   - Custard;
   - Sandwiches;
   - Nachos with cheese;
   - Eggs;
   - Crackers with peanut butter;
   - Bagels with peanut butter or cream cheese;
   - Cereal with half and half;
   - Fruit or vegetables with dips;
   - Yogurt with granola;
   - Popcorn with margarine and parmesan cheese;
   - Bread sticks with cheese sauce.
7. **High-Calorie Recipes:**

   Chocolate Peanut Butter Shake:
   - 1/2 cup heavy whipping cream
   - 3 tablespoons creamy peanut butter
   - 3 tablespoons chocolate syrup
   - 1 1/2 cups chocolate ice cream

   Directions:
   - Put all ingredients into a blender. Mix well.
   - Makes one serving; 1090 calories per serving.
8. **Super Shake:**
   - 1 cup whole milk
   - 1 cup ice cream (1–2 scoops)
   - 1 package Carnation Instant Breakfast

   Directions:
   - Put all ingredients into a blender. Mix well.
   - Makes one serving; 550 calories per serving.
9. **Super Pudding:**
   - 2 cups whole milk
   - 2 tablespoons vegetable oil
   - 1 package instant pudding
   - 3/4 cup non-fat dry milk powder

   Directions:
   - Blend milk and oil. Add pudding mix and mix well. Pour into dishes (1/2 cup servings).
   - Makes four 1/2 cup servings; 250 calories per serving.
10. **Great Grape Slush:**
    - 2 grape juice bars
    - 1/2 cup grape juice or 7-Up
    - 2 tablespoons corn syrup
    - 1 tablespoon corn oil

    Directions:
    - Put all ingredients into a blender. Mix well.
    - Makes one serving; 490 calories per serving.
11. **Calorie Boosters:**

    i. **Egg Yolk or Whole Egg:** Before cooking, add egg yolk or whole egg to foods such as meatloaf, rice pudding, or macaroni and cheese. (To prevent illness, avoid the use of uncooked eggs.)

    ii. **Non-Fat Powdered Milk or Undiluted Evaporated Milk:** Add to beverages (*including* *milk*) or to these foods:

- Creamed soups, yogurt;
- Scrambled eggs, casseroles;
- Pudding mashed potatoes;
- Custard gravies;
- Hot cereal sauces.

iii. **Cream Cheese or Shredded, Melted, Sliced, Cubed or Grated Cheese:** Add to sandwiches, snacks, casseroles, crackers, eggs, soups, toast, pasta, potatoes, rice, or vegetables, or serve as a snack.

iv. **Vegetable Oils, Mayonnaise, Butter, Margarine, or Sour Cream:** Spread mayonnaise or margarine on sandwiches. Mix any of these ingredients with bread, cooked cereals, pasta, potatoes, rice, veggies, pudding, casseroles, soups, and eggs.

v. **Peanut Butter (Creamy or Crunchy):** Spread on bread, crackers, apples, bananas, or celery. Or add to cereal, custard, cookies, or milk shakes.

vi. **Nut "Dust" (Grind Any Type of Nuts in a Blender or Food Processor):** Add to puddings, gravy, mashed potatoes, casseroles, salads, and yogurt cereals.

vii. **Miscellaneous Foods (Limit to One Serving per Day)**

Add:

- Sugar, jelly, jam, preserves;
- Honey;
- Corn syrup;
- Maple syrup.

To:

- Hot cereal;
- Fruit;
- Sweet potatoes;
- Winter squash, cold cereal, fruit salad.

12. **Heartburn:** There are numerous causes of heartburn, such as overindulging, consuming particular foods, taking medications, or having surgery.

    Solutions:

    - Avoid foods that have caused heartburn before. Some foods commonly associated with heartburn are highly seasoned foods, greasy or fried foods, chocolate, alcohol, and beverages that contain caffeine (coffee, tea, and soft drinks).
    - Eat five or six smaller meals a day instead of three large meals. Decreasing the amount of food in your stomach eases digestion and reduces the chances of heartburn.
    - Remain standing or sitting for at least two hours after eating. If you lie down, keep your upper body raised at a 45-degree angle.
    - Eat your last meal several hours before going to bed.
    - Take an antacid one hour after meals to relieve heartburn. You can also try taking antacids before going to bed. If you take antacids frequently, tell your doctor or dietitian.

13. **Changes in How Food Tastes:** What you like to eat is often determined

by how something tastes. Your appetite may be impacted if food starts to taste off; that is, if it starts to taste too sweet, too bland, bitter, or metallic. These tastes are frequently altered by medications.

Solutions:

- Brush your teeth after meals and snacks. Good oral hygiene helps control bad taste. Ask your doctor or dietitian if using a mouthwash would help.
- Cold or room-temperature food might taste better.
- Eat alternatives to red meat. Try turkey, chicken, fish, eggs, or dairy products such as yogurt, cheese, or cottage cheese.
- Use marinades to add flavor to poultry, red meat, or fish. Fruit juice, teriyaki sauce, Italian dressing, beer, or wine will also add flavor.
- Add spices, such as herbs, onions, bacon bits, or almonds to flavor plain foods.
- Use strong seasonings to improve the flavor of meats and vegetables. Rosemary, oregano, basil, tarragon, or mint are good options.
- Eat snacks that leave a refreshing, pleasing aftertaste: fresh fruit, chewing gum, hard candy, cinnamon, or mint-flavored foods or beverages.

14. **Sore Mouth or Throat:** A sore mouth or throat can make eating difficult. Medicines or mouth infections can cause soreness.

Solutions:

- Eat bland, mild-flavored foods. Spicy or salty foods can irritate soreness.
- Eat lukewarm or cold foods. Hot food can irritate soreness.
- Puree foods before you eat them. Most cooked foods can be pureed in a blender or food processor.
- Avoid carbonated beverages or drink them only after they have gone flat. Carbonation can irritate soreness.
- Drink soups or other liquids from a straw or a cup instead of a spoon to keep foods away from sore spots in your mouth.
- Talk with your doctor about using an anesthetic mouthwash to help relieve discomfort.
- Have your doctor examine your mouth to see whether you have a fungal infection. Such infections are treatable and often occur in patients who are ill, especially those taking steroids or antibiotics.
- Avoid rough foods that might be hard to swallow, such as hard breads, toast, popcorn, raw vegetables, nuts, and seeds.
- Eat soft foods that are easy to chew. Try casseroles, meat with gravy, mashed potatoes, cooked cereal, ice cream, eggs, pudding, or cottage cheese.
- Eat foods that are less acidic. Try bananas, canned pears and peaches, applesauce, or fruit nectars. Avoid tomatoes, oranges, grapefruits, and pineapples.

- Drink plenty of liquids all day to keep your throat moist and to help prevent dehydration. Try milk shakes, eggnog, juices, and soups.

15. Dryness in the Mouth: Eating certain foods can be more challenging when one's mouth is dry. Dryness can be brought on by medications, fevers, or oral infections.

Solutions:

- Drink eight or more cups of liquid each day; 10 or more cups if you are feverish.
- Dunk or moisten breads, toast, cookies, or crackers in milk, hot chocolate, or coffee to soften them.
- Take a drink after each bite of food to moisten your mouth and to help you swallow.
- Add sauces to foods to make them softer and more moist. Try gravy, broth, sauce, or melted butter.
- Eat sour candy or fruit ice to help increase saliva and moisten your mouth.
- Don't use a commercial mouthwash. Commercial mouthwashes often contain alcohol that can dry your mouth. Ask your doctor or dentist about alternative mouthwash products.
- Ask your doctor about artificial saliva products. These products are available by prescription.

16. Nausea: Nausea, also known as upset or queasy stomach, is a sick feeling that occasionally results in vomiting. Nausea can result from medications, injuries, constipation, or the flu. There are lots of medications available to treat nausea. Find out if there is a medication that can assist you from your doctor.

Solutions:

- Eat dry foods when you wake up and every few hours during the day. Nausea is often worse on an empty stomach, and dry foods can relieve some of the discomfort. Try pretzels, plain crackers or cookies, dry cereal, or toast.
- Drinking liquids on an empty stomach can add to the feeling of nausea. Try sipping beverages slowly during your meals or drinking 30 to 60 minutes after eating solid foods.
- If the smell of food bothers you, avoid foods with unpleasant or strong odors. Eat somewhere other than the kitchen, where the odors might be strongest.
- Avoid greasy, fried, or spicy foods. These foods take longer to digest and can make you feel bloated, uncomfortable, and more nauseous.
- Avoid large meals and infrequent meals. The smaller and more frequent your meals and snacks are, the more comfortable you will be.
- Eat foods and supplements that are high in calories and protein to maintain your

nutrition when you cannot eat a lot.

- It is important to replace liquids if vomiting occurs. If you can, drink eight or more cups of liquid each day. Add an additional 1/2 cup to 1 cup of liquid for each episode of vomiting.
- Fresh ginger is sometimes helpful in reducing nausea. Do not eat fresh ginger if you are taking anti-coagulant (blood-thinning) medicines, such as warfarin (Coumadin). In addition, do not eat fresh ginger prior to surgery.

17. **Diarrhea:** An increase in the quantity of liquid in the stools, the number of stools, or both can indicate diarrhea. Diarrhea can be brought on by medications, food allergies, stress, and common colds or the flu.

    Extended diarrhea may result in weight loss, weakness, dehydration, and exhaustion. Vital nutrients, including calories, protein, vitamins, water, sodium, and potassium, are lost when you have diarrhea. If you are ill already or are in the process of getting better, this loss could be quite serious. For diarrhea to be properly treated, your doctor has to be aware of its cause. For two days, try the following solutions. Please give your doctor a call if your diarrhea persists after that time. Since fluids and nutrients are rapidly lost, treatment must start before chronic diarrhea becomes harmful.

    Solutions:

    - Drink eight or more cups of liquids per day.
    - For every episode of loose, watery stool, add one to two cups of liquids to the daily eight cups to replace losses.
    - Talk with your doctor or dietitian about increasing or decreasing the amount of fiber you eat.
    - Drink a variety of beverages to help replace lost liquids and nutrients. Try water, coffee, tea, iced tea, lemonade or fruit-flavored drinks, fruit or vegetable juice, broth, milk, or cream soup.
    - Eat soft foods that contain large amounts of liquid, such as sherbet, gelatin, yogurt, and pudding.
    - Use less sugar and fat. Limiting sugar and fat might decrease the amount of water in the intestine and reduce the number of episodes of diarrhea.
    - Ask your doctor whether adjusting your medicines might help relieve the diarrhea. Do not change your medicines without first talking to your doctor.
    - Don't take over-the-counter (non-prescription) drugs for diarrhea without talking to your doctor.

18. **Constipation:** When bowel movements become difficult or rare, usually occurring more than 48 hours apart, it is referred to as constipation. Medication side effects, inactivity, and inadequate hydration

or food intake can all contribute to constipation.

Solutions:

- Drink eight or more cups of fluids per day, such as water, coffee, tea, juice, or flavored beverages.
- Drink something hot as the first beverage in the morning, such as hot water, coffee, tea, or hot apple cider. Hot liquids might stimulate a bowel movement.
- Drink 1/2 to 1 cup of prune juice in the morning to stimulate a bowel movement.
- Increase the fiber in your foods. Try whole grain breads, fresh fruits, whole grain cereals, and fresh vegetables.
- Emphasize fruits that stimulate the bowels, such as watermelon, plums, and other summer fruits, and avoid fruits that constipate, such as bananas.
- Add two to four tablespoons of unprocessed wheat bran to foods and drink plenty of liquids. (Liquids increase the effectiveness of bran). Try bran sprinkled over hot or cold cereal, casseroles, or mixed with applesauce, pancake batter, pudding, muffin batter, milkshakes, or cookie dough.
- Activity such as walking helps normalize bowel function.
- Plan trips to the bathroom immediately after meals since eating is a natural stimulus for having a bowel movement.
- Contact your physician if the constipation persists. Your physician may recommend a laxative or stool softener. Consult your doctor before taking any medication, even over-the-counter (non-prescription) medications, to treat constipation.

19. **Swallowing Problems:** It may be difficult for you to chew and handle solid food if you have weak mouth muscles. It may also be challenging for you to swallow without coughing or choking if there is a delay in the swallowing process in your throat or pharynx (the digestive tube that connects your mouth and esophagus).

Solutions:

- **Positioning:** Sit upright at a 90-degree angle, tilt your head slightly forward, and/or remain sitting or standing upright for 45 to 60 minutes after eating a meal.
- **Dining Environment:** Minimize distractions in the area where you eat. Stay focused on the tasks of eating and drinking. Do not talk with food in your mouth.
- **Amount and Rate:** Eat slowly. Cut your food into small pieces and chew it thoroughly. Do not try to eat more than 1/2 teaspoon of your food at a time.
- **Swallowing:** It may be necessary for you to swallow each bite or sip two or three times. Before inhaling, cough gently or clear your throat if food or liquid gets stuck in

your throat, then swallow once more. If required, repeat.

- **Concentrate on Swallowing Frequently:** Alternating between a food bite and a drink could be beneficial. Reduce the length of the straw to reduce the distance the liquid must travel if you are having trouble sucking liquid up it. Modify the texture and temperature of liquids. Chill the liquids more. Test out some fizzy drinks.
- **Saliva Management:** Drink plenty of fluids. Periodically suck on popsicles, ice chips, lemon ice, or lemon-flavored water to increase saliva, which will increase swallowing frequency.
- **Difficulty Chewing:** If chewing is difficult or tiring, minimize (or eliminate) foods that require chewing, and eat more soft foods. Puree your foods in a blender.
- **Coughing:** If thin liquids cause you to cough, use a liquid thickener. (Your speech pathologist can recommend one for you.) You can also substitute thin liquids with thicker liquid choices such as nectars for juices and cream soups for plain broths.
- **Taking Medicines:** Crush your pills and mix them with applesauce or pudding. Ask your pharmacist for recommendations on which pills should not be crushed and which medicines can be purchased in a liquid form.

The interpretation of dietary, laboratory, anthropometric, and clinical research is known as nutritional assessment. It is employed to ascertain how nutrient intake and utilization affect an individual's or a population group's nutritional status. The fulfillment of the body's

A Closer Look

Human Nutritional Assessment and Survey:

requirements for protective and nutritive substances, as well as how these requirements are reflected in an individual's functional capacity, physical, physiological, and biochemical traits, and overall health, is referred to as nutritional status. Details regarding nutritional status, i.e., nutritional assessments, are necessary to identify potentially critical nutrients (for population groups at risk of deficiency), formulate dietary recommendations, create an efficient public health nutrition (PHN) program to prevent diseases related to nutrition, and track the effectiveness of these interventions. It is essential to continue developing and implementing a harmonized and standardized nutritional assessment methodology to support the recommendations made by current nutrition epidemiology (NE) and PHN research, as well as to collect and compare data against one another. In addition to these key tools, socioeconomic status, cultural norms, and health and vital statistics—ecological factors—should also be considered in order to accurately interpret the findings of nutritional assessment methods.

Nutrition surveys are typically cross-sectional national studies designed to evaluate current nutritional issues, identify populations at risk of chronic malnutrition, assess a population's nutritional status, and provide information for evidence-based nutrition policies. Nutrition surveys can also be used to compare the effectiveness of an intervention by combining information from initial and final evaluations.

Nutritional surveillance planning, carrying out, and assessing public health practices require the continuous, systematic collection, analysis, and interpretation of health-related data. This is known as public health surveillance. Nutritional surveillance studies involve the systematic collection, analysis, and evaluation of data over an extended duration. They can be applied to determine potential nutritional risk factors for malnutrition in a given vulnerable group or the population as a whole. The main goals of nutrition surveillance are to develop, assess, and oversee nutrition intervention programs and policies.

Nutrition screening is used to identify malnourished individuals. It can be carried out on the whole population, on specific subpopulations at risk or on selected individuals. During nutritional screening, simple, cheap, and rapid measurement methods are used.

Nutrition interventions are carried out on population subgroups at risk, which are identified during nutrition surveys or screening. Supplementation and fortification are some examples of nutrition interventions. In order to demonstrate the effectiveness and validity of these interventions, providers need to conduct effective monitoring and evaluation. Three categories of evaluation designs exist. In the most basic, the intervention is implemented for the entire targeted group, and the results are evaluated for suitability by comparing them to predetermined objectives. For the second "plausibility evaluation," quasi-experimental setups are needed, in which one group is given an intervention and the other is either given a placebo or does not receive any treatment at all. The subjects in this design are not randomized, and biases and outside influences are eliminated through multivariate analysis. This method is more costly than the last one. Randomized, controlled, double-blind experimental trials, in which participants are randomized to either the intervention or control group, constitute the third category of evaluating designs. When an intervention using this design is evaluated, particularly when it is well-planned and executed, "probability evaluation" provides the highest level of assurance that the outcome is a direct result of the intervention.

Summary

- Nutrition is the study of how food and drink affects our bodies with a special regard to the essential nutrients necessary to support human health. It looks at the physiological and biochemical processes involved in nourishment and how substances in food provide energy or are converted into body tissues. These nutrients which are the source of energy for our bodies are classed as: carbohydrates, fats, fibre, minerals, proteins, vitamins, and water.
- Nutrition is defined as the processes by which an animal or plant takes in and utilizes food substances. Essential nutrients include protein, carbohydrate, fat, vitamins, minerals and electrolytes. Normally, 85% of daily energy use is from fat and carbohydrates and 15% from protein.
- Food energy, as well as the energy needs of the body, is measured in units of energy called kilocalories. The number of kilocalories in a particular food can be determined by burning a weighed portion of that food and measuring the amount of heat (or kilocalories) it produces.
- A healthy diet is the one which meets the energy requirements and supplies essential macro and micronutrients for supporting the functioning of all vital processes. Growth during infancy is rapid.
- The human body needs the nutrients found in food. These nutrients are classified into six groups: carbohydrates, proteins, fats, vitamins, minerals, and water. Each plays a unique part in maintaining the normal growth and functioning of your body. Together, they are essential to your overall health and wellness.
- Good nutrition aims to achieve and maintain a desirable body composition and high potential for physical and mental work. Balancing energy intake with energy expenditure is necessary for a desirable body weight.
- All foods were not created equal in terms of the kcalories and nutrients they provide. Some foods, such as milk, contribute much calcium to your diet, especially when you compare them with other beverages, such as soft drinks.
- Body composition refers to the proportion of fat and fat-free mass in the body. A healthy body composition is one that includes a lower proportion of body fat and a higher proportion of fat-free mass
- The density of an object is defined as the ratio of its weight to its volume (Density = weight ÷ volume). Two common procedures that estimate body composition based on densitometry are hydrostatic weighing and air displacement plethysmography.
- Water is essential for life, and maintaining hydration is important for physical and mental performance. The human body is largely made of water. Body water content declines with age, from about 75% in babies to 60% in adults.

References

1. Augustin, L., Franceschi, S., Jenkins, D., et al. (2002). Glycemic index in chronic disease: A review. European Journal of Clinical Nutrition, 56, 1049–1071.
2. Benelam, B. (2009). Satiety and the anorexia of aging. British Journal of Community Nursing, 14(8), 332–335. Retrieved September 13, 2009, from Academic Search Complete database.
3. Benton, D. (2008). Micronutrient status, cognition and behavioral problems in childhood. European Journal of Nutrition, 47, 38–50. Retrieved September 12, 2009, from Academic Search Premier database.
4. Blake, J. S. (2008). Nutrition and You. San Francisco, CA: Pearson Benjamin Cummings Publishers.
5. Dwyer, J. (2006). Harrison's Principles of Internal Medicine; Nutritional Requirements and Dietary Assessment. USA: The McGraw-Hill Companies.
6. Payne-Palacio, J. R., & Canter, D. D. (2014). The Profession of Dietetics. Jones & Bartlett Learning.
7. Symmonds, E. M., & Symmonds, I. M. (2004). Essential Obstetrics & Gynaecology. Spain: Churchill Livingstone.
8. Willett, W. C., & Skerrett, P. J. (2005). Eat, Drink, and be Healthy: The Harvard Medical School Guide To Healthy Eating. Free Press (Simon & Schuster).

Chapter 2

TOOLS OF NUTRITION

Contents

Unit Introduction

The field of nutrition science is one that is always developing. The importance of health and wellness has increased due to advancements in dietetic research and practice. The way that food impacts the body's health is known as nutrition. Food is necessary for survival because it gives the body the nutrients it needs to function and stay healthy. Protein, carbohydrates, and fats are examples of macronutrients found in food. These substances not only provide the body with calories to fuel and energy, but also have specific functions in maintaining health. In addition to providing calories, food also contains phytochemicals and micronutrients (such as vitamins and minerals) that are essential for the body to function at its best.

Orientation and Directional Terms

Term	Definition	Illustration
Adequate Intake (AI)	Adequate Intake (AI) is the recommended average daily intake level based on observed or experimentally determined approximations or estimates of nutrient intake by a group (or groups) of apparently healthy people that are assumed to be adequate – used when an RDA cannot be determined.	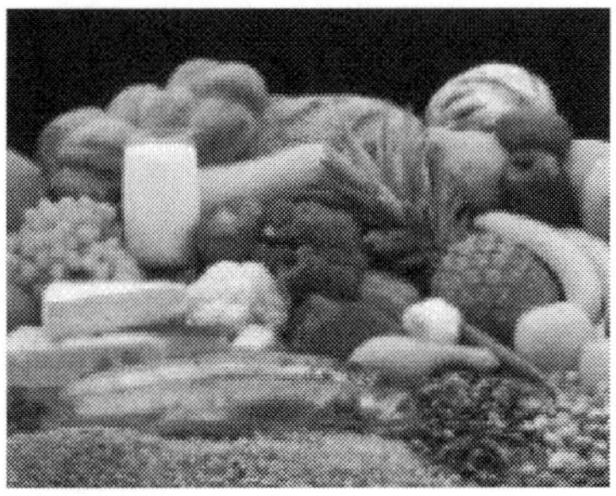
Food composition tables (FCT)	Food composition tables (FCT) are data repository for the content of nutritionally relevant chemical constituents and energy values of foods.	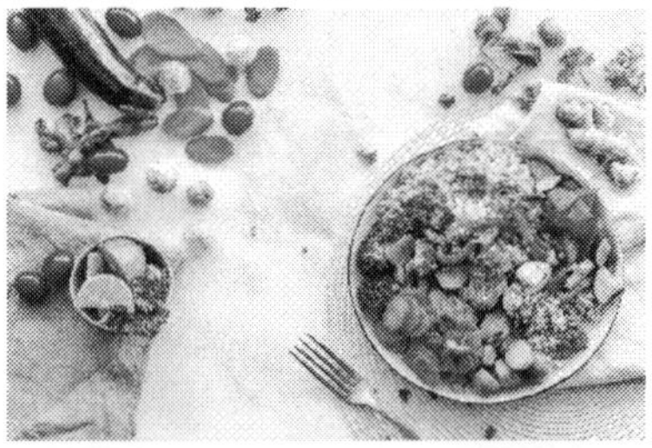
Food diary	A food diary is a daily log of what you eat and drink each day. The diary helps you and your doctor understand your eating habits. It can help you realize what you consume. Once you know this, you can make changes to your diet to improve your weight.	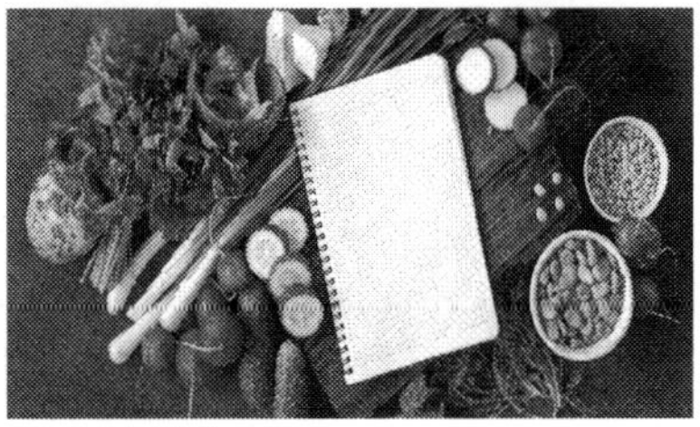
Food Package	Food packaging can be defined as 'a complex and dynamic system aiming to safely prepare foods for transportation, distribution, storage, retailing, handling and end-use, and safely deliver these foods to the consumer in a sound condition (maximum quality) at a minimum cost'	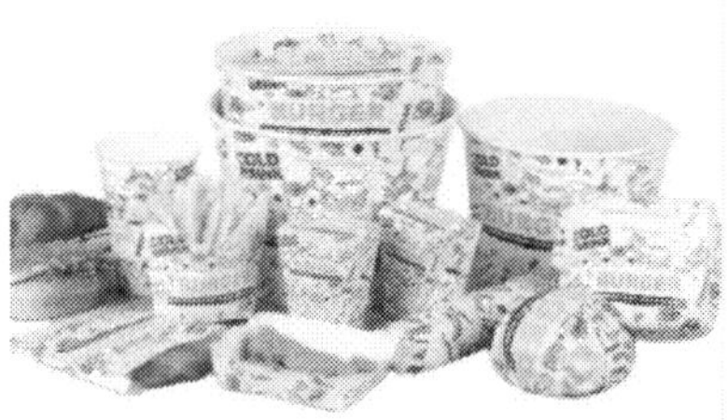
Healthy diet	A healthy diet is a diet that maintains or improves overall health. A healthy diet provides the body with essential nutrition: fluid, macronutrients such as protein, micronutrients such as vitamins, and adequate fibre and food energy.	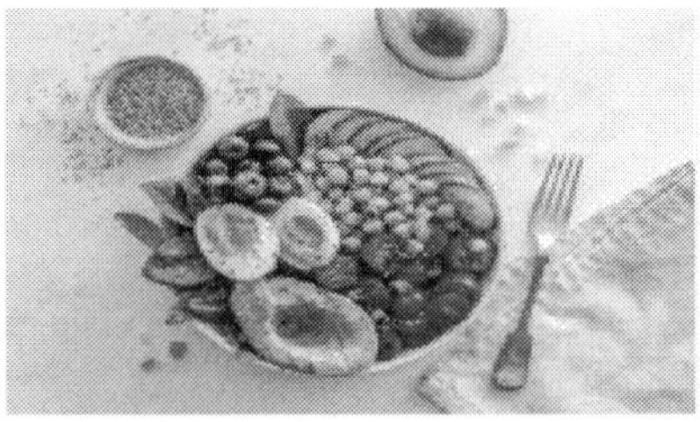

2.1. Food Pyramid

Food pyramids are the ideal tool for quickly visualizing a person's entire diet. When properly designed, food pyramids display the relative amounts of each food group as well as examples of what to eat throughout the day (not just at this one meal!). They also have vibrant, alluring pictures of actual foods. The Food Pyramid aims to simplify the process of eating healthily. Eating a healthy diet entails consuming the right proportions of the vitamins, minerals, fats, proteins, and carbohydrates that your body needs to stay healthy.

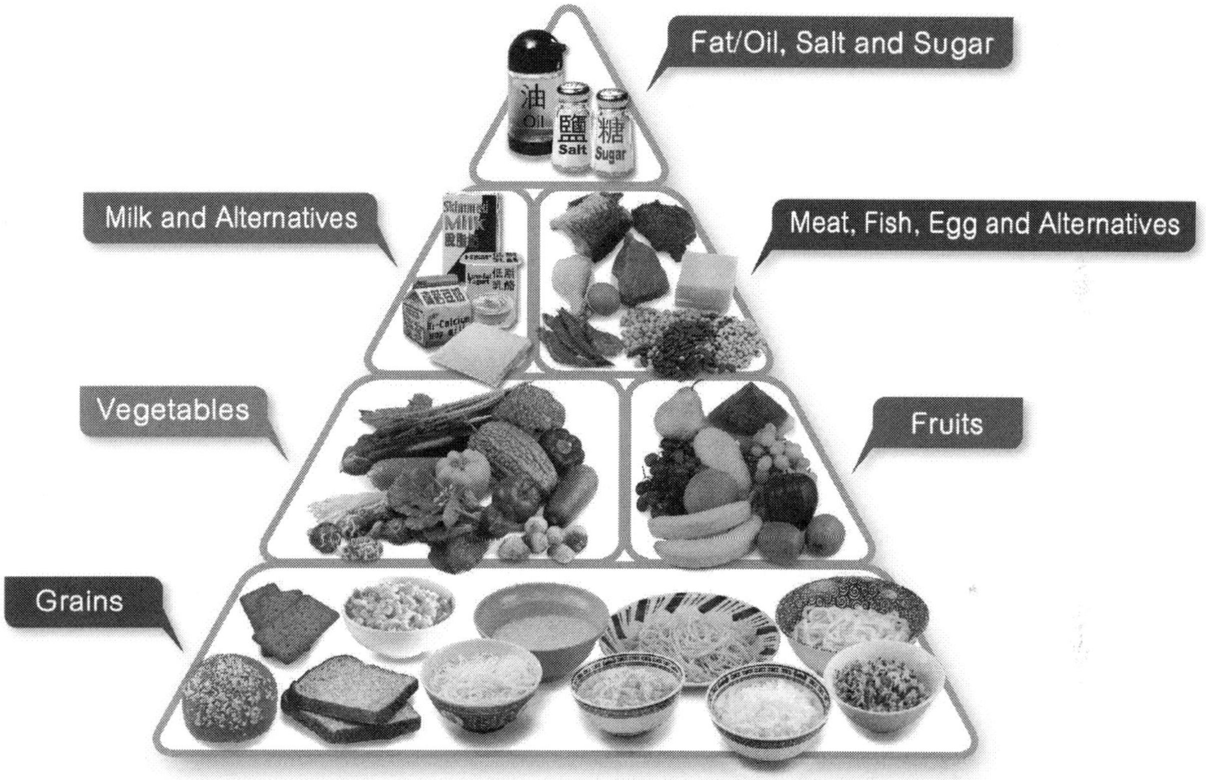

Figure 2.1. *The food pyramid.*

Source: https://www.chp.gov.hk/files/jpg/adult_eng.jpg.

On each shelf of the Food Pyramid, foods that are similar in terms of nutrients are grouped together. This provides you with a variety of food options from which to select a nutritious diet. Getting the correct balance of nutrient-dense foods within your calorie range can be achieved by using the Food Pyramid as a guide. According to studies, we consume an excessive number of calories from foods and beverages on the top shelf of the food pyramid that are high in fat, sugar, and salt. They barely contain any of the vital vitamins and minerals that your body requires. Restricting these is necessary for a healthy diet (Figure 2.1).

2.1.1. Healthy Eating Food Pyramid

Maintaining your health requires a balanced diet. When choosing what to eat, refer to the Healthy

Eating Food Pyramid guide. Grain consumption ought to be the main dietary source. Consume more veggies and fruits. Consume moderate amounts of dairy, eggs, fish, meat, and their substitutes. Cut back on sugar, fat/oil, and salt. Meat should be fattened before cooking. Select low-fat cooking techniques like using non-stick frying pans or steaming, stewing, simmering, boiling, and scalding. Additionally, use less frying and deep-frying. These can support good health and help us achieve a balanced diet.

2.1.2. Eat the Right Food

A single food cannot provide us with all the nutrients we require because different foods have varying nutritional values. A variety of foods from all food groups and within each group are required to meet our daily needs and obtain various nutrients, as per the Healthy Eating Food Pyramid.

2.1.3. Eat the Right Amount

It is not beneficial to our health to eat too much or too little. We require a certain quantity of nutrients daily to stay in good health. Under-nutrition and deficiency symptoms can arise from insufficient food intake, whereas overconsumption of any kind of food can lead to obesity and over-nutrition.

- **Healthy Eating Food Pyramid:**
    - Eat Most – Grains
    - Eat More – Vegetables and fruits
    - Eat Moderately – Meat, fish, egg, and alternatives (including dry beans) and milk and alternatives
    - Eat Less – Fat/ oil, salt, and sugar
    - Drink adequate amount of fluid (including water, tea, clear soup, etc.) every day
- **Healthy Eating Food Pyramid for Children (Aged 2 to 5):**
    - Grains: 1.5–3 bowls
    - Vegetables: at least 1.5 servings
    - Fruits: at least 1 serving
    - Meat, fish, egg, and alternatives: 1.5–3 taels
    - Milk and alternatives: 2 servings
    - Fat/oil, salt, and sugar: eat the least
    - Fluid: 4–5 glasses
- **Healthy Eating Food Pyramid for Children (Aged 6 to 11):**
    - Grains: 3–4 bowls
    - Vegetables: at least 2 servings
    - Fruits: at least 2 servings
    - Meat, fish, egg, and alternatives: 3–5 taels
    - Milk and alternatives: 2 servings
    - Fat/oil, salt, and sugar: eat the least
    - Fluid: 6–8 glasses
- **Healthy Eating Food Pyramid for Teenagers (Aged 12 to 17):**
    - Grains: 4–6 bowls
    - Vegetables: at least 3 servings
    - Fruits: at least 2 servings
    - Meat, fish, egg, and alternatives: 4–6 taels
    - Milk and alternatives: 2 servings
    - Fat/oil, salt, and sugar: eat the least
    - Fluid: 6–8 glasses

- **Healthy Eating Food Pyramid for Adults:**
  - Grains: 3–8 bowls
  - Vegetables: at least 3 servings
  - Fruits: at least 2 servings
  - Meat, fish, egg, and alternatives: 5–8 taels
  - Milk and alternatives: 1–2 servings
  - Fat/oil, salt, and sugar: eat the least
  - Fluid: 6–8 glasses
- **Healthy Eating Food Pyramid for Elderly:**
  - Grains: 3–5 bowls
  - Vegetables: at least 3 servings
  - Fruits: at least 2 servings
  - Meat, fish, egg, and alternatives: 5–6 taels
  - Milk and alternatives: 1–2 servings
  - Fat/oil, salt, and sugar: eat the least
  - Fluid: 6–8 glasses

2.1.4. Benefits of the Food Pyramid

The primary goal of the food pyramid's design is to simplify the process of eating a healthy diet. The food pyramid is crucial because it helps people determine whether they are getting the recommended amounts of essential nutrients like protein, fat, and carbohydrates when beginning a new, healthful diet.

The food pyramid is divided into various sections containing food groups that are typically based on how similar their nutrients are. This genuinely helps you understand the vast range of foods that contain a specific nutrient, providing you with more options. This way, you have access to a wide variety of foods instead of being limited to just one because you require a certain nutrient.

2.1.4.1. Helps You Improve Your Eating Habits

As no one is an expert by birth, everyone who eats healthily now started somewhere. However, getting started is not always simple because it's typically fraught with uncertainty about where to begin, which is why the food pyramid is so important.

The food pyramid can not only assist you in starting a healthy diet, but it can also make it simple for you to maintain it and develop some excellent eating habits, which are essential for becoming healthy. You will not have to overthink what to eat thanks to the food pyramid, which gives you a variety of healthy options to pick from.

We will give you an example to help you understand. Suppose you wish to try this healthy eating thing but are unaware of the food pyramid.

During the preparation of your meal, you realize that it needs more protein to be more balanced. However, since you do not like meat, you now have to find a replacement. You ultimately decide to give up on the whole thing and settle for some junk food because the longer you try to Figure it out, the more discouraged you get. But with the food pyramid, you have more options and new information about how to improve your eating habits by knowing what to eat more of and less of.

2.1.4.2. Can Be Used as a Guide to Help You Eat Better

It is recommended to follow a guide when eating healthy to ensure you are consuming the right proportions. The food pyramid is an ideal choice because of its visually appealing design and clear organization of the five food groups. This guide will help you easily understand how to build balanced and healthy meals.

2.1.4.3. Can Be Used as a Daily Reminder

You can make sure you are constantly reminded to eat healthily by using a food pyramid, but for that to work, it must be displayed in a location you can be certain you will see it every day. Hence, you could always print it out and stick a copy of it somewhere conspicuously where you can't miss it—in your refrigerator, on your office desk, or elsewhere. You can easily download a copy of the food pyramid to your tablet or phone if you enjoy using electronics and gadgets, so you always have easy access to it. With that in place, you're always reminded to eat healthily and to choose different foods for your next meal if you don't want to eat the same things twice. That's pretty great, isn't it? At least you won't be able to use this as an excuse for why you didn't eat a healthy meal that day.

2.1.4.4. Gives You Some Variety

Although we have already discussed this, let's go into further detail. Everyone enjoys having options, which is actually what makes most of the things we do interesting. Eating healthily would be extremely monotonous and depressing if you were to limit yourself to just one food. However, the pyramid gives you a large selection to pick from, which enhances the fun and interest of the experience. Recall that the greatest strategy to maintain a healthy diet is to make it more pleasurable and entertaining.

2.1.4.5. Easy to Understand and Use

It's safe to say that anyone can make use of and gain from the food pyramid. To use it, you don't actually need to be an expert in nutrition. We doubt you will ever have any difficulty understanding it because of its straightforward design.

2.2. Dietary Reference Intakes

The term "dietary reference values" (DRVs) refers to a group of reference values for nutrients, which include the population reference intake (PRI), adequate intake (AI), average requirement (AR), and reference intake range for macronutrients (RI). These values provide guidance to professionals regarding the necessary intake of a nutrient in an otherwise healthy individual or group of individuals. The tolerable upper intake level (UL), or the highest quantity of a nutrient that can be taken in a safe manner for an extended length of time, is also included in DRVs.

The reference values—the Recommended Dietary Allowance (RDA), the AI, the Tolerable UL, and the Estimated Average Requirement (EAR)—combine to form the Dietary Reference Intakes (DRIs). The lowest level of nutrient intake that an individual can sustain to maintain a specific level of nurture is known as a requirement. As a result, special consideration to the selection and rationale of each criterion utilized in the establishment of requirement values is provided throughout this report.

This method is a little different from the one employed by the Food and Agriculture Organization (FAO), International Atomic Energy Agency, and World Health Organization (WHO) Expert Consultation on Trace Elements in Human Nutrition and Health. The level of intake required to prevent pathologically significant and clinically detectable signs of dietary inadequacy is referred to in that report as the "basal requirement." In that report, the term "normative requirement" refers to the amount of intake needed to sustain a desired body store or reserve. In this report, the development of RDAs and AIs instead focuses on the rationale behind the selection of the nutritional adequacy criteria that are used to set requirements. They do not have a normative or basal designation.

All values for EARs, RDAs, and AIs, unless otherwise indicated, indicate the amount of the nutrient or food component to be supplied by foods from diets comparable to those in the US and Canada. Adjustments for variations in nutrient bioavailability may be necessary if the food source of a nutrient is substantially different (as in the diets of some ethnic groups) or if the source consists of supplements.

The recommended intake levels for individuals are known as RDAs and AIs. They ought to lessen the possibility of getting a disease linked to the nutrient in question that has a detrimental effect on function. The DRIs are applicable to the ostensibly healthy population. Achieving the recommended nutrient intakes would not guarantee sufficient nourishment for people who are already malnourished, nor would they suffice for certain disease conditions characterized by elevated nutritional needs. Recommendations for individuals with known diseases that significantly increase nutritional requirements or who are at risk of experiencing side effects from higher intakes must be customized by qualified medical and nutrition personnel. While qualified personnel should make the necessary adjustments for particular situations, the RDA or AI may serve as the foundation for such guidance.

2.2.1. Categories of Dietary Reference Intakes

The average daily nutrient intake of an individual over time is indicated by each type of Dietary Reference Intake (DRI). The amount taken can typically vary significantly day to day without causing harm.

2.2.1.1. Recommended Dietary Allowance

The average daily dietary intake level that is adequate to meet the nutrient requirements of almost all (97 to 98%) healthy individuals in a specific life stage and gender group is known as the RDA. Individuals are supposed to use the RDA as a target for their daily intake. The ability to set an Estimated Average Requirement (EAR) is a prerequisite for the RDA setting process, which is explained below. In other words, no RDA will be set if an EAR cannot be set.

2.2.1.2. Estimated Average Requirement

The daily intake value that is estimated to satisfy the requirement, as determined by the given indicator or criterion of adequacy, of half of the apparently healthy individuals in a life stage or gender group is known as the Estimated Average Requirement (EAR) (*see* Figure 2.2). For nutrient requirements, a normal or symmetrical distribution (where the mean and median are similar) is typically assumed. Half of the individuals in a given group would not have their nutritional needs satisfied at this intake level. For every nutrient, the EAR is generally set using the same procedure. There are few direct data on the needs of children for many of the nutrients, including those in this report. EARs and RDAs for children for these nutrients are therefore derived from extrapolations of adult values.

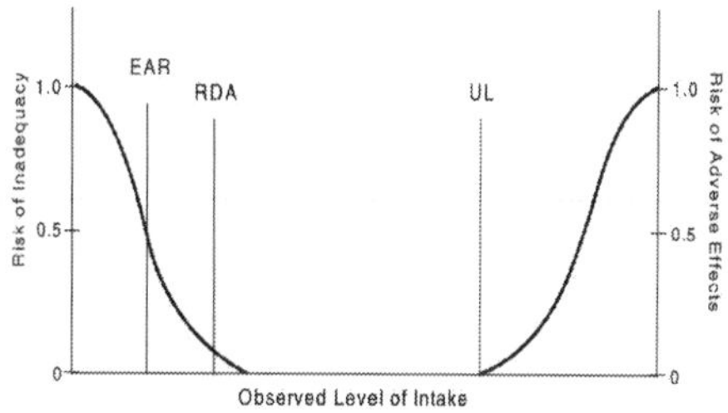

Figure 2.2. *Dietary reference intakes.*

Source: https://dsld.od.nih.gov/daily-values.

2.2.1.3. Method for Setting the Recommended Dietary Allowance When Nutrient Requirements Are Normally Distributed

If the requirement for the nutrient is normally distributed, and the standard deviation (SD) of the EAR is available, the RDA is defined as equal to the EAR plus 2 SDs of the EAR:

$$RDA = EAR + 2\ SD_{EAR}$$

If data about variability in requirements are insufficient to calculate an SD, a coefficient of variation (CV_{EAR}) of 10% will be ordinarily assumed and used to estimate the SD:

$$CV_{EAR} = SD_{EAR}/EAR$$

And

$$SD = (EAR \times CV_{EAR})$$

The resulting equation for the RDA is:

$$RDA = EAR + 2(0.1 \times EAR)$$

$$RDA = 1.2 \times EAR$$

The assumption of a 10% CV is based on extensive data on the variation in basal metabolic rate, (BMR) which contributes about two-thirds of the daily energy needs of many individuals residing and on a similar CV of 12.5% estimated for the protein requirements in adults.

2.2.1.4. Method for Setting the Recommended Dietary Allowance When Nutrient Requirements Are Not Normally Distributed

When one uses factorial modeling to extrapolate the requirement distribution from the distributions of the component parts (e.g. losses, accretion), the individual distributions must be added. This is simple for normal component distributions because the resulting distribution, which has a mean equal to the sum of the component means and a variance equal to the sum of the individual variances, is also normal. The mean value plus two standard deviations is then used to estimate the 97.15% percentile.

It is possible to estimate the EAR and RDA of a nutrient whose requirement is not normally distributed but can be transformed into normality by converting the data, finding the 55th and 97th and half percentiles, and then converting these percentiles back into the original units. Because skewing is typically present, the difference between the EAR and the RDA cannot be used to estimate the CV.

Monte Carlo simulation is used for the summation of the components if normality cannot be assumed for all of the requirement's components. This strategy simulates a sizable population of people (e.g, 100,000) each having a unique need for a specific nutrient. The factorial components, which make up the component parts of nutrient needs, are treated as deriving from separate random distributions to achieve this.

For example, for basal losses of a nutrient, a distribution of expected losses can be generated. For each individual in the simulated population, a randomly selected basal loss value was drawn from that distribution of nutrient losses. This is done for each component of nutrient need, and then these components are summed for each individual yielding the simulated nutrient needs. The total requirement is then calculated for each individual and the median and the 97th and one-half percentile are calculated directly.

Based on established physiology, a distribution of values for the requirement components is modeled. Monte Carlo techniques can be employed to simulate the component distribution. Alternatively, estimates of relative variability can be applied to the component in the simulated population when extensive data sets for comparable populations are available, such as infant growth rates. The objective is to obtain distribution values for each component at each step that represent known physiology or direct observations, as well as values that can be converted into a modellable distribution that can be used to choose members at random to add to the final requirement distribution. The median and 97.5th percentile of the distribution can be directly estimated once the final distribution representing the convolution of components has been determined. It is acknowledged that the Monte Carlo method, in its most basic form, disregards potential correlations between components. To ensure that no source of correlation is overlooked, expected correlation is incorporated into the modeling of the requirement for iron when components are connected to a common variable like growth rate.

Based on established physiology, a model is developed to represent the distribution of values for the requirement components. The distribution of components can be simulated using Monte Carlo techniques, or estimates of relative variability can be applied to the component in the simulated population in cases where extensive data sets for comparable populations (like infant growth rates) are available.

Achieving distribution values for each component that represent known physiology or direct observations, as well as values that can be converted into a modellable distribution that can be used to choose random members to add to the final requirement distribution, is the aim of each stage. It is possible to directly estimate the distribution's median and 97.5th percentile after deriving the final distribution that represents the convolution of components. In its most basic form, the Monte Carlo method is acknowledged to overlook potential correlations between components. But in the case of iron, expected correlation is incorporated into the requirement modeling when elements are connected to a common variable, like growth rate, ensuring that no source of correlation is overlooked.

2.2.1.5. Adequate Intake

An AI, rather than the RDA, is given if there is insufficient scientific data to calculate an EAR. Based on experimentally determined intake levels or approximations of observed mean nutrient intakes by a group (or groups) of healthy individuals, the AI value is calculated.

In virtually every member of a particular population that appears to be in good health, the AIs for children and adults are anticipated to be equal to or greater than the quantity required to maintain a specified nutritional state or criterion of adequacy.

Typical development, the preservation of normal circulating nutrient values, and other facets of general health or nutritional well-being are examples of defined nutritional states.

The AI is set when data are deemed insufficient or inadequate to establish an EAR on which to base an RDA, as is the case in this report for determining the recommended intake of water, potassium, sodium, and chloride. For example, the AI is based on the daily mean nutrient intake supplied by human milk for healthy full-term infants who are exclusively fed human milk.

For young infants, for whom human milk is the recommended sole source of food for almost all nutrients for the first 4 to 6 months. In the case of adults, the AI could be based on information from a single experiment, on estimated dietary intakes in populations that appear to be in good health, or on an analysis of information from various methods that, when considered separately, would not allow for a reasonably confident estimate of an EAR.

2.2.1.6. Similarities Between the Adequate Intake and the Recommended Dietary Allowance

As suggested intake levels for individuals, the AI and RDA are both meant to be utilized as objectives for personal consumption. The values are generally meant to meet the needs of almost every individual in a life stage group. (For infants, the AI is what happens when babies in that age group drink human milk. Bigger babies might have higher demands, which they satisfy by drinking more milk. Similar to RDAs, AIs for kids and teens can be derived from adult values in the event that no additional relevant data are available.

2.2.1.6.1. Differences Between the Adequate Intake and the Recommended Dietary Allowance

Compared to the RDA value, the AI value is far less certain. AIs may differ significantly from and be numerically higher than the RDA because they rely on a higher degree of judgment than is used in estimating the EAR and subsequently the RDA.

Because of this, using AIs requires more caution than using RDAs. Additionally, the expected variation in the nutrient requirement is considered by the formula used to calculate the RDA from the EAR, which is not the case for all AIs.

Data for some nutrients and food ingredients are insufficient to create an RDA or an AI for people who appear to be in good health. This is the case for sulfate, as consumption of the sulfur-containing amino acids methionine and cysteine seems to meet the sulfate requirement. In addition, there is insufficient data to determine the degree to which sulfate inclusion in the diet can reduce the requirements for these essential amino acids.

2.2.1.7. Tolerable Upper Intake Level

The maximum amount of daily nutrient intake that is expected to present no risk of harmful health effects for nearly all individuals in the designated life stage group who appear healthy is known as the Tolerable Upper Intake Level. The possibility of negative effects may rise as intake rises above the UL. The word "tolerable intake" was selected to avoid suggesting a potential positive outcome. Rather, the term is meant to indicate an intake level that is likely to be biologically tolerated. The UL of consumption is not meant to be a recommended level of intake, and there is no proof that consuming a nutrient in amounts above the UL will benefit healthy individuals. The methodology for risk assessment of nutrients was used to conduct an evaluation that served as the basis for the UL. The increased nutrient fortification of foods and the increased use of dietary supplements by a greater number of people at higher dosages necessitated the establishment of upper-limit values. Chronic daily use is covered by the UL. Professionals should first evaluate the characteristics of the individual and group of concern, such as the source of the nutrient, the individual's physiological state, the duration of sustained high intakes, and so forth, before applying very strict ULs, just as they should when applying AIs.

For some nutrients, data are not sufficient for developing a UL for apparently healthy individuals. This indicates the need for caution in consuming amounts greater than the recommended intake; it does not mean that high intakes pose no risk of adverse effects.

There is insufficient evidence to support the safety of regular, long-term intake over the UL. While it is advisable to advise the general public not to routinely exceed the upper limit of tolerance, intake exceeding the UL may warrant further investigation in carefully monitored clinical trials. As long as trial participants have signed informed consent forms regarding potential toxicity and as long as the trials use suitable safe monitoring techniques, clinical trials with doses above the lower limit of toxicity should not be discouraged.

2.2.2. Parameters for Dietary Reference Intakes

2.2.2.1. Life Stage Groups

The life stage groups that follow were selected by considering all of the nutrients that needed to be examined, not just the ones that were covered in this report. There may be more divisions within these groupings in upcoming reports. The analysis may be presented for a larger grouping if there is insufficient data to discern differences in requirements by life stage or gender group.

2.2.2.2. Infancy

Infanthood is divided into two 6-month periods that span the time from birth to 12 months of age. Since intake is fairly constant during the first 6 month, the interval was not further divided. In other words, babies continue to eat the same amount of food relative to their body weight even though they are growing. Growth velocity slows down in the second half of a baby's life, so overall daily nutritional requirements based on body weight may be lower than in the first half. The primary basis for determining the artificial intelligence for nutrients during the first 6 months of life has been determined to be the average intake of a specific nutrient by full-term infants born to healthy, well-nourished mothers and exclusively fed human milk. Because of this, the value utilized is not an EAR, and it is not anticipated that such data will become accessible. The degree to which a baby may exceed its real needs because of consuming human milk in the recommended amounts is unknown, and testing at levels that are known to be potentially insufficient is prohibited by experimental ethics. The infant-fed human milk serves as a model, which is consistent with the methodology used in the most recent RDA and Recommended Nutrient Intakes (RNI) reports to estimate the nutrient allowances of infants. It also backs the advice that, for the first four to 6 months of a normal full-term infant's life, exclusive human milk feeding is the best feeding technique. Generally speaking, no particular thought was given to potential differences in physiological requirements in the first month following birth or to variations in the amount of nutrients ingested from human milk as a result of variations in milk volume and nutrient concentration during the early stages of lactation. This report does not suggest any specific recommended intake to meet the needs of formula-fed infants. Because of a lack of knowledge regarding how the previously published RDAs and RNIs for infants were derived, there has been a great deal of misinterpretation regarding the adequacy of human milk. The previous RDA and RNI values permitted a lower bioavailability of nutrients from nonhuman milk, despite being based on the composition and volume of intake of human milk.

1. **Ages 0 Through 6 Months:** The mean intake of a nutrient from 2 to 6 months of lactation was calculated using consensus values for the nutrient from several reported studies, and an estimated average volume of milk intake of 0.78 L/day was reported from studies of full-term infants by test weighing, a procedure in which the infant is weighed before and after each feeding, to derive the AI value for infants 0 to 6 months. The computed value is the mean because both measures have variations. As

they grow, it is anticipated that babies will drink more human milk.

2. **Ages 7 Through 12 Months:** During the period of slower growth and gradual weaning to a mixed diet of human milk and solid foods from ages 7 through 12 months, there is no evidence of significantly different nutrient needs, except for some nutrients like iron and zinc, for which infants have relatively high requirements. The average volume of milk reported from studies in this age group, 0.6 L/day, plus the specific nutrients provided by the typical intakes of complementary weaning foods consumed by infants of this age, were added to determine the AI values for this age group.

   The lack of information on the total amount of nutrients consumed by infants during their second 6 months of life from a combination of human milk and solid foods is one issue that arises when estimating intake data. Most intake survey data do not specify the source of the milk; however, the reported total intake values suggest that weaning foods were most likely consumed with cow milk or formula derived from cow milk.

3. **Toddlers: Ages 1 Through 3 Years:** An explanation for the biological division of this stage of life can be found in the faster rate of height growth between the ages of one and three and four and five. It seemed appropriate to end this stage of life before the age of 4. There are not enough data to determine DRIs for these early years of life based on indicators of adequate nutrition. Sometimes, data extrapolated from studies of infants or adults 19 years of age and older was used to create DRIs for this age group.

4. **Early Childhood: Ages 4 Through 8 Years:** Ages 4 through 8 or 9 (depending on when each gender's puberty begins) are the appropriate range for biological changes in growth velocity and changing endocrine status. Reasonably good data on nutrient intake and various adequacy criteria (e.g., nutrient balance measured in young children aged 5–7 years) are available for many nutrients, but not for those covered in this report. These data can serve as the foundation for the EARs and AIs applicable to this life stage group.

5. **Puberty/Adolescence: Ages 9 Through 13 Years and 14 Through 18 Years:** The decision was made to start the adolescent age group at 9 years old since the available data support earlier ages for pubertal development. Tanner Stage 2 (the physical marker for the start of increased estrogen secretion) is reached at an average age of 10 points 0 ± 1.8 (standard deviation) years in white girls in the United States.

2.3. Food Exchange

The food items on each list are referred to as "exchanges" since they can be replaced with any other item on the same list. Within each food list, one exchange is roughly equivalent to another in terms of calories, carbs, protein, and fat (Table 2.1).

Table 2.1. *Food Exchange List*

1. **Cereal Exchange**

30 g Provides: Carbohydrate 20 gm, Protein 2 g			
Cereals	**Household Measures**	**Wt/Vol.**	**Calories**
Rice	–	30 g uncooked	100
Wheat flour	–	30 g uncooked	100
Dalia	1/2 katori cooked	30 g uncooked	100
Sago	–	30 g uncooked	100
White flour	–	30 g uncooked	100
Bread	2 slices	40 g	100
Chapati	1.5 [approx. 5–6" diameter]	44 g	100
Jowar roti	0.5	55 g	100
Ragi	–	30 g uncooked	100
Rice flakes	1 katori	30 g uncooked	100
Oatmeal	–	30 g uncooked	100
Vermicelli	1/2 katori cooked	30 g uncooked	100
Corn flakes	–	30 g uncooked	100
Maize dry	–	30 g uncooked	100
Marie biscuit	8 No.	–	100
Monaco biscuit	4 No.	–	100
Idlis	2 No.	–	100
Poha	1/2 katori	–	100
Upma	1/2 katori	–	100
Dosa ordinary	–	–	120
1 Katori-volume 150 ml.			

*katori: bowl.

Source: https://www.iitk.ac.in/hc/food-exchange-list.

2. **Fat Exchange:**

50 g Calories; Fat 5.5 gm			
Fats	**Household Measures**	**Wt.[g].**	**Calori es**
Butter	1 1/2 teaspoon	7.5	50
Ghee	1 teaspoon	5.5	50
Hydrogenated fat [Vanaspati]	1 teaspoon	5.5	50
Oil [coconut, mustard sunflower, corn, groundnut, cotton seed, Til, palm]	1 teaspoon	5.5	50
Cashewnuts	–	10	50
Groundnuts, roasted	–	10	50

Walnuts	–	7.5	50
Pistachio	–	7.5	50
Almonds	–	7.5	50

3. Milk and Milk Products:

50. Calories; Protein 2.5 g			
Milk and Milk Products	**Household Measures**	**Wt./ Vol.**	**Calories**
Curd	2/3 glass	105 g	50
Butter milk	3 glasses	375 ml	50
Cheese	1 ice cube	15 g	50
Milk [buffalo]	1/3 glass	45 ml	50
Milk [cow]	2/3 glass	90 ml	50
Milk, Skimmed*	1 glass	130 ml	50
Milk, Skimmed, powder*	–	15 g	50
Coffee Nescafe + 75 ml milk	–	–	50
[without sugar]	–	–	–
Tea + 75 ml milk	–	–	50
Khoya	–	15 g	50
1 medium glass 150 ml	–	–	–

*provides 5 g protein

4. Vegetable Exchange:

50. Calories; Carbohydrate 10 g			
Vegetables	**Household Measures**	**Wt. (g)**	**Calories**
Beetroot [chukander]	–	75	50
Carrot	1–2 No.	105	50
Colocasia [arbi]	–	45	50
Onion [big]	1 No.	90	50
Onion [small]	2 No.	75	50
Potato	1/2 No.	45	50
Sweet potato	–	30	50
Tapioca	–	30	50
Yam [zimikand]	–	45	50
Broad beans	–	90	50
Cluster beans	–	90	50
Double beans	–	50	50
Jack, Tender	–	105	50
Jackfruit seeds	–	30	50
Leeks	–	60	50
Peas	–	45	50
Singhara	–	45	50
Sambar	1/4 katori	35 ml	50
Cooked vegetable	1/2 katori		50
1 katori: volume 150 ml			

5. Fruit Exchange:

50. Calories; Carbohydrate 10 g			
Fruits	**Size/No.**	**Wt. (ml)**	**Calor ies**
Apple	1 small	75	50
Amla	20 medium	90	50
Banana	1/4 medium	30	50
Cashew fruit	2 medium	90	50
Custard apple	1/4	50	50
Dates	3	30	50
Figs	6 medium	135	50
Grapes	20	105	50
Grape fruit	1/2 big	150	50
Jack fruit	3 medium pieces	60	50
Mango	1 small	90	50

Melon	1/4 medium	270	50
Orange	1 small	90	50
Lemon	1 medium	90	50
Papaya	2 medium	120	50
Peach	1 medium	135	50
Pear	1 medium	90	50
Plums	4 medium	120	50
Pineapple	1 1/2 slices (round)	90	50
Strawberry	40	105	50
Sweetlime	1 medium	150	50
Tomato	4 medium	240	50
Watermelon	1/4 small	175	50

6. Legume and Pulse Exchange:

30 gm Provide: Carbohydrate 15 gm, Protein 6 g			
Pulse [uncooked]	**Household Measures**	**Wt. (g)**	**Calories**
Bengal gram	3/4 katori cooked	30	100
Bengal gram, roasted	–	30	100
Bengal gram-flour [Besan]	–	30	100
Cow gram	1 katori cooked	30	100
Horse gram	–	30	100
Kabuli Channa [white gram]	–	30	100
Lentils	3/4 katori cooked	30	100
Moth beans	–	30	100
Peas, dried	1 katori cooked	30	100
Rajmah [kidney beans]	3/4 katori cooked	60	100
Red gram	3/4 katori cooked	30	100
1 katori-volume 150 ml			

7. Flesh Food Exchange:

70. Calories; Protein 10 g			
Flesh Foods	**Household Measures**	**Wt. (g)**	**Calories**
Egg Hen	2 No.	–	100
Fish	1 piece	60	70
Liver, sheep	–	60	70
Mutton, muscle	3 pieces	60	100
Pork	1 slice	60	70
Prawn	5–7 pieces	60	70
Chicken	1 breast	60	70
Crab	120 g	–	70
Beef	1 slice	60	70

8. Vegetable Exchange:

These Vegetables may be Used as Desired. Carbohydrates and Calories are Negligible			
Leafy Vegetables		**Other Vegetables**	
Bitter gourd [Karela]	Curry leaves	Brinjal	Onion stalks
Amaranth	Fenugreek leaves	Cauliflower	Pumpkin
Brussels sprouts	Mint	Drumstic	Tinda
Cabbage	Spinach	Frenchbeans	Tomato, Green
Coriander leaves	–	Mango, green	–

Drinks*			
	Household Measures	**Vol.**	**Calories**
Orange juice	1 big glass	200 ml.	30
Tomato juice	1 big glass	200 ml	30
Apple juice	1 big glass	200 ml	100
Grape juice	1 big glass	200 ml	80
Mango juice	1 big glass	200 ml	150

Fast Food*			
	Household Measures	**Vol.**	**Calories**
Soft drink	1 bottle	300 ml	120–135
Potato wafers	–	50 g	430
Samosa	1	40 g	130
Veg. cutlet	1	100 g	140
Vada	1	–	150

Cakes and Pastries*		
	Wt/vol.	**Calories**
Cake plain	50 g	150
Chocolate cake	50 g	250
Sponge cake	50 g	150
Pastry	50 g	250–400

Desserts*			
	Household Measures	**Wt/vol.**	**Calories**
Custard	–	150 g	360
Fruit salad	–	150 g	150
Fruit salad with cream	–	150 g	300
Ice cream	–	150 g	380
Carrot halwa	1 medium katori	100 g	600
Badami halwa	–	100 g	570

Sweets*			
	Household Measures	**Wt/vol.**	**Calories**
Coconut burfi	–	25 g	110
Gulabjamun	–	25 g	200
Laddo	–	30 g	160
Rasgulla	–	150 g	140
Jam	2 tablespoons	–	80
Honey	2 tablespoons	–	48

Beverages**		
	Vol.	**Calories**
Beer	150 ml	65
Wine dry	30 ml	30
Wine dessert	30 ml	40
Whisky, brandy, gin, rum	30 ml	65
Vodka	30 ml	65
Ginger ale	30 ml	9

2.3.1. How to Calculate Exchanges Based on Nutrition Information?

Exchanges is a diet plan that counts carbohydrates and caters to the needs of people with diabetes. The goal of incorporating the exchange system into your regular diet is to eat as much food as possible with as little impact on your blood sugar as possible. It is usually easier to Figure out food exchanges by consulting a chart, but knowing how to compute exchanges based on nutritional data can also be helpful.

- **Step 1:** Talk to your doctor or dietician and determine how many calories you should consume each day. This information is essential, as 45 to 65% of your daily calorie intake should come from carbohydrates.
- **Step 2:** Determine the amount of carbs (g) that your calorie intake permits. Divide your range of calories by four, as one gram of carbohydrates is equivalent to four calories. For instance, if your daily caloric intake falls between 720 and 1,040 calories, you will consume 180 to 260 g of carbohydrates.

- **Step 3:** Determine the number of carbohydrate exchanges, or servings, that you can have each day with this. One carbohydrate exchange is equivalent to 15 g of carbohydrates, regardless of the food. To find your exchange range, divide each number by 15 if your daily carbohydrate range is 180 to 260 g. You can have between 12 and 17 carbohydrate exchanges per day in this scenario.
- **Step 4:** Examine food labels, taking note of serving size, total number of servings, and amount of carbohydrates in each serving. If you eat the entire package, you will have consumed 30 g, or two carbohydrate exchanges, if the label specifies that a single serving size is 4 oz and there are three servings (10 g each). Make sure you get the serving size and carbohydrate exchange correct by measuring and weighing the food item.
- **Step 5:** Calculate the grams of carbohydrates in foods without labels by weighing the food, looking up the food factor and applying the formula "food weight x food factor." For example, if you weigh a handful of dry spaghetti and it comes to 2oz, multiply this weight by the food factor for pasta, which is 7.5 g of carbohydrates per ounce. You have 15 g, or one exchange of pasta, in your hand.

2.4. Food Composition Databases (FCDBs)

Food composition databases, or FCDBs, offer comprehensive data on the nutritional makeup of foods, typically originating from a specific nation. Data on the composition of food may be found in a variety of formats eg., either electronic versions, called nutrient databases or databanks, or paper-based versions, called food composition tables. FCDBs offer energy and nutritional values (e.g., protein, vitamins, and minerals) as well as other vital dietary ingredients (e.g., fiber) for every meal on the list. These Figures are estimated from other relevant data or are based on chemical analyses performed in analytical laboratories. Table 2.2 shows an extract from the UK food composition Table 2.2, as an example.

Table 2.2. *Composition of Food per 100 g Edible Portion*

Food	Protein g	Fat g	Carbohydrate g	Energy kcal	Energy kJ
Grapefruit, *raw*	0.8	0.1	6.8	30	126
canned in juice	0.6	Tr*	7.3	30	120
canned in syrup	0.5	Tr*	15.5	60	257
Grapes, average	0.4	0.1	15.4	60	257
Guava, *raw*	0.8	0.5	5.0	26	112

Source: https://www.bezpecnostpotravin.cz/UserFiles/File/Kvasnickova2/EuroFIR_2.pdf.

Information about food composition is vital for many different kinds of tasks in a wide range of professions, such as determining an individual's or a group's energy and nutrient intake.

They are a crucial prerequisite for epidemiological research because they are required to evaluate the impact of diet on health and disease outcomes.

In the end, they support the creation of dietary recommendations for various population groups as well as the planning of menus for medical facilities, jails, schools, and the military.

They have even been applied to the planning of polar expedition food ration requirements. The wide range of applications in a variety of other sectors includes clinical dietetic practice, sports nutrition, the food industry (e.g., product development and food labeling), government food and health departments (e.g., target setting), and nutrition education and health promotion.

2.4.1. Different Uses of Food Composition Databases

Within each of the primary use sectors, the table opposite lists the various applications for food composition databases and tables (Table 2.3). The majority of users can benefit from some general uses of food composition data, such as estimating the nutritional content of foods, comparing foods based on their nutritional composition, and determining which foods are good sources of specific nutrients. Certain applications are specific to a given industry, like creating patient-specific diet plans for clinical settings.

Table 2.3. *Summary Table Showing Different Uses of Food Composition Data, by Field of Work*

	Clinical practice	Research	Public health/ education	Food industry
Estimating/comparing the nutrient content of foods	✓	✓	✓	✓
Identifying sources of particular nutrients	✓	✓	✓	
Analysing individuals' diets	✓	✓		
Devising special diets for patients (e.g. heart disease, coeliac disease)	✓			
Patient information	✓			
Analysing dietary survey data		✓	✓	
Assessing how dietary intake affects health and disease outcomes		✓	✓	
Devising special diets for epidemiological research		✓		
Monitoring food and nutrient availability			✓	
Development of dietary guidelines	✓		✓	
Implementation and monitoring of food legislation			✓	✓
Consumer information and education		✓	✓	✓
Preparing educational materials (e.g. for schools)			✓	
Food labelling and nutrient claims				✓
Product development and reformulation				✓
Marketing of products				✓
Recipe and menu development and analysis		✓	✓	✓
Devising special diets for healthy people with particular needs (e.g. athletes)		✓		
Completing missing values in a dataset	✓	✓	✓	✓

Source: https://www.bezpecnostpotravin.cz/UserFiles/File/Kvasnickova2/EuroFIR_2.pdf.

2.4.1.1. Clinical Practice

2.4.1.1.1. Analyzing the Diets of Patients

In clinical practice, dietary assessment is performed to evaluate a patient's nutritional status or risk. Dietitians typically perform this assessment. After that, dietary recommendations or other nutritional support are made using the results of this assessment. The method used for dietary assessment depends on the characteristics of the patient (e.g., their age, ethnic background, cognitive ability), the clinical circumstances, and the purpose of assessment, which could be any of the following:

- To assess the overall dietary balance;
- To obtain a quantitative estimate of energy and/or specific nutrient intakes;
- To identify nutritional deficiencies or excesses;
- To assess the risk of malnutrition;
- To monitor compliance with dietary advice.

Getting a dietary history, such as a 24-hour recall, in which the patient is asked to recollect all the foods and beverages they consumed over a 24-hour period, is a common technique of dietary assessment used in the clinical setting. This approach has the benefit of being easy to use and fast, which is crucial in clinical practice. The patient 'will not be burdened in any way. A single 24-hour recall can be used to identify significant dietary excesses or deficiencies and can serve as a basis for determining whether more research is necessary, even though it is typically insufficient to provide a quantitative estimate of nutrient intake.

One of the other dietary assessment techniques involves giving the patient a diet diary to fill out over a minimum of three days. This can be help determe whether a patient is following dietary recommendations, tracking the efficacy of a treatment plan, or looking into food intolerances. However, a weighed food record—typically gathered over the course of five to seven days—is necessary to obtain an accurate, quantitative measure of nutrient intake. Though this approach has limitations, primarily involving the patient being more fatigued, it is more accurate than other approaches because gram weights for each food consumed are obtained (see Nelson 2000 for a more thorough discussion of various dietary assessment methods). The patient's energy and nutrient intake can then be ascertained, and whether the diet is fulfilling the patient's nutritional needs by entering the dietary data into a dietary analysis program that makes use of detailed food composition data.

2.4.1.1.2. Devising Special Diets for Patients

Determining the appropriate dietary advice or prescription of a therapeutic diet requires assessing the energy and nutrient intake of the patients. Therapeutic diets are necessary for a variety of clinical conditions. A deep understanding of food composition is necessary for the prescription of therapeutic diets, which must be nutritionally balanced while limiting or controlling the consumption of particular nutrients and/or food components. Table 2.4 provides a list of common clinical conditions that call for therapeutic diets along with the food components that may need to be restricted. Sadly, not all of the components listed in the majority of food composition tables and databases are included in the list (e.g., Monoamines and gluten are typically excluded from lists. In these situations, it might be necessary to obtain this information by consulting additional primary data sources.

Table 2.4. *Clinical Conditions that Require Food Composition Data for the Planning of Therapeutic Diets*

Clinical condition	Food composition information required may include:
Requiring general dietary control	
Diabetes mellitus	Energy, available carbohydrate, fat, protein, fibre
Obesity	Energy, fat
Hypertension	Energy, sodium, potassium, protein
Renal (kidney) disease	Protein, sodium, potassium
Deficiency states	
Anaemia	Iron, folate, vitamin B_{12}
Vitamin deficiencies	Specific vitamins
Metabolic disorders	
Haemochromatosis	Iron
Hyperlipidaemias	Fat, fatty acids, cholesterol
Inborn errors of amino acid metabolism e.g. phenylketonuria	Specific amino acids
Gout, xanthinuria	Purines
Gall bladder disease	Fat, calcium, cholesterol, fibre
Wilson's disease	Copper
Intolerances	
Monosaccharides, disaccharides	Individual sugars (e.g. sucrose, lactose, fructose)
Gluten (and other specific proteins)	Gluten, specific proteins
Migraine	Monoamines
Allergies e.g. nut allergy	Specific protein sources

Source: https://www.bezpecnostpotravin.cz/UserFiles/File/Kvasnickova2/EuroFIR_2.pdf.

The use of food composition data in the development of therapeutic diets has been facilitated by advances in information technology, particularly the development of nutritional analysis and meal planning software.

2.4.1.1.3. Patient Information

A fundamental component of clinical dietetic practice is providing patients with dietary advice and information; this cannot be done without knowledge about the makeup of food. Given that people consume foods rather than nutrients, it is crucial that dietary advice be provided in terms of foods rather than nutrients. This makes food-based dietary guidelines easier for people to understand and adhere to. Giving advice on what foods to eat makes it easier to make sure the diet is balanced overall as well.

In the UK, the Balance of Good Health model is utilized as a guide for healthy eating recommendations for the general population.

This model, represented by a plate shape, visually demonstrates the principles of a balanced diet. The goal of the model is to provide the necessary macro- and micronutrients in alignment with UK dietary reference values and current population dietary goals for optimal health.

The model can be customized to cater to specific groups such as the elderly or individuals from diverse ethnic backgrounds by adjusting the emphasis on various food groups to achieve specific energy or nutrient targets.

For instance, for individuals with anaemia, the model recommends selecting more options from the 'meat and alternatives' group and highlighting other iron-rich foods, along with plenty of fruits and vegetables to increase vitamin C intake (which aids in iron absorption). Additionally, the model is increasingly used as a foundation for managing complex conditions like diabetes or celiac disease.

2.4.1.2. Epidemiological Research

Despite their ever-increasing sophistication and complexity, these studies continue to be essential to nutrition research into the role of food components in health and disease.

Rendering accurate food composition and food intake data is essential to the validity of nutritional epidemiological studies. Consequently, a crucial prerequisite for quantitative nutritional research is an extensive FCDB that is representative of the foods that are readily available.

A method for determining the connections between dietary variables and health in human populations consuming typical food and nutrient intakes is nutritional epidemiology. Identification of putative causes of diseases linked to diet (e.g., diabetes, cancer, and cardiovascular disease) so that changes can be made to them to lessen the burden of illness. In the majority of observational studies in nutritional epidemiology, researchers evaluate variations in the outcome of interest and exposure to determine whether a relationship is present. These studies can be used to identify dietary factors that may be involved in the onset of disease, even though they cannot prove causation.

One way to study the relationship between dietary exposure and disease outcome is through case-control studies, which compare past dietary intake of a specific factor among individuals with and without the disease.

However, these studies may be biased by individuals' ability to accurately recall their diet and potential differences in diet recall between diseased and healthy individuals. In contrast, cohort studies are considered more reliable as they do not rely on memory recall, but they are time-consuming and costly to conduct.

Dietary data collection is a challenging part of nutritional epidemiology – accuracy in the measurement of food and nutrient intake is important to detect true associations. Most cohort or prospective studies use food frequency questionnaires (FFQs) to assess food intake as it would not be practical to use a more detailed method (e.g., 7-day weighed food diary) on a large cohort of participants.

FFQs attempt to assess usual or typical food intake over a longer time period than is usually possible using other dietary assessment methods. Foods are listed in a questionnaire format or multiple response grid and respondents are asked to estimate how often they consume each food and how much they usually consume (using household units) (Table 2.5).

The FFQ is a useful method for assessing the nutrient intake of a population or group or for classifying individuals e.g. into tertiles of intake. However, it is less accurate for estimating the nutrient intakes of individuals.

Table 2.5. *Example of a Section of a Food Frequency Questionnaire (FFQ)*

	Never or < once per month	1-3 days per month	1-2 days per week	3-4 days per week	5-6 days per week	Amount PER DAY on days eaten
White bread and rolls						
Brown/wholemeal/ granary bread and rolls						
Other breads e.g. naan, paratha, chapatti, pitta						
Scones, currant bread, currant buns, teacakes						

Source: https://www.bezpecnostpotravin.cz/UserFiles/File/Kvasnickova2/EuroFIR_2.pdf.

The amount and frequency of foods consumed are recorded and inputted into a specialized data entry program. This program converts food descriptions and portion sizes into weights and links the information to codes for foods in tables of food composition. The resulting data includes the average intake of food, energy, and nutrients on a daily and individual basis. Epidemiologists analyze these patterns to understand the relationship between food and nutrient intake and health outcomes. The use of computerized Food Composition Databases (FCDBs) has greatly benefited epidemiologists and those assessing nutritional status at a population level. These databases can store a large amount of data and make it easier to manipulate, add new values, and calculate and analyze nutrient intakes.

2.4.2. Public Health and Education

2.4.2.1. Monitoring Food and Nutrient Availability

National governments hold responsibility for monitoring and recording the availability of food and nutrients to their populations, and this is carried out at various levels:

2.4.2.1.1. Food Balance Sheets

The information on food balance sheets is derived from statistical data regarding food production, import, and export. In order to compare national food supplies across nations and over time, these data are converted to energy and nutrient availability, giving an aggregated picture of food availability at the national level. These Figures do not give a precise estimate of actual consumption but rather an evaluation of the gross adequacy or inadequacy of the country's food supply, showing where there are excesses or shortfalls.

2.4.2.1.2. Household Expenditure Surveys

Data on food expenditure and purchases at the household level that are translated to nutrient availability are provided by household expenditure surveys. This allows comparisons of food and nutrient availability within a population by income, region, or other household parameters, as well as over time. While food intake is not directly measured by these surveys—rather, food entering the household during the study period is—they are a priceless indicator of trends in food purchases over time.

2.4.2.1.3. Dietary Surveys

The most accurate estimate of food and nutrient intake at the population level is provided by dietary surveys, also known as food consumption surveys. Occasionally, they offer useful supplementary information on dental health, physical activity levels, and nutritional status. Unfortunately, few nations can conduct these surveys regularly due to their high cost and time requirements. Regardless of the level at which food availability data is gathered, an adequate FCDB is necessary for the conversion of food consumption data to nutrient intake data. For FCDBs to be useful in analyzing food and nutrient availability at the national level, they must be current, accessible, and representative of the country's food supplies. Regularly updated food composition tables also offer a way to evaluate long-term shifts in the food supply. For instance, due to modifications in animal husbandry and butchering techniques, the fat and iron content of meat has changed recently in developed nations. Alterations in the food supply can be investigated and tracked by comparing the data on food composition from the present with those from previous food tables.

Examining variations in food composition over time necessitates taking into consideration the fact that, as techniques advance and new technology becomes accessible, nutrient assessment methodology undergoes periodic modifications. Additionally, database compilers may have examined various varieties or samples (e.g., distinct fruit varieties) and employed various techniques for sample preparation (e.g., cooking techniques) so 'there is a chance the results aren't exactly comparable. Therefore, multiple comparison studies would be needed to examine changes in nutrient composition and provide proof of real changes in nutrient levels over time.

High-quality FCDBs that accurately reflect regional cuisines should ideally be created from scratch for every nation or region, but this is prohibitively expensive. As a result, many nations—including the majority of developing nations—have to "borrow" data, which they then combine with local and regional data to create their own national databases. The issue with "borrowing" data from other nations, though, is that local foods 'do not always have the same nutritional makeup as comparable foods from other countries for which data are available. Furthermore, certain products that are sold in some nations may be enhanced or fortified with particular nutrients; as a result, the local applicability of many of the databases that are currently in use is severely restricted. For instance, milk in the US does not usually contain vitamin D from other countries; thus, US data on milk's vitamin D content do not apply to other nations. Similarly, US data on selenium levels would not apply to other countries because US wheat has a naturally higher selenium content than wheat grown in Europe. It would be beneficial if the nations with the most comprehensive databases could fully document how fortification affects nutrient values and offer recipes for composite foods that can be altered to suit local needs.

2.4.2.1.4. Public Health Assessment and Dietary Surveys

Many nations have created national programs, also known as dietary surveys, to evaluate the nutritional status and diet of their populations in light of the growing awareness of the impact of diet on health. The goal of dietary surveys is to offer thorough, cross-sectional data on a population's eating patterns and nutritional status. Dietary survey findings can serve as a foundation for nutrition policy formulation and add to the body of knowledge supporting governmental recommendations for a healthy diet.

2.4.2.1.5. Food Regulations and Food Safety

The availability of sufficient data on the food and nutrient intake of populations in various nations is a prerequisite for many public health nutrition decisions. These include choices about food safety and the augmentation or fortification of foods.

2.5. Nutrition Facts Label

There are various reasons why people read food labels. Regardless of the cause, though, a lot of customers would like to know how to use this information more efficiently and conveniently. The purpose of the following label-building skills is to help you use nutrition labels more easily to quickly and intelligently choose foods that support a healthy diet (Figure 2.3).

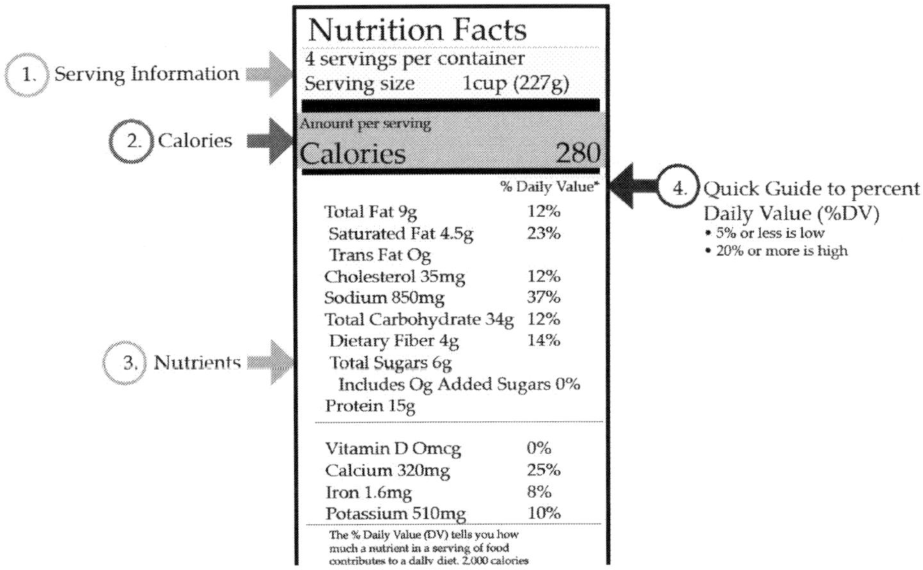

Figure 2.3. *Nutrition facts label.*

Source: https://andersonhousefoods.com/how-to-understand-and-use-the-nutrition-facts-label/.

2.5.1. The Serving Size

The first place to start when you look at the Nutrition Facts label is the serving size and the number of servings in the package. Serving sizes are standardized to make it easier to compare similar foods; they are provided in familiar units, such as cups or pieces, followed by the metric amount, e.g., the number of grams.

Serving Size 1 cup (228g)
Servings Per Container 2

The number of calories and all the nutrient amounts listed on the top portion of the label are influenced by the size of the serving on the food package. Take note of the serving size and, in particular, the quantity of servings included in the food package.

Then ask yourself, "How many servings am I consuming"? (e.g., ½ serving, one serving, or more) In the sample label, one serving of macaroni and cheese equals one cup. If you ate the whole package, you would eat two cups. That doubles the calories and other nutrient numbers, including the %Daily Values, as shown in the sample label (Table 2.6).

Table 2.6. *The Serving Size*

Example	Single Serving	%DV	Double Serving	%DV
Serving size	1 cup (228 g)	–	2 cups (456 g)	–
Calories	250	–	500	–
Calories from fat	110	–	220	–
Total fat	12 g	18%	24 g	36%
Trans fat	1.5 g	–	3 g	–
Saturated fat	3 g	15%	6 g	30%
Cholesterol	30 mg	10%	60 mg	20%
Sodium	470 mg	20%	940 mg	40%
Total carbohydrate	31 g	10%	62 g	20%
Dietary fiber	0 g	0%	0 g	0%
Sugars	5 g	–	10 g	–
Protein	5 g	–	10 g	–
Vitamin A	–	4%	–	8%
Vitamin C	–	2%	–	4%
Calcium	–	20%	–	40%
Iron	–	4%	–	8%

Source: https://www.fda.gov/food/nutrition-facts-label/how-understand-and-use-nutrition-facts-label.

2.5.2. Calories (and Calories from Fat)

An indicator of how much energy a serving of this food contains is its calorie count. Many Americans eat more calories than they require without consuming the recommended amounts of several different nutrients. The calorie section of the label can help you manage your weight (i.e., gain, lose, or maintain.)

A serving of the macaroni and cheese in the example has 250 calories. What is the number of calories from fat in one serving? 110 calories, or nearly half of the total calories in a single serving. If you were to consume the entire contents of the package, that would equal two servings, or 500 calories, of which 220 were fat-based.

General guide to calories:

- 40 Calories is low;
- 100 Calories is moderate;
- 400 Calories or more is high.

When examining a Nutrition Facts label, the General Guide to Calories offers a general point of reference for calories. A 2,000-calorie diet is the foundation of this guide.

2.5.3. The Nutrients: How Much?

Look at the top of the nutrient section in the sample label. It shows you some key nutrients that impact on your health and separates them into two main groups:

2.5.3.1. Limit These Nutrients

The first set of nutrients are those that Americans typically consume in sufficient amounts, if not excessively. They are marked as Limit these Nutrients in yellow. Consuming excessive amounts of fat, trans fat, saturated fat, cholesterol, or sodium can raise your risk of developing heart disease, some types of cancer, or high blood pressure, among other chronic illnesses.

Total Fat 12g	18%
Saturated Fat 3g	15%
Trans Fat 3g	
Cholesterol 30mg	10%
Sodium 470mg	20%

2.5.3.2. Get Enough of These

Dietary fiber, iron, calcium, vitamin A, and vitamin C are insufficiently consumed by the majority of Americans. Getting Enough of these Nutrients is 'what is indicated by the blue highlights. Consuming adequate of these nutrients can enhance your well-being and lower your chance of developing certain illnesses and ailments. For instance, consuming adequate calcium may lower the chance of developing osteoporosis, a disorder that causes brittle bones with age. Consuming a lot of dietary fiber encourages regular bowel movements. A diet low in cholesterol and saturated fat and high in fruits, vegetables, and grain products that contain dietary fiber—especially soluble fiber—may also lower the risk of heart disease.

Dietary Fiber 0g	0%

Vitamin A	4%
Vitamin C	2%
Calcium	20%
Iron	4%

2.5.4. Understanding the Footnote on the Bottom of the Nutrition Facts Label

Note the * used after the heading "%Daily Value" on the Nutrition Facts label. It refers to the Footnote in the lower part of the nutrition label, which tells you the "%DVs are based on a 2,000-calorie diet." This statement must be on all food labels.

But the remaining information in the full footnote may not be on the package if the size of the label is too small.

When the full footnote does appear, it will always be the same.

It doesn't change from product to product, because it shows RDA for all Americans—it is not about a specific food product.

Examine the amounts highlighted in red in the footnote; these are the DV for every nutrient mentioned, and they are determined by the recommendations of public health experts. DVs stand for RDA.

The DVs in the footnote are calculated using a diet of 2,000–2,500 calories. Observe how the DVs for some nutrients (like sodium and cholesterol) vary with calorie intake but not for others.

Percent Daily Values are based on a 2,000 calorie diet. Your Daily Values may be higher or lower depending on your calorie needs.

	Calories:	2,000	2,500
Total Fat	Less than	65g	80g
Sat Fat	Less than	20g	25g
Cholesterol	Less than	300mg	300mg
Sodium	Less than	2,400mg	2,400mg
Total Carbohydrate		300g	375g
Dietary Fiber		25g	30g

2.5.4.1. How the Daily Values Relate to the %DVs

Here is an example showing the relationship between DVs, the %DVs, and dietary guidance. Each nutrient has a DV, %DV, and recommended dietary advice or goal. By following this guidance, you will adhere to the recommended upper or lower limits set by public health experts for the listed nutrients, based on a 2,000-calorie daily diet.

- **Examples of DVs versus %DVs (Table 2.7):**

Table 2.7. *Based on a 2,000 Calorie Diet*

Nutrient	Daily Values (DV)	%DV	Goal
Total fat	65 g	= 100%DV	Less than
Sat fat	20 g	= 100%DV	Less than
Cholesterol	300 mg	= 100%DV	Less than
Sodium	2400 mg	= 100%DV	Less than
Total carbohydrate	300 g	= 100%DV	At least
Dietary fiber	25 g	= 100%DV	At least

Source: https://www.fda.gov/food/nutrition-facts-label/how-understand-and-use-nutrition-facts-label.

- **Upper Limit — Eat "Less Than"**

  The nutrients that have upper daily limits are listed first on the footnote of larger labels and on the example above. Upper limits means it is recommended that you stay below — eatless than — the Daily Value nutrient amounts listed per day. For example, the DV for Saturated fat (in the yellow section) is 20 g. This amount is 100% DV for this nutrient. What is the goal or dietary advice? To eat "less than" 20 g or 100%DV for the day.

- **Lower Limit — Eat "At least"**

  Now, notice that the list of dietary fiber is in the blue section. Dietary fiber has a DV of 25 g, or 100% of the DV. This indicates that consuming this much dietary fiber daily is advised. The section in white represents the DV for total carbohydrates, which is 300 g or 100%DV. This is an approximate amount based on a 2,000-calorie balanced daily diet; it may differ based on your daily intake of protein and fat.

2.5.5. The Percent Daily Value (%DV)

The Daily Value recommendations for important nutrients serve as the basis for the percent %DVs, but they are only applicable to a diet of 2,000 calories per day—not 2,500 calories.

Like most people, you might not be aware of how many calories you eat each day. However, regardless of whether you consume more or less than 2,000 calories, you can still use the %DV as a general guideline.

The %DV helps you determine if a serving of food is high or low in a nutrient. Note: a few nutrients, like *trans* fat, do not have a %DV—they will be discussed later.

The %DV label does all the math; you don't need to know how to calculate percentages to use it. Placing the grams and milligrams on the same daily scale (0–100 %DV) makes the numbers easier to understand. The vertical sum of the %DV column is not 100%. Rather, every nutrient is calculated using 100% of the daily needs for that nutrient (assuming a diet of 2,000 calories).

This allows you to distinguish between high and low intake and to determine which nutrients add significantly—or not—to your daily recommended allowance (upper or lower).

2.5.5.1. Quick Guide to Percent Daily Value

Around 20% or more of the DV is considered high, and 5% or less is considered low.

This guide tells you that 5%DV or less is low for all nutrients, those you want to limit (e.g., fat, saturated fat, cholesterol, and sodium), or for those that you want to consume in greater amounts (fiber, calcium, etc). As the Quick Guide shows, 20%DV or more is high for all nutrients (Figure 2.4).

	% Daily Value*
Total Fat 12g	18%
Saturated Fat 3g	15%
Trans Fat 3g	
Cholesterol 30mg	10%
Sodium 470mg	20%
Total Carbohydrate 31 g	10%
Dietary Fiber 0g	0%
Sugars 5g	
Protein 5g	
Vitamin A	4%
Vitamin C	2%
Calcium	20%
Iron	4%

Figure 2.4. *A quick guide to percent daily value (%DV).*

Source: https://andersonhousefoods.com/how-to-understand-and-use-the-nutrition-facts-label/.

Example: Check the sample nutrition label for the amount of total fat in one serving. Check the Quick Guide to %DV to see how much, if any, 18 %DV is contributing to your 100% DV fat limit. While 18 %DV is still not high compared to 20 %DV, if you ate the entire package (two servings), you would consume twice as much total fat, or 36% of your daily allowance. This amount comes from just one meal, so 'you will have 64% of your daily fat allowance (100% minus 36%) for all the other foods and beverages you consume. This includes snacks and drinks.

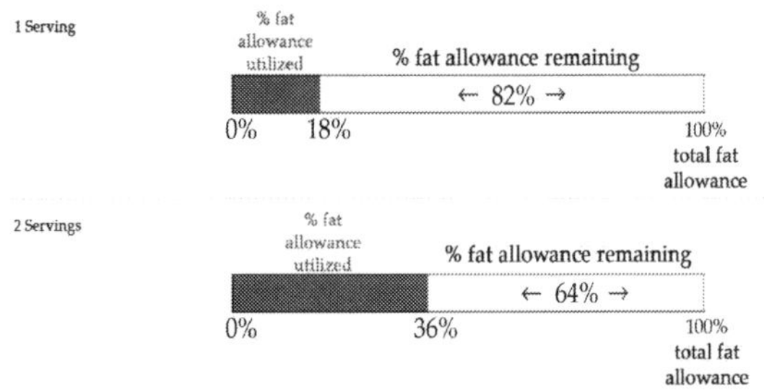

2.5.5.2. Using the Percent Daily Value

1. **Comparisons:** You can also easily make comparisons with the

%DV. One brand or product can be compared to another that is comparable. Just ensure that the serving sizes—particularly the weight (e.g. ounces, milligrams (mg), and grams (g)) of every product. With a few exceptions, such as cereals, serving sizes for similar types of foods are usually consistent, making it simple to determine which foods have more or fewer nutrients.

2. **Nutrient Content Claims:** Use the %DV to help you quickly distinguish one claim from another, such as "reduced fat" vs. "light" or "nonfat." Just compare the %DVs for Total Fat in each food product to see which one is higher or lower in that nutrient--there is no need to memorize definitions. This works when comparing all nutrient content claims, e.g., less, light, low, free, more, high, etc.
3. **Dietary Trade-Offs:** You can use the %DV to help you make dietary trade-offs with other foods throughout the day. You don't have to give up a favorite food to eat a healthy diet. When a food you like is high in fat, balance it with foods that are low in fat at other times of the day. Also, pay attention to how much you eat so that the total fat for the day stays below 100%DV.

2.5.5.3. Nutrients with a Percent Daily Value But No Weight Listed – Spotlight on Calcium

1. **Calcium:** Check the percentage of daily value (%DV) for calcium on food packaging to determine how much a single serving adds to your daily requirement. Keep in mind that foods with 20% or more of the daily value of calcium contribute significantly to your daily total, whereas foods with 5% or less of the daily value contribute slightly.

   Experts advise adult consumers to include 1,000 mg (or 100%DV) of calcium in a daily diet of 2,000 calories or more. This recommendation is frequently expressed in mg, however the Nutrition Facts label only provides a calcium %DV.

   It is recommended that adolescents, particularly girls, take 1,300 mg (130 %DV), and postmenopausal women take 1,200 mg (120 %DV) of calcium daily for specific populations. On food labels, the DV for calcium is 1,000 mg (Figure 2.5).

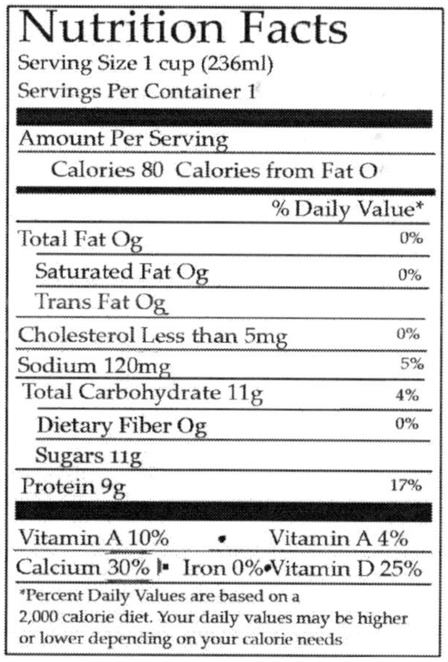

Figure 2.5. *Nutrition-facts.*

Source: https://andersonhousefoods.com/how-to-understand-and-use-the-nutrition-facts-label/.

2. **Don't be Fooled:** You can't assume that a given food category contains a certain amount of calcium, so you should always check the label. For instance, the calcium content of a serving of milk—whole or skim—is usually the same, but the calcium content of an 8-ounce container of yogurt can range from 20 to 45 %DV (Figure 2.6).

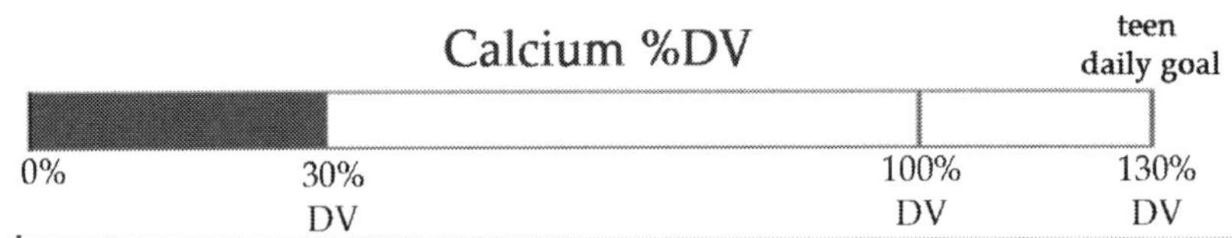

Equivalencies
30% DV = 300mg calcium = one cup of milk
100% DV = 1,000mg calcium
130% DV = 1,300mg calcium

Figure 2.6. *A quick guide to percent daily value (%DV).*

Source: https://www.cooks.com/rec/nutrition/fl_cooks.html.

A Closer Look

"Serving Size" in Nutrition Label:

When reviewing a nutrition label, in addition to analyzing the "1+7" nutritional content, it is important to grasp the portion size that the manufacturer is referring to. The nutritional information on a packaged food item may be provided per 100 g (or 100 ml), "per serving," or "per package."

Serving size describes how much of a certain type of food a person typically eats at each meal occasion. Food manufacturers set the serving sizes; different food types and brands may have different amounts. Consider the following illustration using instant noodles. According to the nutrition label for Noodle A, each package contains two servings, each weighing 45 g. In other words, the manufacturer recommends consuming the entire pack of Noodle A in two separate meals, with each mealtime consuming the same amount of nutrients as indicated on the nutrition label, i.e., energy of 220 kcal, protein of 4 g, etc. The quantity of energy and nutrients consumed will double if the entire package of noodles is eaten in one sitting, i.e., 8 g of protein, and 440 kcal of energy.

If two noodle products have comparable net weights and are intended to be consumed as one serving, it is possible to directly compare their nutritional values on a "per serving" basis. When comparing Noodle B and Noodle C, consuming the entire package of noodles will result in a similar energy intake (344 kcal and 350 kcal, respectively). However, consuming Noodle C will lead to a higher intake of total fat, saturated fat, and sodium.

Occasionally, the serving sizes of various products can vary significantly. In this instance, before comparing, a quick conversion will be required to get their nutritional contents based on the same quantity of food. For example, the serving size of Noodle B is 86 g whereas that of Noodle D is 75 g. The following formula can be used to convert the nutritional content of Noodle D based on a serving of Noodle D to the same weight as a serving of Noodle B:

Nutritional content of 75 g of Noodle D ÷ 75 g x 86 g

After conversion, it shows that consuming 86 g of Noodle D will provide 384 kcal (335 kcal ÷ 75 g x 86 g), which is more than that (344 kcal) provided by 86 g of Noodle B.

Summary

- Food pyramids are the perfect tool for depicting total diet at a glance. Done right – with colorful, enticing images of real foods – food pyramids show examples of what to eat over time (not just at this one meal!) and the relative proportion of each food group.
- Dietary Reference Intakes (DRIs) comprise a set of nutrient-based reference values, each of which has special uses.
- The Recommended Dietary Allowance (RDA) is the average daily dietary intake level that is sufficient to meet the nutrient requirement of nearly all (97 to 98 percent) healthy individuals in a particular life stage and gender group.
- The Tolerable Upper Intake Level (UL) is the highest level of daily nutrient intake that is likely to pose no risk of adverse health effects for almost all apparently healthy individuals in the specified life stage group.
- The word exchange refers to the food items on each list which may be substituted with any other food item on the same list. One exchange is approximately equal to another in carbohydrate, calories, protein and fat within each food list.
- Food composition databases (FCDBs) provide detailed information on the nutritional composition of foods, usually from a particular country. Food composition data may be available in different formats e.g. paper-based, often referred to as food composition tables, or electronic versions, known as nutrient databases or databanks.
- Food balance sheet information is based on statistical data on the production, import and export of foods and is published quarterly by the UN Food and Agriculture Organization.

References

1. Relationship of vitamin B12 deficiency with overweight in male jordanian youth. *Journal of Applied Sciences, 8,* 3060–3063.
2. Cleveland, L. E., Moshfegh, A. J., Alberston, A. M., & Goldman, J. D. (2000). Dietary intake of whole grains. *Journal of the American College of Nutrition, 19*(supp3), 331S–338S.
3. D'Elgin, T. (2005). *What Should I Eat? A Complete Guide to the New Food Pyramid.* New York: Ballantine Books.
4. Fuhrman, J. (2011). *Eat to Live.* Little, Brown (Hachette).
5. Johnson, R. K., & Kennedy, E. (2000). The 2000 Dietary Guidelines for Americans: what are the changes and why were they made? *Journal of the American Dietetic Association, 100,* 769–774.
6. Melnick, M. (n.d.). The USDA ditches the food pyramid for a plate. *Time.* Retrieved July 26, 2016, from link.
7. Messina, V., Melina, V., & Mangels, A. R. (2007). A new food guide: for north american vegetarians. *Canadian Journal of Dietetic Practice and Research, 64*(2), 82–86.

8. Painter, J., Rah, J. H., & Lee, Y. K. (2002). Comparison of international food guide pictorial representations. *Journal of the American Dietetic Association, 102*(4), 483–489.

9. Reyes, R. (2008). Food pyramid frenzy: Lobbyists fight to defend sugar, potatoes and bread in recommended U.S. diet. *Wall Street Journal.* Retrieved December 9, 2006, from link.

10. evidence and examples from the Dietary Approaches to Stop Hypertension (DASH) Trial. *Journal of Food Composition and Analysis, 16,* 313–321.

11. Slimani, N., Charrondière, U. R., van Staveren, W., & Riboli, E. (2000). Standardization of food composition databases for the European Prospective Investigation into Cancer and Nutrition (EPIC): General theoretical concept. *Journal of Food Composition and Analysis, 13,* 567–584.

12. Southgate, D. A. T. (2000). Food composition tables and nutritional databases. In J. S. Garrow, W. P. T. James, & A. Ralph (Eds.), *Human Nutrition and Dietetics.* Churchill Livingstone.

13. Theobald, H. (2004). A whole diet approach to healthy eating. *Nutrition Bulletin, 29,* 44–49.

14. Thomas, B. (2001). *Manual of Dietetic Practice, Third Edition.* Blackwell Science Ltd.

Chapter

ENERGY

3

Contents

Unit Introduction

The science of nutrition studies how food affects health and how the body uses and metabolizes the nutrients it contains to carry out daily tasks (i.e., the kidneys to filter blood, the brain to think, the heart to beat, the lungs to breathe, etc.). This definition includes the amount of energy (measured in kilojoules) required by the body to sustain a healthy weight. Food is how the body receives energy. Body fat is the result of consuming energy (such as carbs, proteins, or fats) and not using it for growth, metabolism, or physical activity. A person's energy requirements depend on a variety of factors, but generally speaking, the more movement there is in the body, the more energy is required.

Orientation and Directional Terms

Term	Definition	Illustration
Basal metabolic rate	Basal Metabolic Rate (BMR) is the number of calories you burn as your body performs basic (basal) life-sustaining function. Commonly also termed as Resting Metabolic Rate (RMR), which is the calories burned if you stayed in bed all day.	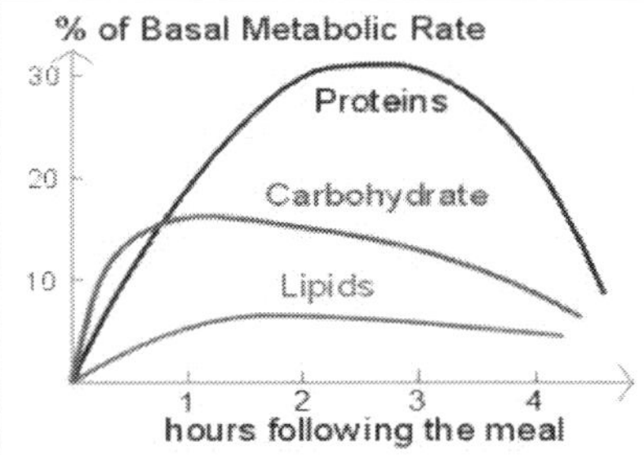
Energy expenditure	Energy expenditure is the sum of the basal metabolic rate (the amount of energy expended while at complete rest), the thermic effect of food (TEF, the energy required to digest and absorb food) and the energy expended in physical activity.	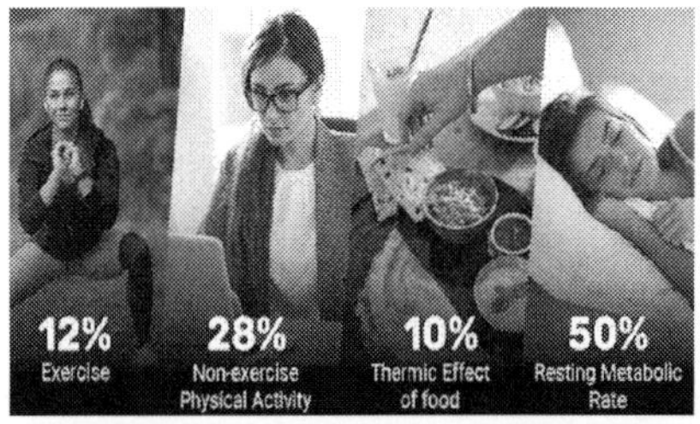
Energy Balance	Energy is another word for "calories." Your energy balance is the balance of calories consumed through eating and drinking compared to calories burned through physical activity.	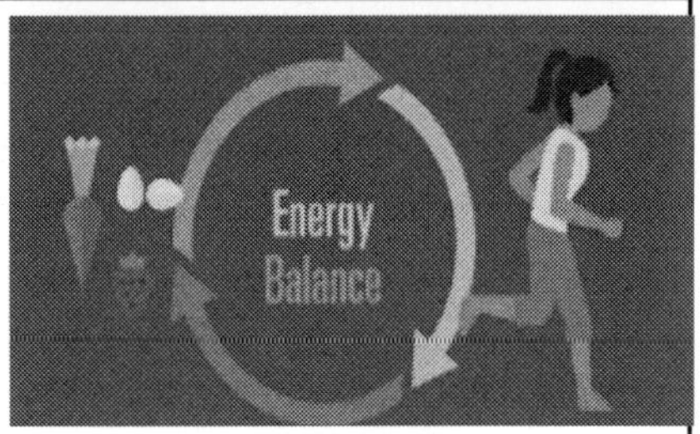
Bioelectric Impedance Analysis (BIA)	Bioelectrical impedance analysis (BIA) is a method for estimating body composition, in particular body fat and muscle mass, where a weak electric current flows through the body, and the voltage is measured in order to calculate impedance (resistance and reactance) of the body.	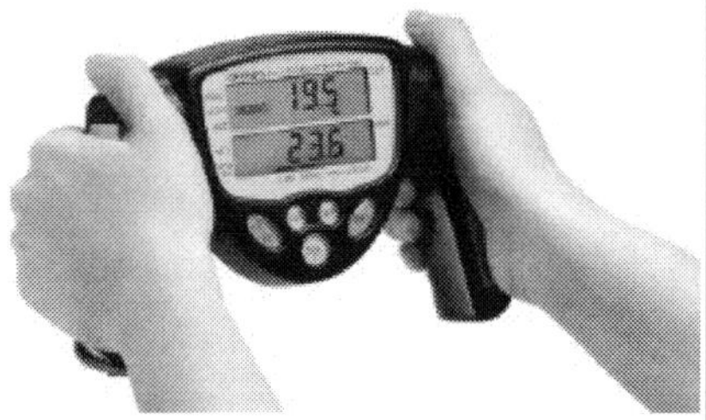
Energy intake	Energy intake is the calorie or energy content of food. Energy expenditure is required for resting metabolic rate to maintain basic physiological functions (e.g. heart beat, muscle function, respiration), metabolise, digest and store food that is consumed, as well as for physical activity.	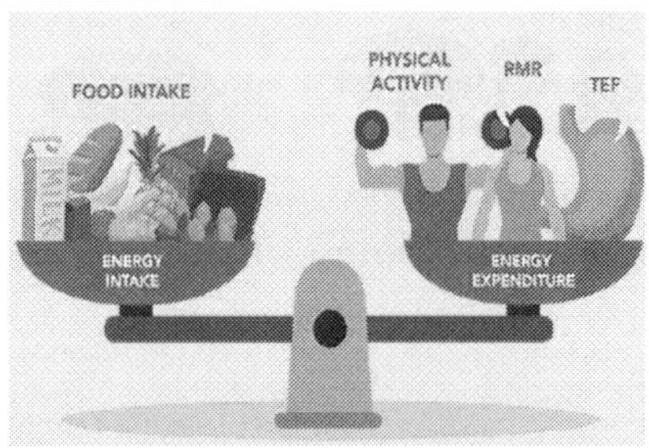

3.1. Energy Balance

The relationship between "energy in" (calories from food and drink) and "energy out" (calories the body uses to meet its daily energy needs) is known as "energy balance." The laws of thermodynamics define this relationship, which determines whether weight increases, decreases, or stays the same. The laws of these creation and destruction state that energy is never truly created or destroyed. Instead, energy is exchanged between different entities.

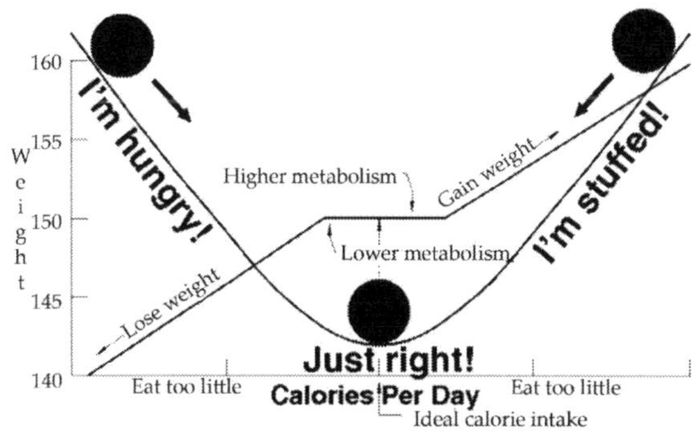

Figure 3.1. *Energy balance.*

Source: https://www.precisionnutrition.com/all-about-energy-balance.

We convert potential energy that is stored within our food (measured in Calories or kcals) into three major "destinations": work, heat, and storage. The body needs energy for maintenance at rest, physical activity, movement, and the digestion, absorption, and transportation of food are all considered forms of "energy out." By tracking how much oxygen we take in, we can determine how much energy we require. We consume food, process it, absorb it, move it around, store it, transfer it, burn it, and then we do it again (Figure 3.1).

3.1.1. Estimated Calorie Requirements

This chart of caloric requirements shows the approximate number of calories required at three different levels of physical activity for different genders and age groups in order to maintain energy balance (and a healthy body weight).

The estimates were calculated using an Institute of Medicine (IOM) equation and are rounded to the nearest 200 calories (Table 3.1).

Table 3.1. *Estimated Calorie Requirements (in kilocalories) for Each Gender and Age Group at Three Levels of Physical Activity*

Gender	Age (Years)	Activity Level		
		Sedentary	**Moderately Active**	**Active**
Child	2–3	1,000	1,000–1,400	1,000–1,400
Female	4–8	1,200	1,400–1,600	1,400–1,800
Female	9–13	1,600	1,600–2,000	1,800–2,000
Female	14–18	1,800	2,000	2,400
Female	19–30	2,000	2,000–2,200	2,400
Female	31–50	1,800	2,000	2,200
Female	51+	1,600	1,800	2,000–2,200
Male	4–8	1,400	1,400–1,600	1,600–2,000
Male	9–13	1,800	1,800–2,200	2,000–2,600

Male	14–18	2,200	2,400–2,800	2,800–3,200
Male	19–30	2,400	2,600–2,800	3,000
Male	31–50	2,200	2,400–2,600	2,800–3,000
Male	51+	2,000	2,200–2,400	2,400–2,800

Source: HHS/USDA Dietary Guidelines for Americans (2005).

- Based on gender, age, and activity level calculations for reference-sized individuals, the Estimated Energy Requirements (EER) from the IOM Dietary Reference Intakes macronutrients report, 2002, are used to determine these levels. The BMI of 21.5 for adult females and 22.5 for adult males is the reference size, as defined by the IOM. It is based on the median height and weight for ages up to and including 18 years of age, as well as the median height and weight for that height.
- Sedentary means a lifestyle that includes only the light physical activity associated with typical day-to-day life.
- Moderately active means a lifestyle that includes physical activity equivalent to walking about 1.5 to 3 miles per day at 3 to 4 miles per hour, in addition to the light physical activity associated with typical day-to-day life.
- Active means a lifestyle that includes physical activity equivalent to walking more than 3 miles per day at 3 to 4 miles per hour, in addition to the light physical activity associated with typical day-to-day life.
- The calorie ranges shown accommodate the needs of different ages within the group. For children and adolescents, more calories are needed at older ages. For adults, fewer calories are needed at older ages.

3.1.2. Why Energy Balance Is So Important?

Energy balance is much more than just a shift in body weight. Your cells' activities also affect the balance of energy in your body. Everything from your metabolism to hormonal balance to the mood is affected when you have a positive energy balance (more in than out) or a negative energy balance (more out than in).

3.1.2.1. Negative Energy Balance

A very negative energy balance can cause a number of problems, such as a decrease in testosterone levels, thyroid hormones, bone mass, metabolism, concentration problems, and decreased physical performance.

Weight loss is nevertheless a result of a negative energy balance. When the body senses a "deficit" in energy, fat stores are tapped to make up the shortfall. The body is incapable of distinguishing between starvation in a poor African village and a rigorous diet under medical supervision at a spa in Beverly Hills. The body simply knows that it isn't receiving enough energy, so it will start to reduce or stop all "non-survival" processes. Find out if someone has a high sex drive by asking them if they have been fasting for two weeks. Not at all.

3.1.2.2. Positive Energy Balance

In addition to causing weight gain, overeating (and/or underexercising) can have negative effects on one's health and cellular fitness. Overeating can lead to several health problems, including plaque accumulation in the arteries, elevated blood pressure and cholesterol, diabetes mellitus, insulin resistance, an increased risk of certain cancers, and more.

Our body weight and general health are determined by the relationship between the number of calories we consume through diet and the amount of energy our bodies expend. The body can adjust very well to a wide range of energy intakes and outputs. Its survival depends on its ability to adapt. Thus, whether or not energy imbalances exist, mechanisms are in place to guarantee stable energy transfer.

3.1.3. Body Mass Index: How to Measure It and Its Limitations?

In comparison to weight alone, body mass index (BMI), which is computed using height and weight data, is a better indicator of body fatness. An individual's BMI can be used to determine if they are underweight (less than 18.5), overweight (more than 25), or obese (more than 30). High BMI values may indicate the impending risk of developing chronic illnesses like Type 2 diabetes, cardiovascular disease, and other diseases.

3.1.3.1. Calculating Body Mass Index

In order to determine your BMI, multiply your weight in pounds by the conversion factor (703 in this case) to convert to metric units, and then divide the result by the square of your height in inches.

$$BMI = [weight\ (lb) \times 703] \div height\ (in)^2$$

Or

$$BMI = [weight\ (kg)] \div height\ (m)^2$$

To see how your BMI indicates the weight category you are in, see Table 3.2 "BMI Categories" or use a chart of weight and height to Figure out your BMI.

Table 3.2. *Body Mass Index (BMI) Categories*

Categories	BMI
Underweight	< 18.5
Normal weight	18.5–24.9
Overweight	25–29.9
Obese	> 30.0

Source: https://chem.libretexts.org/Bookshelves/Introductory_Chemistry/Chemistry_for_Changing_Times_(Hill_and_McCreary)/19%3A_Fitness_and_Health/19.04%3A_Measuring_Fitness.

3.1.3.2. Body Mass Index

- **Limitations:** The body's distribution of fat and fat mass, which are two more indicators of disease risk, are not included in the BMI, which is a relatively straightforward measurement. Muscle mass weighs more than body fat. As a result, BMI may overestimate body fat in individuals who are more muscularally built and underestimate it in those who are overweight or obese. For example, a muscular athlete will weigh more in terms of muscle mass than fat mass for an equivalent height. Though this is an uncommon issue with BMI calculation, the muscular athlete would be less "ideal" and might be classified as more overweight or obese than the couch potato based on their BMIs. Furthermore, even though the individual with osteoporosis may have more fat mass, an older person with osteoporosis (decreased bone mass) will have a lower BMI than an older person without osteoporosis of the same height. Although the BMI of a person is a useful and affordable tool for classification and has a strong correlation with disease risk, additional measurements are required to diagnose obesity and, more precisely, determine the risk of disease.

3.1.4. Body Fat and Its Distribution

3.1.4.1. Measuring Body Fat Content

The weight of a person is composed of water, organs, fat, muscle, and bone tissue. Greater fat mass may be a sign of an increased risk of disease, but fat mass also varies with age, sex, and degree of physical activity.

The greater fat mass in females is partly due to varying hormone levels and is necessary for reproduction. For a female, the ideal fat content ranges from 20 to 30% of her total weight, while for a male, it is between 12 and 20%. There are several methods for calculating fat mass. The skin-fold test is the easiest and least expensive method. To determine body fatness, a health professional measures the thickness of skin on the arms, back, and other areas of the body using a caliper and compares the results to standards. Like BMI, it is a noninvasive and reasonably accurate way to measure fat mass, but it is compared to standards that are primarily based on young to middle-aged adults.

Other methods of measuring fat mass are more expensive and more technically challenging. They include:

1. **Weighing Underwater:** This method calls for a water-filled chamber large enough to accommodate the entire body. A person is weighed outside the chamber initially, and then they are weighed once more while submerged in water. A person with more muscle and bone mass will weigh more in the water than a person with less muscle and bone mass because bone and muscle weigh more than water, but fat does not.
2. **Bioelectric Impedance Analysis (BIA):** The idea behind this device is that fat impedes the body's ability to conduct electricity. The rate at which a tiny amount of electricity moves through the body can be used to calculate the composition of the body. These gadgets, which go by the name "body composition scales," are also offered for home use.

3.1.4.2. Measuring Fat Distribution

The total mass of fat in the body and the distribution of that fat within the body are two indicators of health. As you may have heard, that fat on the hips is preferable to fat in the abdomen.

The body contains different types of fat in different places, and these types of fat behave differently, causing physiological differences depending on the location. Vessel-deposited fat, or visceral fat, indicates the likelihood of developing a disease than total body fat mass. Hormones and inflammatory factors are released by visceral fat, which raises the risk of disease. A measuring tape is the sole instrument needed to calculate visceral fat. Just above the belly button is where the waist circumference measurement is taken. Greater health risks are expected for men with waist circumferences of more than 40 inches and women with waist circumferences of more than 35 inches.

3.2. Balancing Energy Input with Energy Output

Remember that the macronutrients you eat can be stored, transformed into energy, or utilized to create macromolecules. The metabolic pathway of a nutrient depends on the balance of energy. The extra nutrient energy will either be stored or used for growth when you are in a positive energy balance (e.g., during adolescence, gestation, and the healing of wounds). Your body will have to use its stores of energy to meet your needs when you are out of balance with the energy in the universe. When energy intake and expenditure are equal, energy balance is reached. Body weight is maintained in states of energy balance, lost in states of negative energy balance, and gained in states of positive energy balance. It is possible to conceptualize weight as an estimate of the balance of the entire body. Though there are numerous other factors that affect how much energy is consumed and how much is expended, weight is generally a good indicator of energy balance. You have some control over some of these factors, but not all. Let us start by going over the fundamentals of estimating energy intake, demand, and output. Next, we will examine the additional elements that contribute to preserving energy equilibrium and, consequently, body weight.

3.2.1. Estimating Energy Requirement

You must balance the calories you burn each day with the calories you consume from food and drink in order to maintain your current body weight. Here, we will go over how to Figure out how many calories you need each day to meet your energy needs in kg so you can assess if you're getting enough calories from your diet. An algorithm developed by the Institute of Medicine can be used to determine your estimated energy requirement (EER). It considers your height, weight, sex, age, and degree of physical activity (PA).

The EER is a standardized mathematical prediction of a person's daily energy needs in kilocalories per day required to maintain weight. It is calculated via the following formulas:

Adult male: EER = 662 – [9.53 x age (y)] + PA X [15.91 x wt (kg) + 5.39.6 x ht (m)]

Adult female: EER = 354 – [6.91 x age (y)] + PA x [9.36 x wt (kg) + 726 x ht (m)]

3.2.2. Estimating Caloric Intake

You must make a dietary assessment and keep track of the calories you eat to calculate your daily caloric intake (Table 3.3).

Table 3.3. *Physical Activity (PA) Categories and Values*

Activity Level	Men PA Value	Women PA Value	Description
Sedentary	1.00	1.00	No physical activity beyond that required for independent living
Low	1.11	1.12	Equivalent to walking 1.5 to 3 miles per day
Moderate	1.25	1.27	Equivalent to walking 3 to 10 miles per day
High	1.48	1.45	Equivalent to walking 10 or more miles per day

Source: https://pressbooks.bccampus.ca/nutr1100/chapter/estimated-energy-requirements/.

The EER's numerical values were obtained using measurements obtained from an identical-sex, identical-age group with comparable body dimensions and levels of physical activity. To estimate an individual's energy requirements, these standardized formulas are then applied to people with similar characteristics but no measurements. Therefore, as the name implies, an individual's EER is an estimate for an average person with comparable characteristics. Children, women who are pregnant or nursing, and those who are overweight or obese have different EER values. Additionally, keep in mind that the EER is determined for weight maintenance rather than weight gain or loss (Tables 3.4 and 3.5).

Table 3.4. *Estimated Daily Calorie Needs*

Sex	Age (years)	Sedentary	Moderately Active	Active
Child (female and male)	2–3	1,000–1,200	1,000–1,400	1,000–1,400
Female	4–8	1,200–1,400	1,400–1,600	1,400–1,800
	9–13	1,400–1,600	1,600–2,000	1,800–2,200
	14–18	1,800	2,000	2,400
	19–30	1,800–2,000	2,000–2,200	2,400
	31–50	1,800	2,000	2,200
	51+	1,600	1,800	2,000–2,200
Male	4–8	1,200–1,400	1400–1,600	1,600–2,000
	9–13	1,600–2,000	1,800–2,200	2,000–2,600
	14–18	2,000–2,400	2,400–2,800	2,800–3,200
	19–30	2,400–2,600	2,600–2,800	3,000
	31–50	2,200–2,400	2,400–2,600	2,800–3,000
	51+	2,000–2,200	2,200–2,400	2,400–2,800

Source: https://med.libretexts.org/Courses/Folsom_Lake_College/FLC%3A_Nutri_300_(Silva)/01%3A_NUTRI_300_Textbook/09%3A_Energy_Balance_and_Healthy_Weight/9.03%3A_Balancing_Energy_Input_with_Energy_Output.

Table 3.5. *Acceptable Macronutrient Distribution Ranges*

Age	Carbohydrates (% of Calories)	Protein (% of Calories)	Fat (% of Calories)
Young Children (1–3)	65–45	20–5	40–30
Older children/ adolescents (4–18)	65–45	30–10	35–25
Adults (19 and older)	65–45	35–10	35–20

Source: https://med.libretexts.org/Courses/Folsom_Lake_College/FLC%3A_Nutri_300_(Silva)/01%3A_NUTRI_300_Textbook/09%3A_Energy_Balance_and_Healthy_Weight/9.03%3A_Balancing_Energy_Input_with_Energy_Output.

3.2.3. Total Energy Expenditure (Output)

Your daily energy expenditure consists of the calories burned during physical activity, the calories burned during rest (basal metabolism), and the calories burned during food digestion. Total energy expenditure (TEE) is the total of all caloric expenses. Basal metabolism refers to those metabolic pathways necessary to support and maintain the body's basic functions (e.g. breathing, heartbeat, liver, and kidney function) while at rest.

The amount of energy needed by the body to carry out its essential processes over a predetermined amount of time is known as the basal metabolic rate, or BMR. Between 50 and 70% of the energy used each day is used for carrying out the necessities of life. The liver uses the greatest amount of energy out of all the organs (Table 3.6). Regretfully, you are unable to instruct your liver to increase its level of activity to burn more calories and help you lose weight. BMI is influenced by genetics, age, sex, body composition, and nutrition.

For simple reasons, people with larger frames have higher BMRs because they are heavier. Even at rest, muscle mass increases a person's BMR because muscle burns more calories than fat. Women's BMRs are usually lower than men's because they usually have smaller frames and less muscle mass than men. Muscle mass decreases with age, and BMR follows suit. Basal metabolism is also influenced by nutritional status.

For example, calorie restriction during dieting results in a decrease in BMR. This is a result of the body's adaptation to maintain homeostasis, which involves slowing down essential processes to make up for the drop in energy intake. Thyroid hormone levels and body temperature are two more factors that affect BMR (Figure 3.2).

Table 3.6. *Energy Breakdown of Organs*

Organ	Percent of Energy Expended
Liver	27
Brain	19
Heart	7
Kidneys	10
Skeletal muscle (at rest)	18
Other organs	19

Source: https://med.libretexts.org/Courses/Folsom_Lake_College/FLC%3A_Nutri_300_(Silva)/01%3A_NUTRI_300_Textbook/09%3A_Energy_Balance_and_Healthy_Weight/9.03%3A_Balancing_Energy_Input_with_Energy_Output.

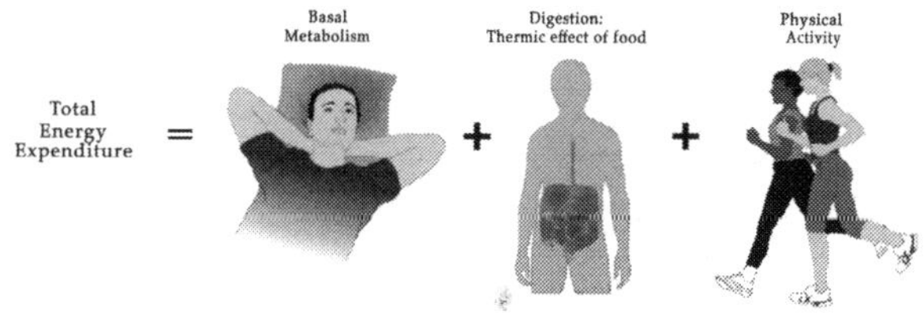

Figure 3.2. *Total energy expenditure.*

Source: https://pressbooks.bccampus.ca/nutr1100/chapter/estimated-energy-requirements/.

The "thermic effect of food" refers to the energy needed for all the enzymatic reactions that occur during food digestion and nutrient absorption; this energy makes up around 10% of daily energy expenditure.

Physical activity during the day requires additional energy. The energy needed for this varies from 15 to 30% of the total energy used, depending on lifestyle. Increasing physical activity is the primary way that an individual can manage TEE.

3.2.4. How to Calculate Total Energy Expenditure?

The availability of calculators has simplified the previously laborious process of calculating TEE. Age, sex, height, weight, and degree of physical activity all affect TEE. The formulas used in the equations are standardized and derived from measurements taken on groups of individuals who share similar characteristics. Web-based TEE calculators require you to log your daily activities and the amount of time spent on them in order to produce accurate results.

3.2.5. Factors Affecting Energy Intake

3.2.5.1. Physiology

Over the past few decades, scientific research has shown that our eating habits are influenced by our genetic makeup and physiological regulation in addition to our personal desires. The primary brain region that regulates appetite is the hypothalamus. Your body detects hunger and fullness through hormonal and neural signals. The unpleasant feeling of being empty, which is known as hunger, is transmitted to the brain by peripheral mechanical and chemical cues. On the other hand, the feeling of being full is known as satiety, and it is also influenced by chemical and mechanical cues received from the peripheral.

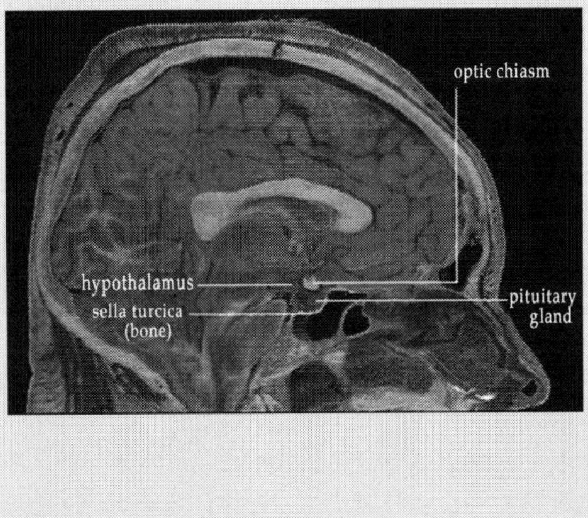

Figure 3.3. *This is a scan of a brain. The hypothalamus contains distinct centers of neural circuits that regulate hunger and satiety.*

Source: https://simple.wikipedia.org/wiki/Hypothalamus.

The brain regions that control hunger and fullness are distributed throughout the hypothalamus (Figure 3.3).

Both hunger pangs and a "growling" stomach are real. The stomach contracts when it is empty, resulting in the distinct "growl" and pang sound. The hypothalamus receives neural signals from the stomach's mechanical movements and subsequently transmits those signals to various brain regions. The conscious desire to eat is the outcome of this. On the other hand, following a meal, the stomach expands and communicates with the brain through a neural signal to cease eating by inducing a feeling of fullness. Additionally, the stomach releases different hormones depending on whether it is full or empty. The hypothalamus and other brain regions receive messages from these hormones signaling them to either find food or stop eating. Intake of food is also regulated by fat tissue. The hormone leptin, which is produced by fat tissue, alerts the hypothalamic satiety center to the body's positive energy balance. The hypothesis that giving leptin to an overweight person would cause them to eat less food was the driving force behind the research and diet pill craze that followed the discovery of 'functions of leptin.

3.2.5.2. Genetic Influences

Genetics undoubtedly influence food intake as well as body fatness and weight. Adopted children usually have similar body fat percentages and weights to their biological parents. Furthermore, compared to fraternal twins, identical twins have a twice higher chance of having similar weights. A few genes, including the one encoding leptin, have been found in the scientific hunt for the genes responsible for obesity. Millions of people are overweight or obese, but the cause is most likely the combination of hundreds of genes and their environment, rather than a single or small number of genes. Although only a small number of people worldwide have been found to have a completely faulty leptin gene, obese people do indeed have mutated versions of the gene coding for leptin.

3.2.5.3. Psychological/Behavioral Influences

You are experiencing a psychological influence on food intake when the aroma of a roasting Thanksgiving turkey and steaming hot pies makes your mouth water. What and how much a person eats is influenced by their opinion of what tastes and smells good. Emotions and mood are linked to food consumption. Obesity and increased food intake are occasionally associated with emotional trauma, compulsive disorders, depression, and low self-esteem. A person's eating habits may be predicted by certain behaviors. Several factors include the quantity of food consumed, the frequency of calorie-dense, salty food snacks, the frequency of TV or computer use, and the frequency of eating out.

3.2.5.4. Societal Influences

Without a doubt, our eating habits and intake are influenced by American society. Over the last few decades, portion sizes have significantly increased. A bagel, for instance, is now larger than it was in the 1960s. Teenagers in America today have enormous access to high-calorie foods and drinks, which has greatly contributed to the country's recent and sharp rise in the prevalence of overweight and obesity in teenagers. Even within the United States, various cultures have distinct eating customs. For example, Americans in the south generally eat more foods high in fat, which may account for why they have higher rates of obesity and overweight than people in the north. (Alaska is an exception due to the state's high rate of obesity and overweight, which is also partially related to diet).

3.3. Measurement of Energy Expenditure of the Body

The quantity of energy (or calories) required for a person to perform a physical function, like breathing, blood circulation, food digestion, or physical movement, is known as energy expenditure. The total calories you burn in a day is known as your total daily energy expenditure, or TDEE. Energy intake, or calorie intake, must be balanced with energy expenditure in order to prevent weight gain. Calories, sometimes known as kilocalories, are the unit of measurement for energy in food. The quantity of heat needed to raise one kilogram of water's temperature by one degree Celsius is known as a kilocalorie. Your total daily energy expenditure, or TDEE, is the total number of calories you burn off for energy every day.

Total daily energy expenditure can vary from person to person depending on body size, gender, body composition, genetics, and activity level. The total energy expenditure for a small sedentary woman may be 1800 calories or less per day. But the TDEE for a large man may be 2000 calories or more. The oxidation of macronutrients in food provides the energy needed by the human body to sustain its organic and vital functions. Energy expenditure (EE) can be defined as the process of producing energy through the combustion of energy substrates (proteins, lipids, carbohydrates, and alcohol), which results in the production of carbon dioxide (CO_2) and the consumption of oxygen (O_2). Adenosine triphosphates (ATPs), high-energy molecules, store the remaining chemical energy that is lost as heat and in urine.

The total amount of energy an organism needs each day is called TEE, and it is calculated by adding the three factors of basal energy expenditure (BEE), diet-induced thermogenesis (DIT), and physical activity (PA). Predictive equations, bioelectrical impedance (BIA), doubly labeled water (DLW), indirect and direct calorimetry (IC and DC), and other techniques are used for EE measurements. The EE determination is crucial for modifying each person's nutritional offer because it considers their specific health conditions and the amount of energy they require for physical activity. The majority of these techniques have been applied extensively in human research for various therapeutic purposes (such as obesity and enteral and parenteral nutrition). However, due to disparate findings from the literature, opinions regarding the applicability of some of them are divided. Thus, this review highlights the benefits and drawbacks of various energy expenditure estimation techniques while outlining the components of energy expenditure.

3.3.1. Description of Methods

Energy expenditure can be measured using one of the three approaches:

1. In indirect calorimetry, oxygen consumption and/or carbon dioxide production is measured and converted to energy expenditure using formulae.
2. In direct calorimetry, the rate of heat loss from the subject to the calorimeter is measured.
3. A number of non-calorimetric techniques have been used to predictthe energy expenditure by extrapolation from physiological measurements and observations.

The accuracy, reproducibility and reliability of the measurements obtained using these various techniques vary enormously as the complexity and cost of the techniques themselves.

3.3.2. Indirect Calorimetry

There are five main methods for utilizing indirect calorimetry to measure energy expenditure.

3.3.2.1. Total Collection Systems

In this instance, used air is gathered in a transportable, flexible bag or an airtight, rigid framework.

3.3.2.1.1. Rigid Total Collection System

A system that is rigid for total collection is the Tissot Gasometer. The device consists of an inverted glass bell with a capacity of 100–1000 liters and an internal circulation fan that is suspended over water. All air is removed from the bell. Subsequently, the subject exhales via a mouthpiece and a nonreturn valve into the bell, which fills with exhaled air gradually and rises above the water seal. For a maximum of two hours, the height attained by the bell is recorded every minute. Additionally, the composition of expired air is periodically measured from the bell to ascertain the amount of oxygen consumed and/or carbon dioxide produced.

3.3.2.1.2. Flexible Total Collection System

A system for flexible total collection is the Douglas bag. It consists of a 100–150 liter polyvinyl chloride (or other leak-proof material) bag. Tubing connects the top of the bag to a three-way valve, which can be rotated to admit atmospheric air, seal the bag, or admit expired air through tubing that is connected to a respiratory valve. This method involves rolling up the bag to release its contents, rotating the three-way valve to seal it, and then rotating the valve again to open the circuit to ambient air. The three-way valve is turned to allow the expired air to be released for 10 to 20 minutes while the subject inhales through the mouthpiece. The three-way valve is turned to seal the bag at the end of the timed collection period. Two valves—one at the mouthpiece and the other closer to the bag—are used in an alternate valve arrangement. You can extend the duration of the measurement by using multiple bags. Following the collection of the expired air, the volume of the expired air in the bag is measured (using a mass flow meter, for example), and the concentrations of oxygen and/or carbon dioxide are determined by analyzing a sample. The error of energy expenditure measurements made with Douglas bags can be very small (less than 3%), but it can rise significantly under ideal circumstances if the apparatus is not well-maintained, the volume, oxygen, and/or carbon dioxide measurements are not accurate, and/or the operator is inexperienced or unskilled.

3.3.2.2. Open-Circuit Indirect Calorimeter Systems

Depending on the setup chosen and the needs of the experiment, open-circuit systems can be used to record energy consumption over a period of hours or days. The subject inspires air in an open-circuit system, and the expired gases are subsequently examined. Open-circuit systems come in two varieties: expiratory collection systems, in which a subject draws air from the atmosphere and exhales it into a measurement unit through a non-return valve, and ventilated open-circuit systems, in which a subject breathes into a container through which air is drawn.

3.3.2.2.1. Ventilated Open-Circuit Systems

Ventilated open-circuit systems typically consist of parts to mix and gather used air, gauge system flow, analyze gas concentrations, and circulate air. There are wide variations in the techniques used to gather expired air. Collecting expired air with a mouthpiece, mask, transparent hood, or canopy is the simplest method. It is possible to conduct measurements for several hours at a time. The most intricate method involves placing the subject inside a known-volume room or chamber with advanced sensing equipment to measure physical activity. Measurements can be taken for up to several days using a room or chamber.

Ventilated open-circuit indirect calorimeters share similar basic components regardless of how the expired air is collected. A pump is used to extract expended air from the collection device; precise measurement of this flow rate is essential. Following the mixing of the expired air with a fan or mixing chamber, a sample of the expired air is dried and its concentrations of carbon dioxide and/or oxygen are measured. A mass spectrometer can be used to measure gas concentrations instead of paramagnetic or infrared analyzers, which are typically used to analyze carbon dioxide and oxygen. The accuracy of these calorimeters is confirmed by burning known masses of chemical standards, such as ethanol or butane, inside the system and calculating what percentage of the burned mass is detected by the calorimeter. Indirect calorimeters with vented open circuits are precise to within 0.2% of the real thing.

Response times for room or chamber systems can range from 5 to 30 minutes, for ventilated hoods or canopies, 2 minutes, and for masks or mouthpieces, less than 30 seconds, depending on the software, air mixing, and room volume. Systems that use hoods, canopies, and masks are frequently set up as "metabolic carts," allowing the equipment to be easily moved on wheels. Finally, inspired carbon dioxide concentrations should not go above 1%12 since doing so may result in an increase in respiratory effort.

3.3.2.2.2. Expiratory Collection Open-Circuit Systems

Numerous open-circuit expiratory collection systems exist. This method has the advantage of allowing for the portable design of the calorimeter, which makes it possible to measure energy expenditure in free-living individuals. These devices typically consist of a mask or mouthpiece that is attached to a one-way valve that allows expired air to enter the instrument. A tiny amount of the expired air is diverted to a gas storage reservoir, which is examined at the conclusion of each measurement period, based on the flow rate of expired air through the valve, which is measured. These devices allow for sporadic measurements to be made for up to two days. This idea has been modified in several ways, such as by drawing air through the system at a set pace. Modern portable calorimeters are more accurate, durable, and dependable than ever, thanks to technological advancements, and they should continue to provide valuable field data in the future.

3.3.2.2.3. Confinement System (Respiratory Chambers)

The subject is placed inside a gas-tight sealed container of known volume (e.g., 16 m^3), and oxygen consumption and carbon dioxide production are estimated from changes in the concentrations of these gases in chamber air over time. The period of observation may be prolonged by periodically flushing the chamber with fresh air. A number of confinement systems have been constructed with errors of 2% and response times of 50 minutes. Currently, confinement systems are rarely used.

3.3.2.3. Closed-Circuit Systems

A sealed respiratory gas circuit is used in closed-circuit systems to measure gaseous concentrations over time. Expiratory air was extracted from a sealed 5 m^3 chamber in one conformation. Following the absorption of carbon dioxide and water vapor, oxygen was added back into the air stream, allowing it to re-enter the chamber. The amounts of reintroduced oxygen and carbon dioxide absorbed were used to calculate energy expenditure. Spirometer use was one small-scale application of this strategy. An oxygen-containing bell is the source of inspiration for a spirometer; water vapor and carbon dioxide that has expired are then absorbed before the expired air is reintroduced to the bell. The bell is hung over water with its height decreasing in direct proportion to the amount of oxygen consumed. These days, closed-circuit systems are hardly ever used.

3.3.3. Direct Calorimetry

It is outside the purview of this paper to describe every variation of direct calorimeter in detail. The instruments typically cost over $1,000,000 to build and operate, necessitating the employment of a full-time technician. Beyond less expensive and complex indirect calorimeters, they offer little to most investigators and require a great deal of expertise to set up and maintain. Direct calorimetry is used in highly specialized laboratories where measurements of direct heat loss have particular significance. The heat that the body loses is measured by direct calorimeters. About 80% of the total heat loss is accounted for by convective and radiative heat losses, with the remaining 20% coming from evaporative heat loss. In humans, conductive heat loss is minimal. Isothermal, heat sink, and convection systems are the three main categories of direct calorimeters. There have been instances where these strategies have been combined.

3.3.3.1. Isothermal Systems

A layer of insulating material lines the chamber of an isothermal calorimeter. The layer's exterior is in thermal equilibrium with the chamber wall, which is kept at a constant temperature by circulating fluid, and its interior is in thermal equilibrium with the chamber's interior. The non-evaporative heat loss from the subject in the calorimeter is proportional to the temperature gradient across the insulating layer. These instruments have a response time of less than five minutes and a measurement error of 1% when operated by an optimal operator.

3.3.3.2. Heat Sink or Adiabatic Systems

These calorimeters are made up of a chamber where a liquid-cooled heat exchanger extracts the lost heat from the subject. A "zero temperature gradient wall" is created when the rate of heat extraction is controlled to produce an equal temperature difference between the inner and outer chamber walls.

These instruments have a response time of 10–30 minutes and a 1–2% measurement error. A "suit calorimeter" was developed using this idea. The subject could wear the suit for up to 48 hours, and it weighed less than 10 kg. This device reduced evaporative heat loss, but the measurement error was less than 3%.

3.3.3.3. Convection Systems

These calorimeters are made up of an insulated chamber that has a controlled air flow rate. The flow rate, the air's specific heat capacity, and the rise in temperature of the ventilating air leaving the chamber are used to calculate the amount of heat lost by a subject inside the chamber. These instruments have a response time of 10–20 minutes and a 1–2% measurement error.

3.3.4. Non-Calorimetric Methods for Measuring Total Energy Expenditure

Energy expenditure is estimated by non-calorimetric methods through extrapolation from energy expenditure-related variables. These techniques are frequently benchmarked against calorimetric techniques.

3.3.4.1. Isotope Dilution, Doubly Labeled Water

In the doubly labeled water method, stable, non-radioactive isotopes (D_2O^{18}) are used to label or "tag" both the hydrogen and the oxygen in the water. Estimating carbon dioxide production and energy consumption can be done by eliminating administered D_2O^{18}. This basic idea of the technique is as follows. In body water, O_2 of expired CO_2 is in equilibrium with O_2:

$$CO_2 + H_2O \leftrightarrow H_2CO_3$$

As a result, if O_2 in body water is marked with the tracer O^{18}, the label will spread throughout circulating H_2CO_3 and expired CO_2 in addition to body water. The concentration of O_2 label in body water will gradually drop as CO_2 expires and bodily water is lost through respiration, perspiration, and urine. If tracer D_2 is used to tag H_2 in body water, the label will only spread throughout the circulating H_2O and H_2CO_3. As body water is lost over time, the concentration of H_2 label will gradually drop (part of the hydrogen may, however, get portioned into body fat or protein). Therefore, the differences in the elimination rates of the O_2 and H_2 tracers will represent the elimination rate of CO_2 if both O_2 and H_2 in body water are tagged with known amounts of tracers simultaneously.

Orally administered doubly labeled water is typically administered to subjects following the collection of baseline urine, saliva, or blood samples. After giving the body's water space enough time to fully mix the isotopes, samples of blood, saliva, or urine are taken over the course of 7 to 21 days. These samples are utilized in mass spectroscopy measurements of D_2 and O^{18} enrichments. Then, changes in body water's D_2

and O^{18} concentrations over time are computed, along with CO_2 production and energy use. Using this method, energy expenditure can be measured with an error of 6–8% over a period of 7–21 days. If samples are regularly collected throughout the measurement period as opposed to being collected just before and after, this error can be somewhat reduced.

3.3.4.2. Physiological Measurements

3.3.4.2.1. Heart Rate Monitoring

Heart rate and energy expenditure in humans are significantly correlated, at least when no exercise is involved. Heart rate monitors can be used for measurements over a period of several days and are lightweight, non-invasive, and non-restraining. Heart rates of free-living subjects have been recorded using a variety of devices with differing degrees of complexity.

The conceptual drawback of this strategy is that, for a given individual, heart rate and energy expenditure do not correlate linearly because cardiac stroke volume varies with changes in posture and heart rate.

Regarding the slope, intercept, and curve characteristics of the relationships between heart rate and energy expenditure, there is a significant inter-individual variance. Moreover, variations in covariables that influence heart rate—like emotion—also have an effect on the relationship between "heart rate/energy expenditure." As a result, when a unique regression equation is created to link heart rate to energy expenditure for each individual, the accuracy of heart rate prediction of energy expenditure is increased. For every subject, some researchers employ multiple regression equations. Heart rate monitoring can be used to estimate energy expenditure during light activity; at best, the mean (±95% confidence limits) error is 3 ± 20%.

3.3.4.2.2. Integrated Electromyography

Muscular activity is an energy expenditure component that can be measured with integrated electromyography. This measurement records the total electrical muscle activity from multiple muscle fibers over the course of the measurement period. But different muscle groups and fibers have different strength/force relationships, so measuring a variety of muscle groups is necessary to obtain a representative assessment of whole-body activity. These restrictions render this method unworkable.

3.3.4.2.3. Pulmonary Ventilation Volume

Pulmonary ventilation volume measurement, which involves measuring the volume of gas exchanged directly over time, can be used to estimate energy expenditure, but it is not a practical method to use for longer than very brief periods.

3.3.4.2.4. Thermal Imaging

Detecting human heat loss to the environment through thermal imaging was made more difficult in the early studies due to limited precision and accuracy as well as the complexity of data processing. Future research, especially in the field of thermoregulation, appears to be promising given the use of automated, high-resolution, fast-response thermal imaging in more recent studies.

3.4. Basal Metabolism

Everything your body does to create and repair tissues, generate energy, and keep you healthy is referred to as metabolism. The term "basal metabolism" only describes the minimal amount of energy required by your body to function while at rest. It excludes the extra energy needed to sustain even a minimal level of activity while you are awake and moving around. The quantity of calories your body burns for energy even while you are asleep is known as your basal metabolism. The functions necessary for life, such as breathing, blood pumping, and body temperature regulation, are supported by this energy. Additionally, your body requires continuous energy to maintain proper fluid balance and the necessary components for metabolism. For instance, without a certain potassium and sodium concentration, your muscles and nerves cannot function. The Linus Pauling Institute estimates that 20 to 40% of your resting energy is spent monitoring and controlling these two minerals.

3.4.1. Factors Affecting Basal Metabolism

Your basal metabolism is influenced by multiple factors. Some people are genetically predisposed to having a higher metabolic rate. Your metabolic rate is influenced by the ratio of muscle to fat since muscles burn three times as many calories as fat, even when you are sleeping. Age matters because as we age, our bodies lose muscle mass, which slows down our metabolism. Your metabolism can slow down by up to 30% if you don't eat enough calories to meet your minimum energy requirements. For every 0.5°C above normal body temperature, a fever raises the body's metabolic rate by 7%. The metabolic rate can decrease by 30 to 40% if the thyroid gland isn't producing enough hormones.

3.4.2. Basal Metabolic Rate

A formula based on your age, weight, and height can be used to determine your BMR, but this method only yields an estimate. You must take into account all of your unique circumstances, use specialized tools, and take measurements under stringent guidelines, like right after a restful night's sleep or during a fast, in order to determine the exact rate. Of the calories your body uses, the BMR only contributes to about 70%. Your BMR, degree of physical activity, and the calories burned during food digestion and nutrient absorption all contribute to your overall energy expenditure.

3.4.3. Changing Basal Metabolic Rate

A useful tool that comes with knowing about basal metabolism is the demonstration that you can control your metabolic rate by maintaining a healthy weight and building muscle. Your metabolism is slowed down and calories are conserved when you follow a restricted diet. This is why resistance training—which involves using muscles against external resistance through exercises like lifting weights, climbing stairs, sit-ups, push-ups, and leg lifts—is a great way to gain or preserve muscle mass. If you are currently inactive or have any health conditions that restrict activity, speak with your healthcare provider before starting resistance training.

A Closer Look

Energy Drinks and Supplements:

Energy drinks and supplements have gained widespread popularity as quick-fix solutions for enhancing energy levels, focus, and performance. However, taking a closer look reveals both potential benefits and risks associated with their consumption. These products typically contain ingredients such as caffeine, taurine, B-vitamins, amino acids, and herbal extracts, which are purported to increase alertness, combat fatigue, and improve physical and cognitive performance. Caffeine, a central nervous system stimulant found in most energy drinks, enhances alertness and cognitive function, and temporarily boost energy levels. Taurine, an amino acid commonly included in energy drinks, has been suggested to support cardiovascular health and aid in exercise performance. Additionally, B-vitamins play essential roles in energy metabolism, while amino acids like L-carnitine and L-arginine are believed to enhance endurance and muscle recovery. Despite these potential benefits, the excessive consumption of energy drinks and supplements can pose various health risks. High levels of caffeine in these products may lead to adverse effects such as increased heart rate, elevated blood pressure, insomnia, nervousness, and gastrointestinal discomfort. Furthermore, excessive intake of certain vitamins, minerals, or herbal extracts may cause toxicity or interact with medications, leading to adverse health outcomes. Moreover, energy drinks are often high in sugar and calories, which can contribute to weight gain, tooth decay, and metabolic disorders when consumed in excess. Additionally, the marketing of energy drinks and supplements often targets young adults and athletes, promoting unrealistic performance-enhancing claims without sufficient scientific evidence. Consequently, individuals may be misled into believing that these products are safe and effective, leading to overconsumption and potential harm. To mitigate these risks, consumers must essentially approach energy drinks and supplements with caution and moderation. They should read product labels carefully, be aware of their own tolerance to caffeine and other ingredients, and avoid combining these products with alcohol or other stimulants. Moreover, individuals should prioritize obtaining nutrients and energy from whole foods and beverages, rather than relying solely on supplements or highly processed energy drinks. Finally, consulting with a healthcare professional or registered dietitian can help individuals make informed decisions about the appropriate use of energy drinks and supplements based on their unique health needs and goals. In conclusion, while energy drinks and supplements may offer temporary boosts in energy and performance, their consumption should be approached judiciously to minimize potential risks and maximize benefits.

Summary

- "Energy balance" is the relationship between "energy in" (food calories taken into the body through food and drink) and "energy out" (calories being used in the body for our daily energy requirements).
- Body mass index (BMI) is calculated using height and weight measurements and is more predictive of body fatness than weight alone. BMI measurements are used to indicate whether an individual may be underweight (with a BMI less than 18.5), overweight (with a BMI over 25), or obese (with a BMI over 30).
- Total body-fat mass is one predictor of health; another is how the fat is distributed in the body. You may have heard that fat on the hips is better than fat in the belly—this is true. Fat can be found in different areas in the body and it does not all act the same, meaning it differs physiologically based on location.
- The amount of energy you expend every day includes not only the calories you burn during physical activity, but also the calories you burn while at rest (basal metabolism), and the calories you burn when you digest food. The sum of caloric expenditure is referred to as total energy expenditure (TEE).
- Energy expenditure is the amount of energy (or calories) that a person needs to carry out a physical function such as breathing, circulating blood, digesting food, or physical movement. Your total daily energy expenditure (TDEE) is the total number of calories you burn each day. To prevent weight gain, energy intake or calorie intake must be balanced with energy expenditure.

References

1. Bernstein, L. M., Grossman, M. I., Kryzwicki, H., Harding, R., Berger, R. M., McGary, V. E., Francis, E., & Levy, L. M. (1955). Comparison of various methods for determination of metabolizable energy value of a mixed diet in humans. *U.S. Army Med. Nutr. Lab. Rep. No. 168,* Fitzsimons Army Hospital, Denver, 49 pp.
2. Calloway, D. H., & Zanni, E. (1980). Energy requirements and energy expenditure of elderly men. *American Journal of Clinical Nutrition, 33,* 2088–2092.
3. DHHS (U.S. Department of Health and Human Services). (1988). *The Surgeon General's Report on Nutrition and Health.* U.S. Government Printing Office, Washington, D.C., 727 pp.
4. Durnin, J. V. G. A. (1986). Energy requirements of pregnancy: An integration of the longitudinal data from the 5-country study. In *Nestlé Foundation Annual Report,* pp. 147–154. Nestlé Foundation, Lausanne, Switzerland.
5. Durnin, J. V. G. A., & Passmore, R. (1967). *Energy, Work, and Leisure.* Heinemann Educational Books, London, 166 pp.
6. Elmstahl, S. (1987). Energy expenditure, energy intake and body composition in geriatric long-stay patients. *Comprehensive Gerontology A1,* 118–125.
7. Forsum, E., Sadurkis, A., & Wagner, J. (1988). Resting metabolic rate and body composition of healthy Swedish women during pregnancy. *American Journal of Clinical Nutrition, 47,* 942–947.

8. Garrow, J. S. (1978). *Energy Balance and Obesity in Man,* 2nd ed. Elsevier/North-Holland Biomedical Press, New York, 243 pp.

9. Garrow, J. S., & Blaza, S. (1982). Energy requirements in human beings. In A. Neuberger & T. H. Jukes (Eds.), *Human Nutrition,* pp. 1–21. MTP Press, Lancaster, U.K.

10. Gustafson, D., Rothenberg, E., Blennow, K., Steen, B., & Skoog, I. (2003). An 18-year follow-up of overweight and risk of Alzheimer Disease. *Archives of Internal Medicine, 163*(13), 1524–1528.

11. Harris, J. A., & Benedict, F. G. (1919). A biometric study of basal metabolism in man. *Publication No. 279.* Carnegie Institution, Washington, D.C.

12. Hill, J. O., Wyatt, H. R., Reed, G. W., & Peters, J. C. (2003). Obesity and the environment: where do we go from here? *Science, 299,* 853–855.

13. Hytten, R. E., & Leitch, I. (1971). *The Physiology of Human Pregnancy,* 2nd ed. Blackwell Scientific Publications, Oxford, 599 pp.

14. Institute of Medicine. (2011). *Dietary Reference Intakes for Calcium and Vitamin D.* Washington, DC: The National Academies Press.

15. Johnson, R. E. (1963). Caloric requirements under adverse environmental conditions. *Fed. Proc., 22,* 1439–1446.

16. McGandy, R. B., Barrows, C. H. Jr., Spanias, A., Meredith, A., Stone, J. L., & Norris, A. H. (1966). Nutrient intakes and energy expenditure in men of different ages. *J. Gerontol., 21,* 581–587.

17. Merrill, A. L., & Watt, B. K. (1955). *Energy Value of Foods, Basis and Derivation.* Agricultural handbook no. 74. human nutrition research branch, Agricultural research service, U.S. Department of Agriculture. U.S. Government Printing Office, Washington, D.C.

18. NCHS (National Center for Health Statistics). (1979). *Dietary Intake Source Data.* DHEW Publ. No. 79–1221. NCHS, Hyattsville, MD.

19. Newby, P. K., Muller, D., Hallfrisch, J., Qiao, N., Andres, R., & Tucker, K. L. (2003). Dietary patterns and changes in body mass index and waist circumference in adults. *American Journal of Clinical Nutrition, 77*(6), 1417–1425.

20. NRC (National Research Council). (1986). *Nutrient Adequacy: Assessment Using Food Consumption Surveys.* Report of the subcommittee on criteria for dietary evaluation, food and nutrition board, Commission on life sciences. National Academy Press, Washington, D.C., 146 pp.

21. NRC (National Research Council). (1989). *Diet and Health: Implications for Reducing Chronic Disease Risk.* Report of the committee on diet and health, Food and Nutrition Board. National Academy Press, Washington, D.C., 750 pp.

22. Oliveira, G. A., et al. (2003). Students' misconception about energy yielding metabolism: Glucose as the sole metabolic fuel. *Advances in Physiological Education, 27,* 97–101. doi:10.1152/advan.00009.2003.

23. Prentice, A. M., Lucas, A., Vasquez-Velasquez, L., Davies, P. S. W., & Whitehead, R. G. (1988). Are current dietary guidelines for young children a prescription for overfeeding? *The Lancet, 2,* 1066–1069.

24. Roberts, S. B., & Young, V. R. (1988). Energy costs of fat and protein deposition in the human infant. *American Journal of Clinical Nutrition, 48,* 951–955.

25. Sadurkis, A., Kabir, N., Wagner, J., & Forsum, E. (1988). Energy metabolism, body composition, and milk production in healthy swedish women during lactation. *American Journal of Clinical Nutrition, 48,* 44–49.

26. Southgate, D. A. T., & Durnin, J. V. G. A. (1970). Calorie conversion factors: an experimental reassessment of the factors used in calculation of the energy value of human diets. *British Journal of Nutrition, 24,* 517–535.

27. Tanner, J. M. (1984). Physical growth and development. In J. O. Forfar & G. C. Arneil (Eds.), *Textbook of Paediatrics, Vol. 1,* pp. 278–330. Churchill Livingstone, Edinburgh.

28. Thomson, A. M., Hytten, F. E., & Billewicz, W. Z. (1970). The energy cost of human lactation. *British Journal of Nutrition, 24,* 565–572.

29. Todd, K. S., Hudes, M., & Calloway, D. H. (1983). Food intake measurement: problems and approaches. *American Journal of Clinical Nutrition, 37,* 139–146.

30. USDA (U.S. Department of Agriculture). (1984). *Nationwide Food Consumption Survey. Nutrient Intakes: Individuals in 48 States, Year 1977–78.* Report No. I-2. Consumer nutrition division, Human nutrition information service. U.S. Department of Agriculture, Hyattsville, MD, 439 pp.

31. USDA (U.S. Department of Agriculture). (1988). *Nationwide Food Consumption Survey. Continuing Survey of Food Intakes of Individuals. Women 19–50 Years and Their Children 1–5 Years, 4 Days, 1986.* Report no. 86-3. Nutrition monitoring division, human nutrition information service. U.S. Department of Agriculture, Hyattsville, MD, 82 pp.

32. van Raaij, J. M. A., Schonk, C. M., Vermaat-Miedema, S. H., Peck, M. E. M., & Hautvast, J. G. A. J. (1989). Body fat mass and basal metabolic rate in Dutch women before, during, and after pregnancy: a reappraisal of energy cost of pregnancy. *American Journal of Clinical Nutrition, 49,* 765–772.

33. WHO (World Health Organization). (1985). *Energy and Protein Requirements. Report of a Joint FAO/WHO/UNU Expert Consultation.* Technical report series 724. World Health Organization, Geneva, 206 pp.

Chapter

4

MACRONUTRIENTS

Contents

Unit Introduction

Greater amounts of macronutrients (in the gram range) are required. They typically consist of protein, fat, carbohydrates, and water. Energy-providing nutrients are another name for macronutrients, which include water. Calorie-based, energy is necessary for the body to create, maintain, and repair new tissue as well as to conduct nerve signals and control bodily functions.

Macronutrients are the main nutrients that make up the foods we eat. There are three, and you've probably heard of them before (Figure 4.1):

- Carbohydrates;
- Protein; and
- Fat.

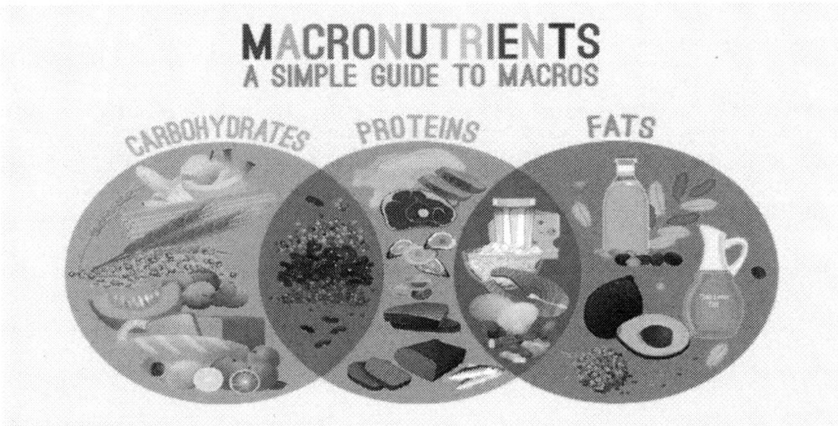

Figure 4.1. *Macronutrients.*

Source: https://avitahealth.org/wp-content/uploads/2022/03/macronutrients.jpg.

Orientation and Directional Terms

Term	Definition	Illustration
Dietary fiber	Dietary fibre is found in wholegrain cereals and fruit and vegetables. Fibre is made up of the indigestible parts or compounds of plants, which pass relatively unchanged through our stomach and intestines. Fibre is mainly a carbohydrate.	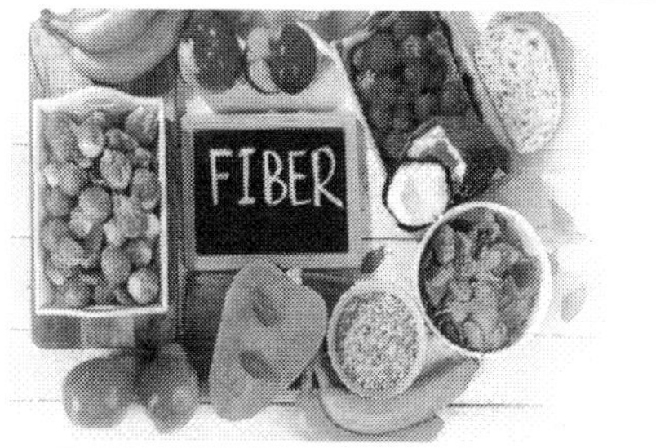
Deoxyribonucleic acid	Deoxyribonucleic acid is a molecule composed of two chains that coil around each other to form a double helix carrying the genetic instructions used in the growth, development, functioning and reproduction of all known living organisms and many viruses.	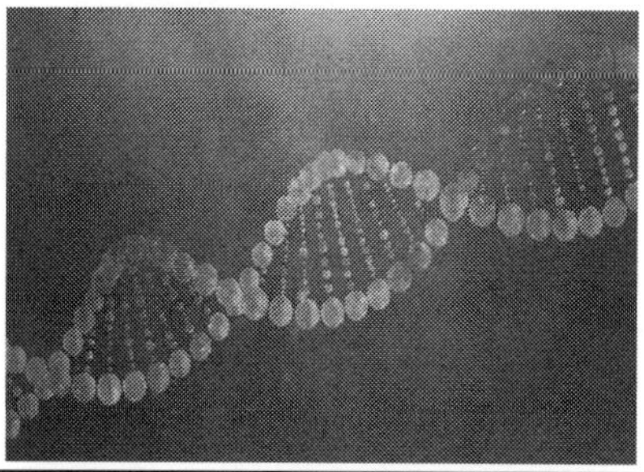
Blood glucose	Blood glucose literally refers to the amount of glucose in your blood. This glucose comes from whatever you eat and drink plus the stores of glucose that sit within your liver and muscles.	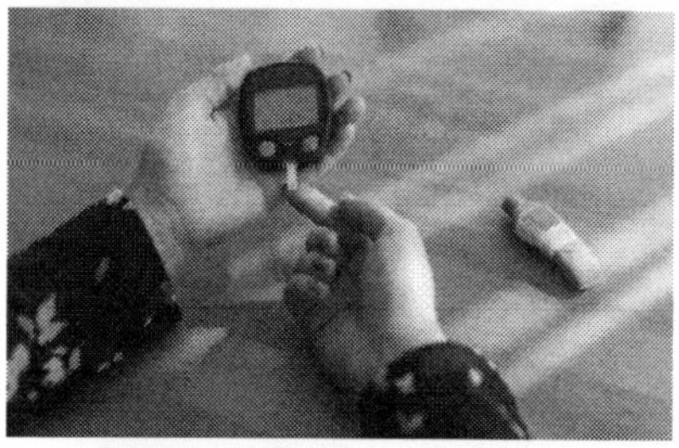
Vegetarianism	Vegetarianism is the practice of abstaining from the consumption of meat (red meat, poultry, seafood, and the flesh of any other animal), and may also include abstention from by-products of animal slaughter.	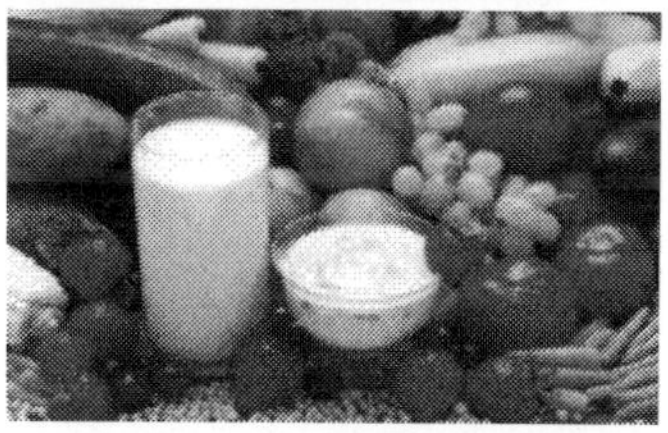
Fatty acid	A fatty acid is a carboxylic acid with a long aliphatic chain, which is either saturated or unsaturated. Most naturally occurring fatty acids have an unbranched chain of an even number of carbon atoms, from 4 to 28.	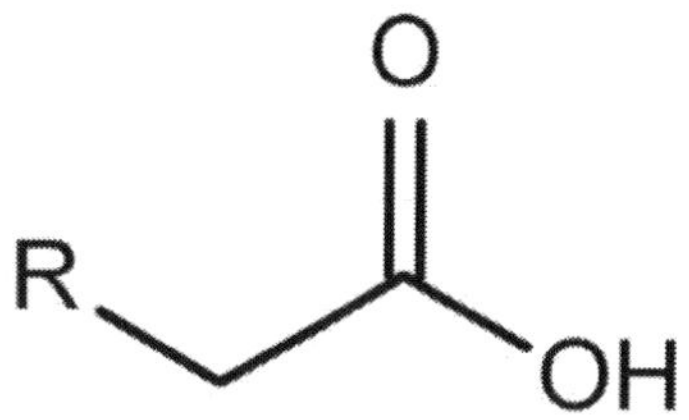

4.1. Carbohydrates

Among the three macronutrients are carbohydrates. As a result, they serve as a vital energy source for the body as a whole and are the energy source of choice for all nerve cells, including brain cells. Literally, the word "carbohydrate" refers to "hydrated carbon." Hydrogen and oxygen combine to form water (H_2O), and an object is said to contain water when it meets certain criteria. As a result, the chemical abbreviation for carbohydrates, CHO, stands for carbon, hydrogen, and oxygen atoms. Carbohydrates are mostly found in plant foods like grains, fruits, and vegetables. Photosynthesis is the process by which plants produce glucose, the most prevalent type of carbohydrate. Chlorophyll, a green pigment found in plants, absorbs sunlight during photosynthesis, providing the energy required to power the production of glucose. Glucose is a carbohydrate that is created when carbon dioxide from the leaves and water that is taken up by the roots of plants combine. Glucose is continuously stored by plants and used to power their own growth. The stored glucose is then metabolized, absorbed, and used by our bodies when we eat plant-based foods.

4.1.1. Functions

Carbohydrates are primarily responsible for supplying energy, with each gram of carbohydrate providing 4 calories. To ensure a constant supply of energy, the body stores about half a day's worth of carbohydrates in the liver and muscles in the form of glycogen. Additionally, carbohydrates play a crucial role in protein-sparing action, as consuming enough carbohydrates (at least 50–100 g/day) allows proteins to focus on their primary function of building and repairing body tissues.

An appropriate intake of carbohydrates is necessary for healthy fat metabolism. An abnormally high amount of fat is metabolized to help meet the energy requirement if enough carbohydrates are not availableavailable. When there is an urgent need for energy, the cells do not fully oxidize fat, which results in the production of substances known as ketones. Acids called ketones build up in the blood and urine, disrupting the body's acid-base equilibrium. We refer to this state as ketoacidosis. It can be brought on by starvation, extremely low-carb diets, or IDDM (insulin-dependent diabetes mellitus), commonly known as type 1 diabetes. It may result in death or a coma. When the body consumes enough carbohydrates, it is shielded from ketones. This is sometimes referred to as carbohydrates' antiketogenic effect. Another crucial role for carbohydrates in the diet is to supply fiber. Vegetables, fruits, and grains all contain dietary fiber. Fiber produces large, soft stools that pass through the large intestine rapidly.

4.1.2. Food Sources

Carbohydrates are mostly found in plant foods, such as fruits, vegetables, cereal grains, and sugars. Milk is the only significant animal source of carbohydrates. Almost everywhere in the world, cereal grains and their derivatives are staple foods. In many parts of the United States, Africa, Asia, and Latin America, rice is the staple grain. The foundation of the diets of Americans and Europeans is wheat and the variety of breads, pastas, and breakfast cereals made from it. In Europe and the US, rye and oats are frequently used in breads and cereals. Cereals also include certain proteins, minerals, and vitamins. A portion of these nutrients are lost during processing. Food manufacturers in the US frequently include the minerals iron and the B vitamins thiamine, riboflavin, and niacin to their finished products in order to make up for this loss. The product is then referred to as enhanced. A grain is said to be fortified when a nutrient is added that it did not previously contain. The fortification of cereal grains with folic acid to prevent neural tube defects is one example of fortification.

Vegetables high in carbohydrates (in the form of starch) include potatoes, beets, peas, lima beans, and corn. Green leafy vegetables provide dietary fiber. They are all also a good source of minerals and vitamins. Fruits supply vitamins, minerals, fiber, and fruit sugar. Table sugar, syrup, honey, and other sugars, as well as foods high in sugar, like candies and desserts, supply carbohydrates in the form of sugar with minimal other nutrients and store fats. Consequently, the foods that contain them in large quantities are referred to as low-nutrient-dense foods.

4.1.3 Difference Between Simple and Complex Carbohydrates

There are two types of carbohydrates: simple and complex. Complex carbohydrates have hundreds or thousands of molecules, while simple carbohydrates only have one or two molecules.

4.1.3.1. Glucose, Fructose, Galactose, and Ribose Are Monosaccharides

In our diet, glucose, fructose, and galactose are the three most prevalent monosaccharides. Six carbon atoms, 12 hydrogen atoms, and six oxygen atoms make up each of these monosaccharides (Figure 4.2).

Significant variations in the degree of sweetness among these three monosaccharides arise from minuscule structural variations. Glucose usually binds to other sugars to form complex carbohydrates and disaccharides instead of occurring in food on its own. Glucose is an essential energy source for all cells in our bodies and the preferred energy source for the brain.

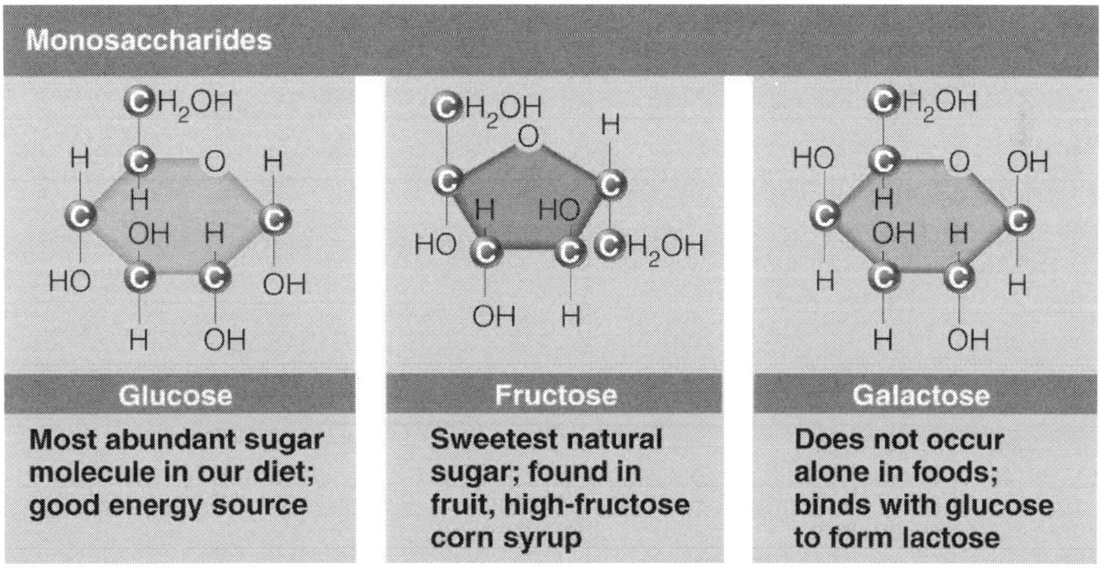

Figure 4.2. *The three most common monosaccharides. Notice that all three monosaccharides contain identical atoms: 6 carbon, 12 hydrogen, and 6 oxygen. It is only the arrangement of these atoms that differs.*

Source: https://www.fdli.org/wp-content/uploads/2019/09/11-12-A-Scientific-Look-at-Impact-of-Sugar.pdf.

Fructose, known as the sweetest natural sugar, is found in fruits and vegetables. It is also referred to as levulose or fruit sugar. High-fructose corn syrup, made from corn, is a common ingredient in processed foods like soft drinks, desserts, candies, and jellies. Galactose is typically found paired with glucose to form lactose, a common disaccharide. Ribose, a five-carbon monosaccharide, is not commonly found in diets but is produced by our bodies from food and is present in DNA and RNA.

4.1.3.2. Lactose, Maltose, and Sucrose Are Disaccharides

Lactose, maltose, and sucrose are the three disaccharides most frequently present in food (Figure 4.3). One glucose molecule and one galactose molecule make up lactose, also known as milk sugar. It is interesting to note that human breast milk tastes sweeter than cow's milk because it contains more lactose. Two glucose molecules make up maltose, also known as malt sugar. It usually occurs in foods in combination with other molecules rather than on its own. A byproduct of our bodies breaking down these bigger molecules is maltose. The left over sugar after fermentation in the making of beer and liquor products is called maltose. The anaerobic process known as fermentation produces adenosine triphosphate (ATP) by breaking down an organic material into simpler forms with the help of an agent, such as yeast. As a result, maltose is created when sugar breaks down anaerobically to produce alcohol. Contrary to popular assumption, after the fermentation process, very little maltose is left in alcoholic beverages; as a result, they are poor sources of carbohydrates.

One glucose molecule and one fructose molecule make up sucrose. Sucrose is sweeter than lactose or maltose because it contains fructose. A large portion of the sweet flavor found in honey, maple syrup, fruits, and vegetables comes from sucrose. The sucrose in sugarcane and sugar beets is refined to create table sugar, brown sugar, powdered sugar, and numerous other products.

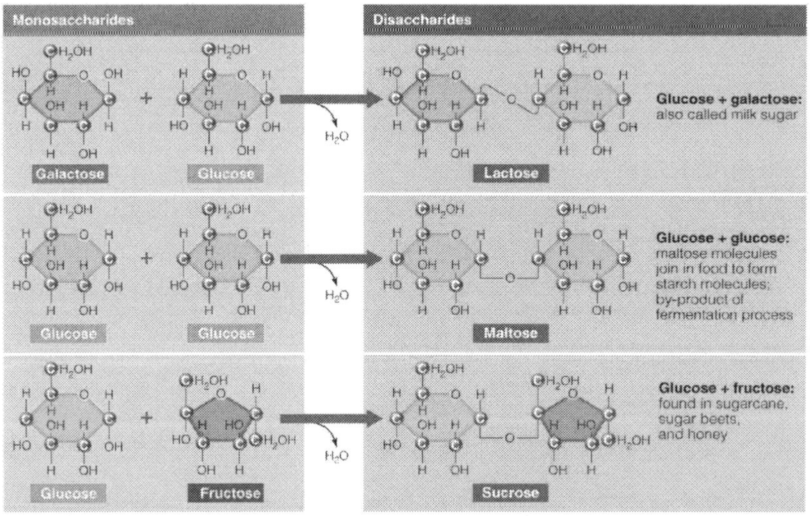

Figure 4.3. Galactose, glucose, and fructose combine in different arrangements to make the disaccharides lactose, maltose, and sucrose.

Source: https://www.fdli.org/wp-content/uploads/2019/09/11-12-A-Scientific-Look-at-Impact-of-Sugar.pdf.

One carbon on each monosaccharide and an oxygen bond holds the two monosaccharides that make up a disaccharide together. In nature, this bond exists in two different forms: alpha and beta. An alpha bond between a glucose and a fructose molecule creates sucrose. An alpha bond also produces the disaccharide maltose. On the other hand, a beta bond between a glucose and a galactose molecule creates lactose. Humans can readily digest alpha bonds while finding it extremely difficult or possibly impossible to digest beta bonds. The disorder known as lactose intolerance is brought on by a lack of the enzyme lactase, which is required to break the beta bond found in lactose. This deficiency affects a large number of people. High-fiber foods also contain beta bonds, which makes the digestion of the majority of fibers difficult.

4.1.3.3. Complex Carbohydrates Include Oligosaccharides and Polysaccharides

The second main type of carbohydrates are the complex carbohydrates, and they are primarily made up of lengthy chains of glucose molecules. In theory, complex carbohydrates are any carbohydrates that contain three or more monosaccharides. Oligosaccharides, derived from the word "few," are carbohydrates containing three to 10 monosaccharides. Raffinose and stachyose are two oligosaccharides that are most frequently present in our diets. Galactose, glucose, and fructose combine to form raffinose. Beans, cabbage, broccoli, brussels sprouts, and whole grains are common foods that contain it. Glucose and fructose are the two galactose molecules that make up stachyose. Numerous beans and legumes contain it.

The raffinose family of oligosaccharides (RFOs) includes the sugars raffinose and stachyose. These RFOs enter the large intestine undigested because humans lack the enzymes necessary to break them down. They are fermented by bacteria in the large intestine, where they release hydrogen, carbon dioxide, and methane as byproducts. Alpha-galactosidase, an enzyme required to degrade RFOs in the digestive system, is present in the product Beano. As a result, this product may assist in lessening the gas produced in the stomach after consuming beans and other vegetables. Hundreds to thousands of glucose molecules make up the majority of polysaccharides (poly, meaning "many"). Most fibers, starch, and glycogen are examples of polysaccharides.

4.1.3.4. Starch Is a Polysaccharide Stored in Plants

Instead of storing glucose as individual molecules, plants store it as starch-forming polysaccharides. There are two types of starch: amylopectin and amylose. Amylopectin is highly branched, while amylose is a straight chain of glucose molecules. Foods containing starch contain both types of starch. Since amylopectin has more open branches than amylose, it has a greater surface area and is, therefore, exposed to more digestive enzymes. This causes it to be digested more quickly than amylose, which in turn causes it to raise blood glucose more quickly.

Legumes (peas, beans, and lentils), tubers (potatoes and yams), and grains (wheat, rice, corn, oats, and barley) are all excellent food sources of starch. The complex starch molecules found in plants are not exactly usable by our cells. Rather, the body needs to convert them into glucose, a monosaccharide, so that we can use it to meet our energy requirements. Most starches that have alpha bonds connecting the many glucose units are readily absorbed by our bodies; starches with beta bonds are essentially indigestible and are referred to as resistant. Resistant starch is technically categorized as a kind of fiber. Our intestinal bacteria produce butyrate, a short-chain fatty acid, when they ferment resistant starch. Resistant starch consumption may be advantageous because some studies have shown that butyrate can lower the risk of cancer. More resistant starch is found in legumes than in grains, fruits, or vegetables. This characteristic, along with their high fiber and protein content, makes legumes a nutritious food.

4.1.3.5. Fiber Is a Polysaccharide That Gives Plants Their Structure

Fiber is made up of lengthy polysaccharide chains, just like starch, but the bonds holding fiber molecules together are difficult for the body to break. This indicates that most fibers do not provide any energy to our diet because they pass through the digestive system undigested and unabsorbed. But fiber also provides a host of other health advantages. Currently, there are several ways to define fiber.

Recently, the Food and Nutrition Board of the Institute of Medicine proposed three distinctions: dietary fiber, functional fiber, and total fiber:

- Dietary fiber is made up of the indigestible plant components that support the stems, leaves, and seeds of plants. You could consider dietary fiber to be the "skeleton" of the plant.
- Non-digestible forms of carbohydrates that are produced in a lab or extracted from plants and have been shown to have health benefits are known as functional fiber. Functional fiber comes in the form of fiber supplements and is added to food. A few sources of functional fiber include cellulose, guar gum, pectin, and psyllium, some of which you may find on nutrition labels.
- Total fiber is the sum of dietary fiber and functional fiber.

4.1.3.6. Soluble Fibers

Water dissolves soluble fibers. They are also fermentable, meaning that the bacteria in the colon can readily break them down and viscous, gelling when moist.

Berries, beans, oat products, and citrus fruits contain soluble fibers. Studies indicate that soluble fiber consumption on a regular basis lowers blood glucose and cholesterol levels, which in turn lowers the risk of type 2 diabetes and cardiovascular disease.

Examples of soluble fibers include the following:

- Galactosaccharide chains and other monosaccharides are found in pectin. Many fruits and berries contain pectin in their intracellular tissues and cell walls. They can be separated and added to foods like yogurt and jams to thicken them.
- Galactose, glucuronic acid, and other monosaccharides are found in gums. Gums are a broad class of viscous polysaccharides. They are thickening, gelling, and stabilizing agents that are usually separated from seeds. Common gums added to food are gum arabic and guar gum.
- Galactose, mannose, and other monosaccharides are found in mucilages, which resemble gums. Psyllium and carrageenan are two examples. Psyllium is the seed husk of psyllium plants, sometimes called flea or plantago seeds. The source of carrageenan is seaweed. Mucilage serves as stabilizers in food.

4.1.3.7. Insoluble Fibers

Fibers classified as insoluble usually do not dissolve in water. Since these fibers are typically non-viscous, colon bacteria cannot ferment them. They are typically present in many vegetables and whole grains like rye, brown rice, and wheat. These fibers are known to encourage regular bowel movements, ease constipation, and lower the risk of diverticulosis, a bowel disorder, but they are not linked to lower cholesterol levels. Examples of insoluble fibers include:

- Lignins are fibers that don't contain carbohydrates. Carrots and the seeds of fruits and berries contain lignins, which are present in the woody portions of plant cell walls. Brans, or the outer husk of whole grains like wheat, oats, and rye, and other whole grains also contain lignins.
- Cellulose serves as the primary structural ingredient in plant cell walls. Comprised of glucose units arranged in a chain, cellulose features beta bonds that distinguish it from amylose and render it indigestible by humans. This substance is abundant in whole grains, fruits, vegetables, and legumes, and can also be derived from wood pulp or cotton. In food production, cellulose is utilized as an agent for anti-caking, thickening, and texturizing.
- Among the monosaccharides found in hemicelluloses are glucose, mannose, and galacturonic acid. The cellulose in plant cell walls is surrounded by hemicelluloses, which can be found in whole grains and vegetables, and they are the main part of cereal fibers. While hemicelluloses are mostly insoluble, some are also categorized as soluble.

4.1.4. How Do Our Bodies Break Down Carbohydrates?

The main objective of carbohydrate digestion is to convert polysaccharides and disaccharides into monosaccharides, which can subsequently be converted to glucose. Glucose is the form of sugar that our bodies use for energy (Figure 4.4).

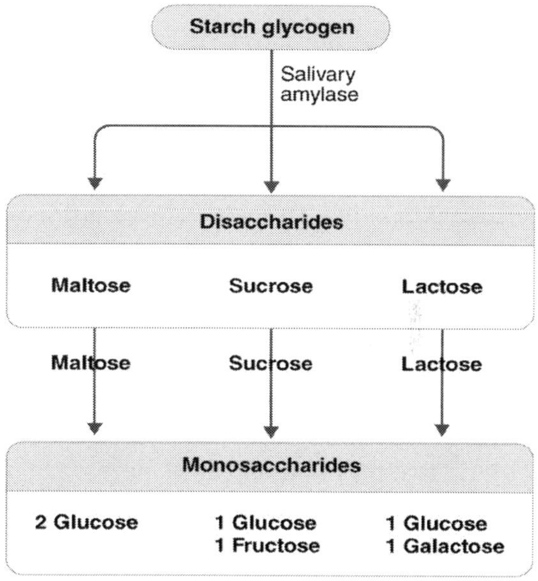

Figure 4.4. *A review of carbohydrate digestion and absorption.*

Source: https://cdn1.byjus.com/wp-content/uploads/2019/09/Digestion-and-Absorption-2.png.

4.1.4.1. Digestion Breaks Down Most Carbohydrates into Monosaccharides

Digestion of carbohydrates starts in the mouth. When you chew, saliva and the starch in the food combine to form a paste. An enzyme called salivary amylase is found in saliva and works to break down starch into smaller pieces, which in turn produces the disaccharide maltose. Notice that the next time you eat bread, it tastes sweeter; this is a sign that the starch is breaking down into maltose. Disaccharides do not undergo oral digestion. Carbohydrate digestion stops as soon as the food bolus exits the mouth and reaches the stomach. This is because salivary amylase is rendered inactive by stomach acid. In the small intestine, most of the digestion of carbohydrates takes place. The pancreas secretes pancreatic amylase, an enzyme that enters the small intestine along with the contents of the stomach. Amylase in the pancreas keeps breaking down any leftover starch into maltose. Disaccharides are converted into monosaccharides by additional enzymes that are present in the microvilli of the mucosal cells lining the digestive tract. The enzyme maltase converts maltose to glucose. The sucrase enzyme breaks down sucrose into glucose and fructose. Lactose is broken down by the enzyme lactase into glucose and galactose. The suffix "ase" is used to identify enzyme names. All monosaccharides are absorbed into the mucosal cells lining the small intestine after the breakdown of carbohydrates has finished, where they pass through and enter the bloodstream. Glucose and galactose are taken up by the enterocytes Through active transport, involving a carrier protein that has been saturated with sodium. The energy needed for this process comes from the ATP breakdown. Since fructose is absorbed through facilitated diffusion, no energy is needed. Fructose absorbs more slowly than either glucose or galactose. Because of its slower rate of absorption, fructose remains in the small intestine for a longer period and osmotically absorbs water. When fructose is consumed, this not only causes a lesser rise in blood glucose but may also cause diarrhea.

4.1.4.2. The Liver Converts Most Non-Glucose Monosaccharides into Glucose

Fructose and galactose are transformed into glucose in the liver after the monosaccharides enter the bloodstream. If glucose is required right away for energy, it is released into the bloodstream and can reach the cells to supply energy. The body stores glucose as glycogen in the muscles and liver if it is not immediately required for energy. Depending on the body's energy requirements, enzymes in the liver and muscles breaks down glucose molecules into glucose (a catabolic, or destructive) process or combines them to form glycogen (an anabolic, or building) process. The muscles can store roughly 120 g (480 kcal) of glycogen, while the liver can hold 70 g (280 kcal). Our bodies use the glycogen stored in the liver to sustain blood glucose levels and meet the needs of all of our cells, including the brain, spinal cord, and red blood cells, in between meals (Figure 4.5).

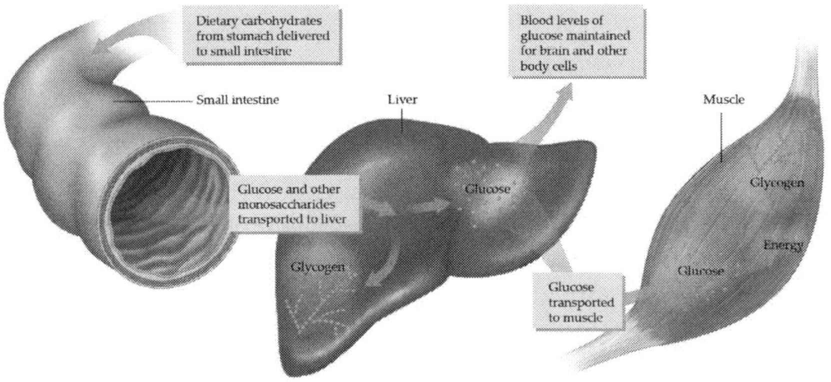

Figure 4.5. *Glucose is stored as glycogen in both liver and muscle. The glycogen stored in the liver maintains blood glucose between meals; muscle glycogen provides immediate energy to the muscle during exercise.*

Source: https://www.amazon.in/Nutree-Pure-Diabe-90-Ayurvedic-Supplements/dp/B079KCSPD1.

Our muscles constantly receive energy from the glycogen stored in them, especially during vigorous exercise. A technique known as glycogen, or carbohydrate, loading allows endurance athletes to store 2- to 4-times as much muscle glycogen as they would normally. Any extra glucose is turned into glycogen in the muscles and liver, where it is stored for times when the body needs energy. Any extra glucose can be stored as fat in adipose tissue after the liver and muscles have used up all their stored carbohydrates.

4.1.4.3. Fiber Is Excreted from the Large Intestine

The small intestine of humans lacks the enzymes necessary to break down fiber. As a result, undigested fiber travels through the small intestine and into the colon, or large intestine. Some previously undigested carbohydrates are fermented by bacteria, producing a few short-chain fatty acids like acetic acid, butyric acid, and propionic acid as well as gases like sulfur, hydrogen, and methane. These short-chain fatty acids provide energy to the cells that make up the large intestine. Fermented fibers are thought to yield between 1 and 2.5 kcal/g. This is less than the 4 kcal/g that come from digested and absorbed carbohydrates in the small intestine; the reason for this difference is that the colon's fermentation of fibers is an anaerobic process, which produces less energy than the aerobic digestion of other carbohydrates. It goes without saying that the fibers that are completely undigested give our bodies no energy.

4.1.4.4. A Variety of Hormones Regulate Blood Glucose Levels

To ensure that the brain and other cells receive enough glucose, our bodies control blood glucose levels within a very specific range. The body needs a variety of hormones to maintain blood glucose levels, including insulin, glucagon, epinephrine, norepinephrine, cortisol, and growth hormone. Our blood glucose level rises after we eat. However, unless glucose can enter the cells of the nerves, muscles, and other tissues, it cannot aid in their normal function in our blood. The size of glucose molecules prevents them from passing through our tissues' cell membranes on their own. The hormone insulin, which is secreted by the pancreatic beta cells, is necessary for glucose to enter. Insulin is carried by the blood to tissues of the body, where it activates unique cell-resident carrier proteins known as glucose transporters. When insulin reaches the cell membrane, it prompts glucose transporters to move to the cell's surface, where they help move glucose through the membrane and into the cell. Therefore, insulin can be compared to a key that unlocks the cell membrane's gates and allows glucose to be transported into the interior of the cell, where it can be used as an energy source. Moreover, insulin encourages the muscles and liver to absorb glucose and store it as glycogen.

Your blood glucose level drops after a period without eating. The pancreatic alpha cells are stimulated to release glucagon, another hormone, in response to the drop in blood glucose. In contrast to insulin, glucagon causes the liver to release glucose into the bloodstream, where it is subsequently absorbed by the cells and used as an energy source. For the liver to promote gluconeogenesis, or "generating new glucose," the synthesis of glucose from amino acids, glucagon also helps the body break down proteins into amino acids.

Other hormones that raise blood sugar levels include growth hormone, cortisol, norepinephrine, and epinephrine. When blood glucose levels are low, the adrenal glands and nerve endings release adrenaline and norepinephrine. They work by enhancing the rate of breakdown of glycogen by the liver, which raises the amount of glucose released into the blood. Moreover, they boost gluconeogenesis.

These two hormones are also in charge of our "fight or flight" response to danger; they are secreted when we require a quick energy boost. The adrenal glands secrete growth hormone and cortisol, which influence fat, muscle, and liver tissue. Cortisol reduces the amount of glucose used by muscles and other body organs and increases gluconeogenesis. Growth hormone increases the amount of fatty acids that are stored in our adipose tissue, increases the liver's production of glucose, and reduces the muscles' absorption of glucose. Normally, these hormones' effects cancel each other out and keep blood sugar levels within normal bounds. A change in this balance may result in diseases like hypoglycemia or diabetes.

4.1.4.5. The Glycemic Index Shows How Foods Affect Our Blood Glucose Levels

The ability of a food to increase blood glucose levels is indicated by its glycemic index. Foods with a high glycemic index cause blood sugar levels to rise quickly. This in turn sets off a significant insulin surge that could result in a sharp decrease in blood sugar levels. Blood sugar swings from foods with a low glycemic index are mild to moderate. Foods are frequently compared to the glycemic effect of pure glucose when determining their glycemic index values.

Predicting the glycemic index of a food is not always simple. Contrary to popular belief, foods high in simple sugars do not always have a higher glycemic index than foods high in starches. Compare the glycemic index of apples and instant potatoes, for example. Despite being starchy, instant potatoes have a glycemic index value of 83, compared to an apple's value of only.

The amount of fat and fiber in the meal, along with the type of carbohydrate and how it is prepared, can all influence how quickly the body absorbs it. Particularly, we consume the majority of our food as part of a meal. The overall meal's glycemic index takes precedence over the order of the individual foods. Some nutrition experts think the glycemic load is a better indicator of a food's impact on glucose response than the glycemic index of a person. The total grams of carbohydrates in a food multiplied by the glycemic index of that specific carbohydrate is its glycemic load. For example, carrots are known to have a comparatively high glycemic index of roughly 68, but they only have a 3 glycemic load. This is because a serving of carrots contains relatively little total carbohydrates. Because of their low glycemic load, eating carrots is not likely to result in a noticeable increase in insulin or glucose levels.

Glycemic load and glycemic index are important concepts to understand because foods and meals with a lower glycemic load are better for people with diabetes because they will not cause sharp swings in blood sugar levels. Because they typically contain more fiber—and since fiber is known to help lower blood fat levels—they may also lower the risk of heart disease and colon cancer. According to recent research, individuals who follow lower-glycemic diets are more likely to have normal blood glucose levels and higher levels of the good blood lipid high-density lipoprotein (HDL), and lower levels of the bad blood lipid low-density lipoprotein(LDL), which is linked to an increased risk of heart disease. Low-glycemic diets, both in terms of index and load, are linked to a lower risk of prostate cancer. Both the glycemic load and the glycemic index are still debatable despite some promising research findings. Many nutritionists believe that there is insufficient data to support their health benefits. Furthermore, a lot of people think that the glycemic index and load concepts are too complicated for people to use in their everyday lives. Some researchers maintain that the prevention and treatment of many chronic diseases depend heavily on assisting people in selecting foods with a lower glycemic index or load. People are advised to eat a variety of fiber-rich, less processed carbohydrates, such as fresh vegetables, whole-wheat bread, and beans and lentils until this controversy is resolved. These types of carbohydrates are known to have a lower glycemic load and to contain a multitude of essential nutrients.

4.1.5. Digestion and Absorption

Monosaccharides are simple sugars that can enter the bloodstream straight from the intestine. These sugars include glucose, fructose, and galactose. Fructose and galactose are converted to glucose in the liver after they are transported there. The cells then receive glucose from the blood. Disaccharides like lactose, maltose, and sucrose need to be broken down further. Prior to being absorbed into the bloodstream, they need to be changed into simple sugar glucose. The digestibility of polysaccharides varies, and they are more complex. Starch is converted to the intermediate product dextrin after the cellulose wall is broken down; maltose is then converted to glucose. When starch is cooked, it becomes dextrin. For instance, toasting bread results in a golden-brown color and a sweeter flavor due to the conversion of starch to dextrin. Starch is first broken down in the mouth by the salivary amylase enzyme, which converts starch to dextrin. The food is combined with gastric juices in the stomach, where the second phase occurs. The final stage takes place in the small intestine, where pancreatic amylase's enzyme action converts the digestible carbohydrates to simple sugars, which are then absorbed into the bloodstream.

4.1.5.1. Metabolism and Elimination

Before cells can begin to undergo metabolism, all carbohydrates are converted to simple sugar glucose. Glucose can be oxidized once the blood has delivered it to the cells. The amount of glucose entering the cells is often greater than what the cells can utilize. In these situations, glucose is transformed into glycogen, which is then stored in the muscles and liver. (After that, only the liver breaks down glycogen, releasing glucose when needed for energy. When the body consumes more glucose than it can use right away or store as glycogen, the excess glucose is turned into fat and stored as adipose (fatty) tissue.

The hormone insulin, which is secreted by the pancreatic islets of Langerhans and keeps blood glucose levels between 70 and 110 mg/dl normal, is primarily responsible for controlling the process of glucose metabolism. In case of insufficient or no insulin secretion, the blood glucose level rises too high. Blood glucose levels above 126 mg/dl are referred to as hyperglycemia, and they are typically a sign of diabetes mellitus. Insulin injections or an oral hypoglycemic tablet must be used to control blood sugar if dietary control is not successful. Hypoglycemia is a condition in which blood glucose levels are abnormally low (less than 70 mg/dl). If a person waits too long between meals or if their pancreas secretes too much insulin, they may experience a mild case of hypoglycemia. Fatigue, trembling, perspiration, and headaches are among the symptoms. Energy is produced when glucose is oxidized. Carbon dioxide and water are the only byproducts of the metabolism of carbohydrates, except for cellulose. It is an incredibly effective nutrient.

4.1.5.2. Dietary Requirements

While there is no set daily requirement for carbohydrates, the Food and Nutrition Board of the National Research Council suggests that half of an individual's energy intake should come from carbohydrates, with a preference for complex carbohydrates. It is recommended that only 10% of energy should come from simple carbohydrates. Fatigue and weight reduction can arise from even a slight carbohydrate deficit. A severely low-carb diet may result in ketoacidosis, a metabolic state in which the liver enters a fasting state after using up all its stored glycogen. At this point, the liver uses the energy from fat that has been mobilized to create glucose. Ketones are byproducts of fat metabolism that accumulate in the blood and are subsequently eliminated by the kidneys. One needs a minimum of 50–100 g of carbohydrates daily to avoid these effects.

In the US, a significant health issue is the prevalence of obesity. Some people think that eating too many carbohydrates is the main factor contributing to obesity. Most of any excess carbs are converted to glycogen and stored as adipose tissue. Furthermore, an overabundance of sugar-derived carbohydrates can suppress appetite for more vital nutrients. An excessive amount of carbohydrates can lead to flatulence, tooth decay, and irritation of the stomach lining.

4.1.5.3. Considerations for the Health Care Professional

Healthcare providers may have a difficult time teaching patients about carbohydrates. Some people need to be educated on the nutritional distinctions between whole wheat toast and Danish pastry, baked potatoes and potato chips, and fresh peaches and fruit cocktails in a can. A lot of people will need to be educated about dietary fiber's definition, sources, and benefits. While sugar can be consumed in moderation by some, it cannot be overindulged by others. All will necessitate the health care provider to be accepting, understanding, and patient.

4.2. Proteins

A macronutrient called protein is necessary for the development of muscle mass. Though it can also be found in other foods like nuts and legumes, it is also found in animal products. Large molecules called proteins are necessary for our cells to operate correctly. Amino acids make up what they are. Our bodies rely on proteins for both structure and function. They are necessary for the regulation of the body's tissues, cells, and organs. The building blocks of every body cell are proteins. Body protein content reaches the adult level of roughly 18% of body weight by the time a child reaches 4 years of age. For healthy growth and development, as well as for the preservation of one's health, one must consume enough proteins each day. The names of proteins make sense. Originating in Greek, the word protein signifies "of primary significance" (Figure 4.6).

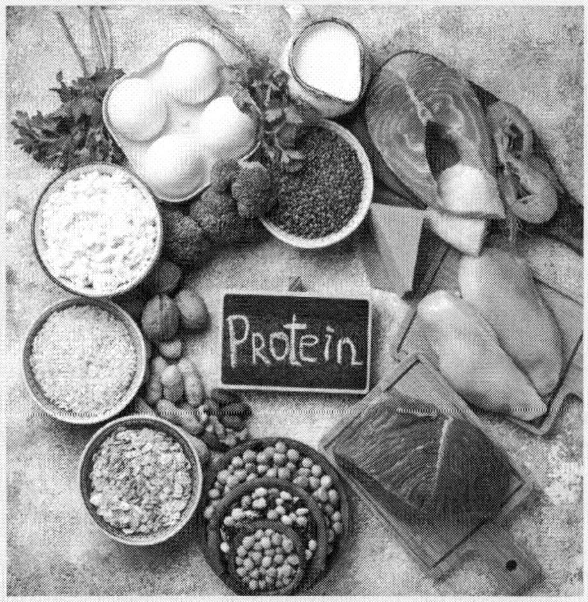

Figure 4.6. *Eating just a little more protein can enhance your health.*

Source: https://scitechdaily.com/images/Foods-Rich-in-Protein-777x777.jpg.

4.2.1. Functions

In addition to building and mending bodily tissue, proteins are essential for controlling a number of bodily processes and supplying energy in the event that the diet is deficient in fat and carbohydrates.

4.2.1.1. Building and Repairing Body Tissue

Building and mending body tissues is the main job of proteins. This is made feasible by the inclusion of the right kind and quantity of amino acids in the diet. Additionally, certain amino acids released into the blood are recycled to create new and repair other tissue during the breakdown of cells during metabolism (catabolism) (anabolism). The recycled amino acids are used by the body just as effectively as those that come from food.

4.2.1.2. Regulating Body Functions

Proteins play a crucial role in the body as they are vital for the production of hormones and enzymes needed to regulate metabolism and aid in digestion. Additionally, proteins help to maintain proper fluid and electrolyte levels, preventing conditions such as edema. They are also important for building antibodies and supporting a healthy immune system.

4.2.1.3. Providing Energy

When there is not enough fat and carbohydrate in the diet, proteins can supply energy. Four calories are contained in one gram of protein. However, this is not a wise way to use proteins. They cost more than carbohydrates overall, and the majority of complete proteins also include cholesterol and saturated fats.

4.2.2. Food Sources

Foods derived from plants and animals both contain proteins (Table 4.1). The best complete protein sources are found in animal food sources. Meats, seafood, poultry, eggs, milk, and cheese are among them. Animal-based foods contain high biologic value proteins, but they also contain cholesterol and saturated fats. Thus, it is important to choose complete proteins wisely from low-fat animal foods like fish, lean meats, and low-fat dairy. In case hyperlipidemia is a concern, consuming more than two or three whole eggs per week is advised.

Table 4.1. *Rich Sources of Proteins*

COMPLETE PROTEINS		INCOMPLETE PROTEINS	
Meats	Eggs	Corn	Grains
Fish	Milk	Peanuts	Nuts
Poultry	Cheese	Peas	Sunflower seeds
		Navy beans	Sesame seeds
		Soybeans	

Source: https://www.brainkart.com/article/Food-Sources-of-Proteins_32704/.

Compared to proteins in animal foods, those in plant foods are incomplete and have a lower biologic quality. Plant-based diets are nonetheless significant providers of protein. Corn, grains, nuts, sesame seeds, sunflower seeds, and legumes like split peas, chickpeas, navy beans, and soybeans are a few examples of plant foods high in protein.

Analogs, such as as textured soy protein, and tofu, can be made from plant proteins. Soy protein and other ingredients are combined to create meat substitutes, or analogs, from soybeans that mimic different types of meat. Alternatives to meat include canned, dried, or frozen foods. An excellent source of protein, iron, and B vitamins is an analog.

Tofu is a versatile dairy-free cheese alternative made from soy milk, known for its ability to take on the flavors of other ingredients when cooked.

It is a source of high-quality proteins and B vitamins, with low sodium content. Textured soy protein and tofu are affordable and nutritious substitutes for meat. Lacto-ovo and lacto-vegetarian diets can easily meet their protein needs through a variety of dairy products, enriched grains, nuts, and legumes. Strict vegetarians who avoid all animal products must include protein-rich options like soybeans, soy milk, and tofu in their diet.

4.2.3. How Are Proteins Made?

The necessary amino acids are chosen by the body from the "pool" of all amino acids that are constantly present in the bloodstream to synthesize proteins.

4.2.3.1. Amino Acids Bond to Form a Variety of Peptides

The amine group of one amino acid binds to the acid group of the other in a special kind of chemical bond known as a peptide bond, as shown in Figure 4.7. As a byproduct of the process, a water molecule is released. A dipeptide is made up of two amino acids, and a tripeptide is made up of three amino acids. A polypeptide is made up of 10 or more amino acids that are linked together, whereas an oligopeptide is a string of four to nine amino acids. A polypeptide chain can fold into any of the many intricate shapes that give proteins their intricate structure as it gets longer.

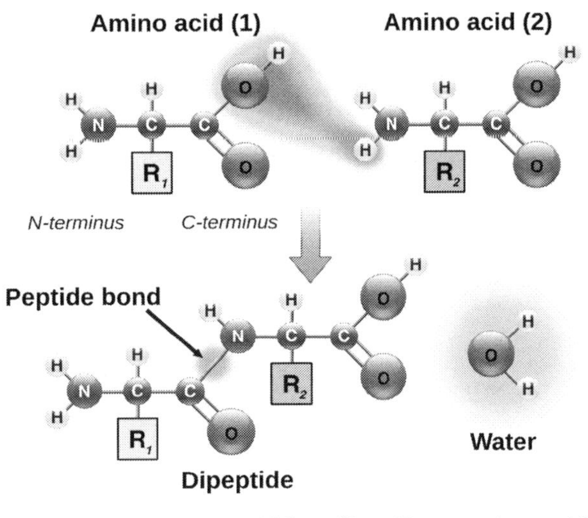

Figure 4.7. *Amino acid bonding. Two amino acids join to form a dipeptide. By combining multiple amino acids, proteins are made.*

Source: https://upload.wikimedia.org/wikipedia/commons/thumb/6/6d/Peptidformationball.svg/400px-Peptidformationball.svg.png.

4.2.3.2. Genes Regulate Amino Acid Binding

We are all unique because each of us received a distinct set of genes from our parents. Every protein molecule in our bodies has a unique amino acid sequence that is encoded by our genes. Subtle variations in the amino acid composition can result in notable variations in the proteins that are synthesized. Each of us has distinct physical and physiological traits that are caused by these variations in proteins. The process by which cells use their genes to make proteins is known as gene expression.

4.2.3.2.1. The Structure of Genes

A gene is a segment of DNA that acts as a template to produce a specific protein during synthesis, also known as expression. Nucleotides are the basic units of DNA. They consist of a pentose sugar called deoxyribose with a phosphate group forming a "backbone," and one of the four nitrogenous bases—adenine (A), guanine (G), cytosine (C), or thymine (T)—attached to it. These nucleotides are found in DNA molecules in two long, parallel chains that are coiled into a double helix. Since nucleotides only differ in their nitrogenous bases, the exact sequencing of nucleotides along these chains accounts for the astonishing variability of DNA.

The hydrogen bonds that bind the nitrogenous bases of nucleotides together keep them together in chains. Only the complementary base of each base can form a bond; for example, A always bonds to T and G always bonds to C. The genetic instructions are transferred from DNA to the resulting protein according to the complementary nature of bases.

4.2.3.2.2. Transcription and Translation

In reality, the ribosome location in the cytoplasm where proteins are synthesized. DNA, however, never exits the nucleus. Therefore, for gene expression to happen, the DNA needs to replicate itself, or create an identical copy that can be transported to the cytoplasm. DNA replication guarantees that the genetic data utilized to construct the protein is the same as the genetic data in the original gene. DNA provides the blueprints for constructing each protein in the body through the process of replication. Information from DNA is copied, or transcribed, by a unique molecule in cells and transported to the ribosomes. Messenger RNA, sometimes known as messenger ribonucleic acid, is this molecule. A, G, C, and U (which stands for uracil, which replaces the thymine found in DNA) are the four nitrogenous bases of RNA, which is a single strand of nucleotides instead of DNA. Additionally, as its name implies, ribose, a pentose sugar, rather than deoxyribose, is present. Transcriptional information from the base sequence of the DNA is copied by mRNA to its own base sequence. After that, the mRNA separates from the DNA and exits the nucleus, delivering its genetic "message" to the cytoplasmic ribosomes.

The language of the mRNA nucleotide sequences is translated into the language of amino acid sequences, or proteins, once the genetic information reaches the ribosomes. When mRNA binds to ribosomal RNA (rRNA) at the ribosomes, its nucleotide sequences are distributed to transfer RNA (tRNA) molecules, resembling assembly line part orders. The tRNA molecules now travel throughout the cytoplasm in search of the precise amino acid that corresponds to their "order." Subsequently, they move their amino acid to the ribosome, where it is assembled into proteins. Following the loading of the amino acids onto the ribosome, tRNA facilitates the movement of each amino acid into its correct location. After the new protein's synthesis is completed, it is freed from the ribosome and has the option of remaining functional or undergoing additional cellular modification. The structure and functionality of a given protein are determined by the correct arrangement of amino acids. Errors in the correct nucleotide sequencing of the DNA or in the translation of this sequencing can result in genetic abnormalities.

While every cell in our body contains the DNA necessary to make every protein, not every gene is expressed, and not every cell produces every kind of protein. For instance, the DNA needed to produce the hormone insulin is present in every cell. However, only pancreatic cells express the insulin gene, which is necessary for the production of insulin. Different nutrients and our physiological needs both affect how genes are expressed. For example, different proteins that clot blood are produced in response to a cut in the skin that causes bleeding. Alternatively, the gene for the protein ferritin, which stores iron, will be expressed if we eat more iron than we require, allowing us to store the extra iron. Our health is significantly influenced by our genetic composition and the way our genes are expressed.

4.2.3.3. Protein Turnover Involves Synthesis and Degradation

To function correctly, our bodies need new proteins all the time. To create the building blocks for new proteins, proteins must be broken down and synthesized. This process is known as protein turnover. The process enables the cells to adapt to the ever-changing requirements of physiological processes. For example, skin cells need to be constantly replaced because they only survive for around 30 days. The body's supply of amino acids, which is drawn from both the amino acids we eat and the ones our bodies release when other cells break down, can provide the building blocks required to create these new skin cells. The body uses its supply of amino acids to make new ones as well as other substances like fat, glucose, and urea.

4.2.3.4. Protein Organization Determines Function

Protein structure have been categorized at four levels. The primary structure of a protein refers to the sequence of amino acids in the protein.

As the polypeptide chain containing different amino acids twists and turns, it forms a spiral shape known as the secondary structure of the protein. Stability in the secondary structure is achieved through hydrogen bonds or disulfide bridges connecting different parts of the protein. This spiral then folds into a unique three-dimensional shape, known as the tertiary structure, which is essential for the protein's function. Additionally, multiple polypeptides can bond together to create a larger protein with a quaternary structure, which can be either globular or fibrous. One cannot overstate how crucial a protein's shape is to its functionality. Muscle fibers, for instance, have protein strands that are substantially longer than they are wide. This structure is crucial for allowing the contraction and relaxation of muscles. On the other hand, red blood cells are made of globular proteins that give rise to the shape of flattened discs with indentations in the middle, resembling tiny doughnuts. Red blood cells can change shape, flow freely through even the smallest capillaries to carry oxygen, and then return to their original shape thanks to their structure and the flexibility of their proteins (Figure 4.8).

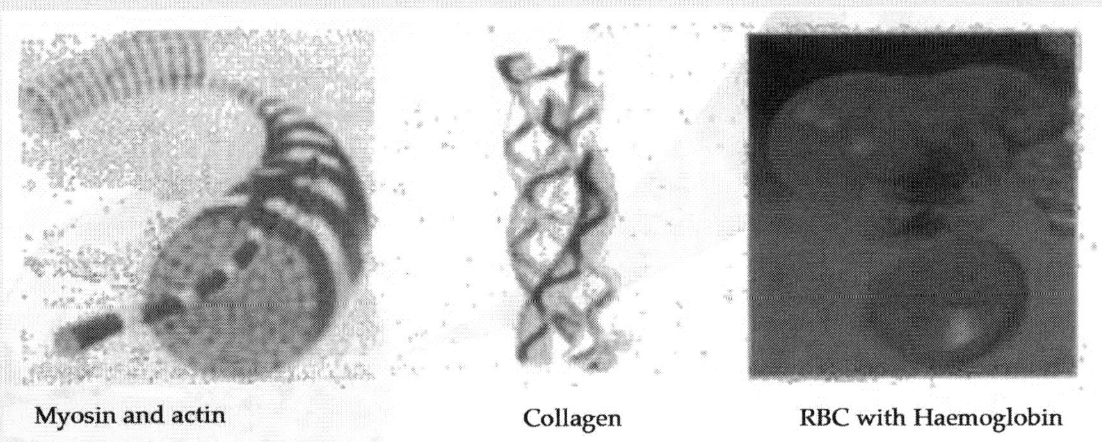

Figure 4.8. *Levels of protein structure.*

Source: https://www.brainkart.com/article/Introduction-to-the-World-of-Proteins_21284/.

4.2.3.5. Protein Denaturation Affects Shape and Function

When proteins come into contact with heat, bases, acids, heavy metals, alcohol, and other harmful substances, they can uncoil and lose their structure, and the process is called denaturation, which characterizes alteration in the structure of proteins. The stiffening of whipped egg whites, the curdling of milk upon the addition of lemon juice or another acid, and the solidification of eggs during cooking are common instances of protein denaturation. Proteins retain their primary structure unaffected by denaturation. But a protein's function is also gone when it is denatured. For example, it is detrimental when a crucial enzyme becomes denaturated as a result of heat or acidity because it can no longer function as intended. When there is a high fever or when the blood pH is not within the normal range, this kind of denaturation can happen.

Denaturation is beneficial in certain situations. For example, during digestion, proteins become denaturated, which facilitates the breakdown of these proteins into amino acids and their absorption into the bloodstream from the digestive tract.

4.2.3.6. Protein Synthesis Can Be Enhanced by Mutual Supplementation

Many people think that in order to get all the proteins we need, we have to eat meat or dairy products. Not at all! Picture a rice and bean meal. Beans have sufficient levels of isoleucine and lysine but low levels of cysteine and methionine. Rice has enough methionine and cysteine but not enough isoleucine or lysine. Rice and beans together provide a complete protein source. When two or more incomplete protein sources are combined to create a complete protein, the process is known as mutual supplementation. The two foods involved are referred to as complementary foods because they each provide complementary proteins that when combined, provide all nine essential amino acids. These foods do not have to be consumed at the same meal. As was already mentioned, food and shed cells provide the body with free amino acids, which are then maintained in the blood. The amino acids in a protein that we eat that may be complementary become part of the amino acid pool. Complete proteins can then be synthesized by combining these free amino acids. However, since partially completed proteins cannot be stored for later use, it is best to eat complementary-protein foods on the same day. For individuals following a vegetarian diet, especially those who do not eat any animal products at all, mutual supplementation is crucial.

4.2.4. Digestion and Absorption

When food is ground into tiny pieces by the teeth in the mouth, the mechanical digestion of protein starts. The stomach is where chemical digestion starts. For the stomach to be ready for the enzyme pepsin to start breaking down proteins into polypeptides, hydrochloric acid is used. Trypsin, chymotrypsin, and carboxypeptidase are the three pancreatic enzymes that carry out the remaining chemical digestion of the polypeptides once they get to the small intestine. Finally, the proteins are broken down into amino acids by intestinal peptidases. Following digestion, the villi in the small intestine absorb the amino acids, which are then transported by the blood to every bodily tissue. They are utilized there to create necessary proteins.

4.2.5. Dietary Requirements

The amount of protein that an individual needs depends on their size, age, sex, and mental and physical health. More body cells need to be maintained in an oversized person than in a small one. For every pound of body weight, a growing child, a pregnant woman, or a nursing mother require more protein than the typical adult. The body absorbs fewer amino acids when digestion is inefficient, which increases the body's need for protein. It is sometimes believed that the elderly are like this. Extra proteins are typically needed to produce antibodies and replace lost tissue following surgery, severe burns, or infections. Furthermore, emotional trauma can increase nitrogen excretion by the body, which increases the need for foods high in protein.

The National Research Council of the National Academy of Sciences considers the average adult's daily requirement to be 0.8 g of protein for each kilogram of body weight. To determine your requirement, do the following:

1. Divide body weight by 2.2 (the number of pounds per kilogram).
2. Multiply the answer obtained in step 1 by 0.8 (gram of protein per kilogram of body weight).

Table 4.2 provides an idea of the amount of protein in an average day's diet.

Table 4.2. *Protein in an Average Diet for 1 Day*

Meal Time	Food Group	Raw	Cooked Recipe	Servings Amounts
Breakfast	Milk	100 ml	Milk or	1/2 Cup
	Sugar	10 g	Tea or	2 Cups
			Coffee	1 Cup
	Cereals	50 g	Breakfast Item	
	Pulses	20 g		
Lunch	Cereals	100 g	Rice	1 Cup
			Pulkas	2 Nos.
	Pulses	20 g	Dhal	1/2 Cup
	Vegetables	100 g	Veg. curry	1/2 Cup
	Vegetables	50 g	Veg. salad	7-8 Slices
	Milk	100 ml	Curd	1/2 Cup
Tea	Cereals	50 g	Snack	
	Milk	50 ml	Tea	1 Cup
	Sugar	10 g		
Dinner	Cereals	100 g	Rice	1 Cup
			Phulkas	2 Nos.
	Pulses	20 g	Dhal	1/2 Cup
	Vegetables	100 g	Veg. curry	1/2 Cup
	Milk (Curd)	50 ml		
	Vegetables	50 g		
	Fruit	100 g	Seasonal	1 Medium

Source: https://www.brainkart.com/article/Dietary-Requirements-of-Proteins_32709/.

4.2.5.1. Protein Excess

People in the developed world have an easy, time-consuming more protein than their bodies need. This ought to be avoided for a variety of reasons. Complete protein meals often contain cholesterol and saturated fats, which can cause heart disease and provide excess calories. Long-term high-protein diets appear to be linked to both colon cancer and high calcium excretion, which causes the bones to lose calcium and may exacerbate osteoporosis, according to some studies. Consuming too much protein can cause people to ignore the equally important fruits and vegetables, and too much protein can overload the kidneys and liver, which convert nitrogen to urea, making it harder for them to eliminate too much urea.

4.2.5.2. Protein and Amino Acid Supplements

Supplements containing protein and amino acids are taken for a variety of purposes, including "bulking up" for athletes, nail growth, and body protein sparing during weight loss. Muscle is built through weightlifting, not by protein bars or supplements. Extra protein has never been known to affect fingernails, and dieters should follow MyPyramid's recommendations for a balanced diet. Meals high in quality protein have a higher bioavailability than pricey supplements. A single amino acid is never found naturally in food and can be toxic to the body. The human body was meant to function on food, not supplements. If a single amino acid is advised, it is imperative to consult a doctor prior to using the amino acid.

4.2.5.3. Nitrogen Balance

The nitrogen balance can be used to discuss protein requirements. This happens when the quantity of nitrogen taken in and expelled is equal. When the intake of nitrogen is greater than the excretion of nitrogen, a positive nitrogen balance occurs. This shows that new tissue is growing, and it happens during pregnancy, in growing children, in athletes developing more muscle, and in the process of rebuilding tissues following physical trauma from illness or injury. A negative nitrogen balance suggests that there is a loss of protein. Fever, wounds, burns, starvation, and immobilization are some of the possible causes.

4.2.5.4. Protein Deficiency

People who go for extended periods without getting enough protein will experience muscle wasting and develop extremely thin arms and legs. A shortage of albumin, a protein found in blood plasma, can also lead to edema, which looks extremely swollen. When enough protein is consumed, the water is expelled. It is possible for people to lose weight, energy, and appetite, and for wounds to heal very slowly. Edematous patients experience depression and lethargy. Children who have been egregiously neglected as well as the elderly, destitute, or disabled exhibit these symptoms. To prevent protein deficiencies, vegetarians and vegans in particular, must carefully consider the kinds and amounts of protein in their diets.

4.2.5.5. Protein Energy Malnutrition (PEM)

Foods high in protein and energy are deficient in those with protein energy malnutrition (PEM). In developing nations where there are persistent shortages of foods high in protein and energy, this kind of condition is not uncommon. Youngsters who do not get enough protein don't reach their full growth potential. Pregnant women who consume inadequate amounts of protein may give birth to children who are mentally permanently handicapped. Two deficiency diseases in children are brought upon by an extremely low intake of either protein, energy, or both. Very young children who do not get enough energy and protein from their diets, along with enough vitamins and minerals, are susceptible to marasmus, a condition caused by severe malnutrition.

The baby with marasmus does not have edema, but it does look malnourished. The skin is thin and wrinkled, and the hair is lifeless and dry. Kwashiorkor is another protein deficiency illness that can afflict both adults and children. When there is an abrupt or recent shortage of food high in protein, like during a famine, kwashiorkor develops.

This illness leads to the accumulation of fat in the liver, and the deficiency of hormones and protein causes edema, painful skin lesions, and alterations in skin and hair pigmentation. The rate of mortality in patients with kwashiorkor is high. Those who recover from these deficiency illnesses may experience irreversible mental retardation. It is true that starving young children has a high ultimate cost. A few indicators to help differentiate marasmus from kwashiorkor are listed in Table 4.3.

Table 4.3. *Differentiating Marasmus and Kwashiorkor*

MARASMUS	KWASHIORKOR
Total surface fat (TSF)* and midarm circumference (MAC) decreased	TSF and MAC within normal limits
Weight decreased	Weight possibly within normal limits
Visceral proteins (albumin) within normal limits or decreased	Visceral proteins decreased
Immune function within normal limits	Immune function decreased
Dull, dry hair	Reddish-color hair
Emaciated, wrinkled appearance	Puffy appearance
Lack of protein and total energy	Edema

Source: https://www.brainkart.com/article/Dietary-Requirements-of-Proteins_32709/.

4.2.6. How Much Protein Should We Eat?

Many people are very concerned about getting enough protein in their diet. Really, among athletes and physically active people, the lack of protein in their diets is one of the most frequent worries. Protein in food is usually not a concern because eating a sufficient and varied diet allows us to readily obtain the necessary amount of protein for our bodies.

4.2.6.1. Nitrogen Balance Is a Method Used to Determine Protein Needs

A highly specialized process called nitrogen balance is used to assess an individual's protein requirements. Since the body excretes nitrogen when recycling or utilizing proteins, one can use the balance to determine whether one's protein intake is sufficient to meet one's needs. The nitrogen-balance technique, usually limited to experimental labs, measures the intake and excretion of nitrogen over a two-week period. The study participant is fed a standardized diet whose nitrogen content has been measured and recorded. The individual must eat every food item offered. Laboratory technicians measure the nitrogen content of the subject's urine and feces directly because most nitrogen is expelled in these bodily fluids. Little amounts of nitrogen are expelled through the skin, hair, and bodily fluids like mucus and semen; however, the measurements are estimated due to the difficulty of obtaining nitrogen expelled through these routes. Technicians then combine the nitrogen measured in the subject's urine and feces with the estimated nitrogen losses. The difference between nitrogen intake and nitrogen excretion is then used to calculate nitrogen balance. Positive nitrogen balance refers to a state in which an individual consumes more nitrogen than they excrete. This state, which happens during times of growth, pregnancy, or recovery from an illness or protein deficiency, shows that the body is either retaining or adding protein. Individuals in negative nitrogen balance excrete more nitrogen than they take in. This shows that the body is losing protein, which happens when a person is starving following an extremely low-energy diet. This is because the body metabolizes body proteins for energy when energy intake is insufficient to meet demands over an extended period. Urine and feces contain the nitrogen that is expelled from these proteins. Negative nitrogen balance can also happen because of severe burns, infections, high fevers, and injuries resulting in substantial blood loss. Individuals in these circumstances need to eat more protein in their diet. When nitrogen intake and nitrogen excretion are equal, a person is said to be in nitrogen balance. This suggests that consumption of protein meets needs for protein. In a state of nitrogen balance are healthy adults who are not pregnant.

4.2.6.2. Recommended Dietary Allowance for Protein

The RDA for protein is 0.8 g/kg of body weight per day. Because more protein is required during periods of growth and development, children, adolescents, and pregnant or lactating women have higher protein needs. Vegetarians and those who lead active lives may also have greater protein requirements.

4.2.6.3. Too Much Dietary Protein Can Be Harmful

A high protein diet may raise your chance of developing health issues. Heart disease, bone loss, and kidney disease are the three medical conditions that have drawn the most attention lately.

4.2.6.3.1. High Protein Intake Is Associated with High Cholesterol

Elevated blood cholesterol levels are linked to high-protein diets primarily comprising animal products. This is most likely because animal products contain saturated fat, which is known to raise blood cholesterol and increase the risk of heart disease. According to one study, eating a diet high in whole grains, fruits, and vegetables and meeting the RDA for protein helped people with heart disease feel better. But when some of the study participants decided to follow a high-protein diet, their risk factors grew worse. Furthermore, studies have demonstrated that vegetarians have a significantly lower risk of heart disease.

4.2.6.3.2. High Protein Intake May Contribute to Bone Loss

Nutritionists have been concerned about high-protein diets because they increase calcium excretion, but how might a high-protein diet cause bone loss? This could be as a result of the higher concentration of sulfur amino acids (methionine and cysteine) in animal products. The blood becomes more acidic because of the metabolism of these amino acids, and the bone loses calcium in an attempt to buffer the acids. It's hotly debated whether eating a lot of protein actually causes bone loss, even though it can increase calcium excretion. A low protein diet leads to bone loss, which raises the risk of osteoporosis and fractures. Increased consumption of soy and animal protein has been demonstrated to protect bone in middle-aged and older women. At this point, it does not seem like there is enough concrete evidence to conclude that eating more protein makes healthy individuals lose bone.

4.2.7. Can a Vegetarian Diet Provide Adequate Protein?

Vegetarian diet comprises only plant-based foods, such as fruits, grains, and nuts, is known as vegetarianism. Approximately 4 million adults in the US are vegans, meaning they do not consume any animal products, including dairy and eggs, out of an estimated 7 million vegetarian adults. A large number of vegetarians attend college; some young adults who choose to adopt a vegetarian lifestyle do so after moving away from home and accepting responsibility for their eating habits.

4.2.7.1. Types of Vegetarian Diets

Vegetarian diets come in almost as many varieties as there are vegetarians. Some self-described vegetarians frequently consume fish and fowl. Others eat a lot of eggs, milk, and cheese but abstain from animal flesh. Others completely shun anything derived from animals, including milk, eggs, and even byproducts like gelatin pudding and candies. The flexitarian diet, which is a kind of "vegetarian" diet that has recently attracted a lot of media attention, is characterized by a person who eats mostly plant-based foods, eggs, and dairy products but occasionally indulges in red meat, poultry, and/or fish.

4.2.7.2. Why Do People Become Vegetarians?

The most common responses are included in subsections.

4.2.7.2.1. Religious, Ethical, and Food-Safety Reasons

Some people decide based on their spiritual or religious beliefs. While some religions forbid or restrict the eating of animal flesh, generalizations should be avoided.

For instance, while some Hindu sects prohibit eating meat, many other Hindus routinely eat small amounts of meat, poultry, and fish, as can be seen by looking at the menu at any Indian restaurant. Vegetarianism is practiced by many Buddhists and some Christians, such as Seventh Day Adventists. A lot of vegetarians base their decision to become vegetarians on their personal philosophy. These individuals believe that the methods used in the contemporary animal industries are cruel, so they believe it is morally and ethically wrong to eat animals or any products derived from them (such as dairy or egg products). While they may eat milk and eggs, they only buy them from family farms where they believe the animals are treated humanely. Concerns regarding meat handling procedures are also very real since tainted meat has occasionally entered our food supply. For instance, tainted meat in hamburgers served at a fast-food restaurant was ultimately linked to a severe outbreak of bloody diarrhea in 1982. The recent mad cow disease outbreak is one beef-related worry that has swept through Europe.

4.2.7.2.2. Ecological Benefits

Numerous individuals opt for vegetarianism due to worries about the impact of meat industries on the worldwide environment. As a result of the substantial demand for meat in advanced nations, meat production has shifted from small-scale family farms to the more expansive system of agribusiness. Critics highlight the environmental consequences of agribusiness, such as extensive water and grain usage to feed animals, methane emissions and other waste produced by animals, and expanded land use to sustain livestock.

4.2.7.2.3. Health Benefits

Some people adhere to vegetarianism due to its numerous health advantages. A varied and balanced vegetarian diet can lower the risk of many chronic diseases, according to research that has been conducted over a number of years.

Health benefits include:

- Reduced intake of fat and total energy reduces the risk for obesity. This may in turn lower a person's risk for type 2 diabetes.
- Lower blood pressure, which may be due to a higher intake of fruits and vegetables. People who eat vegetarian diets tend to be nonsmokers, drink little or no alcohol, and exercise more regularly, which are also factors known to reduce blood pressure and help maintain a healthy body weight.
- Reduced risk of heart disease, which may be due to lower saturated fat intake and a higher consumption of antioxidants that are found in plant-based foods.
- Fewer digestive problems such as constipation and diverticular disease, perhaps due to the higher fiber content of vegetarian diets.
- Reduced risk of some cancers. Research shows that vegetarians may have lower rates of cancer, particularly colon cancer. Many components of a vegetarian diet could contribute to reducing cancer risks, including higher fiber and antioxidant intakes, lower dietary fat intake, lower consumption of carcinogens (cancer-causing agents) that are formed when cooking meat, and higher consumption of soy protein, which may have anticancer properties.
- Reduced risk of kidney disease, kidney stones, and gallstones. The lower protein contents of vegetarian diets, plus the higher intake of legumes and vegetable proteins such as soy, may be protective against these conditions

4.2.7.3. Challenges of a Vegetarian Diet

A vegetarian diet has numerous benefits but also comes with a lot of drawbacks. Restricting the consumption of meat and dairy products increases the risk of consuming insufficient amounts of specific nutrients, particularly for individuals following a vegan, macrobiotic, or fruitarian diet. It is easier for vegetarians to get these nutrients when they eat dairy and/or egg products. Those who struggle with disordered eating may use vegetarianism as a justification to cut out a lot of foods from their diets rather than eating a wide variety of healthful non-animal foods.

4.3. Fat

The body requires fat as a vital nutrient to function. Maintaining optimal health requires consuming the appropriate amount and type of dietary fat, according to experts. On the other hand, eating too little or too much fat can have negative health effects.

4.3.1. Function of Fat

The property that sets lipids apart from other large and diverse groups of substances is their insoluble nature in water. A salad dressing comprises olive oil, a lipid, and vinegar, and primarily water. Shaking the bottle spreads the oil but does not dissolve it, which is why it quickly separates again. All living things, including bacteria, plants, and humans, contain fats. The reason you can't wash your face with water alone is because of their presence in your skin; you need a soap to dissolve the insoluble fats in your skin before you can wash them off. We concentrate on dietary fats as well as some lipids produced by the body.

The body and food contain a wide variety of fats. Within the body, fats are found as steroids in bile salts, sex hormones, and other substances. They are also combined with phosphorus in cell membranes and stored in adipose tissues, which shield and insulate organs. Foods contain both fats and oils as forms of fats. The difference between these two types of oil is that while oils like olive oil are liquid at room temperature, fats like butter and lard are solid. When discussing the lipid content of diets and foods, the term "fats" is used in dietary guidelines, food labels, and other nutrition information meant for the public. Commonly, foods and the body's cells and tissues contain three different types of fats. Triglycerides, phosphor fats, and sterols are these. Let us examine each in turn.

4.3.1.1. Triglycerides Are the Most Common Food-Based Lipid

Triacylglycerols, another name for triglycerides, make up 95% of the fat that we eat and similarly store the majority of our body fat in this form. Three fatty acids are joined to a three-carbon glycerol backbone to form a triglyceride, as indicated by the prefix tri. Extended sequences of carbon atoms connected to hydrogen atoms and one another constitute fatty acids.

They are classified as acids because one end of their chains has an acid group, or carboxyl group. As an alcohol made up of three carbon atoms, glycerol is the backbone of a triglyceride molecule. Triglycerides are formed by one fatty acid attaching to each of these three carbons.

Triglycerides are categorized according to three factors: the number of carbons in each fatty acid, the degree of saturation (the amount of hydrogen bonded to each carbon atom in the fatty acid chain), and their shape, which is sometimes dictated by the way they are processed commercially.

Each of these elements has an impact on how the body uses triglycerides and how they impact our overall health.

4.3.1.2. Triglycerides Vary in Chain Length

The quantity of carbons that each fatty acid has attached to the glycerol backbone varies; this is known as the fatty acid's chain length:

- Short-chain fatty acids are usually fewer than six carbon atoms in length.
- Medium-chain fatty acids are 6 to 12 carbons in length.
- Long-chain fatty acids are 14 or more carbons in length.

A fatty acid's carbons can be counted starting from the carbon of the carboxyl end (COOH), also known as the α-carbon (alpha or first carbon), or from the carbon of the terminal methyl group (CH_3), also known as the ω-carbon (omega or last carbon). Because it influences how fats are metabolized and utilized by the body, fatty acid chain length plays a significant role in lipid digestion and absorption processes. Short- and medium-chain fatty acids, for instance, are metabolized, transported, and broken down more quickly than long-chain fatty acids. Compared to short- or medium-chain fatty acids, long-chain fatty acids are typically more prevalent in nature and, consequently, in our diet. We will go into greater detail on fat digestion and fatty acid absorption soon.

4.3.1.3. Triglycerides Vary in Level of Saturation

The kinds of bonds that make up the fatty acids can also change in triglycerides. A fatty acid is referred to as saturated fatty acid (SFA) if there is not a single double bond forming any part of its length. This is due to the fact that every carbon atom in the chain is hydrogen-saturated, meaning that the maximum amount of hydrogen is bound to each atom. Coconut oil, palm kernel oil, butter, cheese, whole milk, cream, lard, and beef fat are a few foods that are high in saturated fats. If two carbon atoms are joined by a double bond within the chain, hydrogen is excluded by this double bond. Monounsaturated fat is the result of one part of the molecule having less hydrogen than the other. At room temperature, monounsaturated fatty acids (MUFAs) are typically liquid. Cashew nuts, peanut oil, canola oil, and olive oil are foods high in monounsaturated fatty acids. Polyunsaturated fatty acids (PUFAs) are fat molecules with more than one double bond because they have even less hydrogen in them. Polyunsatu-rated fatty acids, which come from canola, corn, safflower, and cottonseed oils, are also liquid at room temperature.

The kinds of fatty acids that are present in food vary. For instance, 80 to 90% of the energy in plant fats comes from monounsaturated and polyunsaturated fats, compared to 40 to 60% in animal fats for the same amount of energy. MUFAs and PUFAs are both abundant in most oils, as you can see. Saturated fats are typically found in smaller amounts in diets heavy in plant foods than in diets high in animal products.

4.3.1.4. Carbon Bonding Affects Shape

Toothpicks come in packs of 200 or more in small boxes, but how many could you fit in the same box if you broke them into V shapes anywhere along their length? Very few, as the bent toothpicks would jumble together and take up much more space. Similar to straight toothpicks, saturated fat molecules always form rigid, straight chains because they lack double carbon bonds. These chains pack tightly because they do not have any kinks in them. Saturated fats are solid at room temperature because of this, including the fat found in meats.

While unsaturated fats have a kink along their length due to each double carbon bond. As a result, they are liquid at room temperature and cannot firmly pack together to form something like a stick of butter. Both polyunsaturated and monounsaturated fatty acids have the fluid and flexible properties that are crucial for fatty acids that are incorporated into cell membranes and those that carry substances through the bloodstream. There are two possible shapes for unsaturated fatty acids: trans and cis. Prefix trans signifies across or opposite, while cis indicates a location on the same side.

In lipid chemistry, these terms describe the positioning of the hydrogen atoms around the double carbon bond, as follows:

- In a cis fatty acid, the two hydrogen atoms of the double bond are on the same side. Because of this arrangement, the double carbon bond on the cis molecule has a noticeable kink. Cis fatty acids are generally found in nature, and thus in foods like olive oil.
- In a trans fatty acid, on the other hand, the hydrogen atoms are joined on the opposite diagonal side of the double carbon bond. Trans fatty acid fats become more rigid and straighter due to this positioning, much like saturated fats. While some trans fatty acids can be found in full-fat cow's milk, most trans fatty acids are made commercially by modifying the fatty acid while food is being processed. Hydrogen is introduced to fatty acids in the process of hydrogenating oils, like safflower or corn oil. The monounsaturated and polyunsaturated fatty acids in the oil undergo this process, which breaks their double bonds and inserts more hydrogen on their diagonally opposite sides. By straightening out the molecules, this process increases the oil's solidity and saturation at room temperature. Corn oil margarine, then, is a fat derived from corn oil that has been partially hydrogenated. Trans fatty acids are present in hydrogenated margarines in higher amounts than in butter. Because the extra hydrogen lowers the tendency of the carbon atoms in the fatty acid chains to undergo oxidation, the hydrogenation of fats helps foods containing these fats, like cakes, cookies, and crackers, to resist rancidity.

4.3.1.5. Some Triglycerides Contain Essential Fatty Acids

The function of a fatty acid in the body is determined by its length (number of carbons) and the location of its double bonds. As previously mentioned, the carbons of a fatty acid can be numbered starting from either the α-carbon of the beginning carboxyl group (α [alpha] is the first letter in the Greek alphabet) or the carbon of the terminal methyl group, known as the ω-carbon (ω [omega] is the last letter in the alphabet). The carbons from the ω-carbon have been numbered using this numbering system. The body is unable to add double bonds before the ninth carbon from the ω-carbon during the synthesis of fatty acids.

EFAs are vital for development and health because they are the building blocks of eicosanoids, which are significant biological molecules. Since eicosanoids are derived from fatty acids with 20 carbon atoms, their name is derived from the Greek word eicosa, which means "twenty." They consist of leukotrienes, thromboxanes, and prostaglandins. Eicosanoids are produced in almost all body cells and are among nature's most powerful regulators of cellular function. They support the regulation of blood coagulation, vasodilatation and constriction, vascular permeability, secretory activity, and motility of the gastrointestinal tract. A balance between the different eicosanoids is necessary to ensure that the right amount of blood clotting or blood vessel dilatation/constriction takes place. The abundance of the EFAs available as precursors and the enzymes within each pathway determine which eicosanoids the body synthesizes. In our diet, linoleic acid and alpha-linolenic acid are the two essential fatty acids.

4.3.1.5.1. Linoleic Acid

Vegetable and nut oils like sunflower, safflower, corn, soy, and peanut oil contain linoleic acid, also referred to as omega-6 fatty acid. You are probably consuming enough of this important fatty acid in your diet if you use vegetable oils or margarines made from vegetable oil. The body converts linoleic acid to arachidonic acid, which is a building block for several eicosanoids.

4.3.1.5.2. Alpha-Linolenic Acid

The importance of alpha-linolenic acid, or omega-3 fatty acid, was not realized until the middle of the 1980s. It is mostly present in canola oil, walnuts and walnut oil, soybeans and soybean oil, dark green, leafy vegetables, and flaxseeds and flaxseed oil. Perhaps you've read news articles about the health advantages of omega-3 fatty acids, which are present in a lot of fish. Fish, shellfish, and fish oils contain two types of omega-3 fatty acids: docosahexaenoic acid (DHA) and eicosapentaenoic acid (EPA). Lean fish like cod or flounder are lower in EPA and DHA than fish that are naturally higher in oil, like salmon and tuna. According to research, diets rich in EPA and DHA promote the body's production of prostaglandins and thromboxanes, which lower blood clotting, plasma triglycerides, and inflammation—all of which lower a person's risk of heart disease.

4.3.1.6. PhosphoFats Combine Fats with Phosphate

Phosphorus fats are present in our diets in addition to the triglycerides we just talked about. For instance, they are widely found in egg yolks, peanuts, and soybeans. They are also found in processed foods that contain emulsifiers, which are additives that keep food blended. The first and second carbons of a glycerol backbone, to which fatty acids are attached, and the third carbon of another compound, which contains phosphate, make up phospho fats. Due to the solubility of phosphates in water, phosphor fats also have this property, which allows them to aid in the bloodstream's fat transportation. The hydrophobic (lipid-avoiding) end of the phosphoFats, or their phosphate "head," and the hydrophilic (water-attracting) end, or their lipid "tail," are what make them special. This characteristic aids in the regulation of material transport into and out of the cell by the cell membrane. Moreover, phosphoFats aid in the digestion of dietary fats. Bile is created in the liver by the combination of phosphor fats called lecithins, bile salts, and electrolytes.

4.3.1.7. Sterols Have a Ring Structure

Sterols are a type of lipid that the body produces and is present in both plant and animal foods. However, they differ greatly from triglycerides or phosphor fats in terms of their multiple rings. Sterols are present in plants, but their absorption is poor. The most prevalent sterol in the diet, dietary cholesterol, appears to be blocked from being absorbed by plant sterols. The main form of cholesterol in food is cholesterol esters, which are cholesterol ring structures with a fatty acid attached. The fatty portion of animal products, including butter, egg yolks, whole milk, meats, and poultry, contains endogenous (dietary) cholesterol. Low- or reduced-fat dairy products, yogurt, and cheeses, as well as lean meats, are low in cholesterol. Since the body constantly produces cholesterol, primarily in the liver, adrenal cortex, reproductive tissues, and intestines, eating it is not necessary. Because cholesterol is a component of every cell membrane and functions in concert with phosphor and fatty acids to preserve membrane integrity and regulate fluidity, its continuous production is essential. The neural cells that comprise the brain, spinal cord, and nerves are especially rich in it. Both endogenous and exogenous cholesterol are used by the body to produce various important sterol compounds, such as vitamin D, adrenal hormones, and sex hormones (estrogen, androgens like testosterone and progesterone), as well as bile salts, which are the main component of bile and aid in the emulsification of fats in the stomach before digestion. Therefore, cholesterol is vital to human health even though it has a bad reputation.

4.3.2. Fats in the Body

Very low-fat diets are out. Why do so many people find them difficult to adhere to, boring, limiting, and tasteless? Furthermore, because fat slows down digestion, a lot of people on low-fat diets struggle with hunger all day long or consume so many low-fat foods that their calorie intake becomes too high to lose weight. Dietary fat functions vital functions in the body. Whether it comes from a stick of butter or a spoonful of peanut butter, every gram of fat has nine kcal. For those unable to consume large amounts of food, this caloric density is crucial and can save lives during times of scarcity. High-fat foods are beneficial for the sick, elderly, and those with extremely low appetites. Little children also require fat to provide enough calories for growth because their small tummies cannot hold large volumes of food.

1. **Fats are an Energy Reserve:** Your body can store an infinite amount of energy as fat tissue, but it can only store a limited amount of glucose as glycogen for energy. This was necessary in the past when food was scarce, but it is a problem in our world of excess calories now. This stored energy is used when you sleep, when you don't eat as much, and when you exercise.
2. **Fats Provide Essential Fatty Acids (EFA):** Chemically speaking, fatty acids vary in the length of their carbon chains, the location of carbon-carbon double bonds, and the degree of saturation (the number of hydrogen atoms bound to carbon). Each fatty acid has a distinct function due to these important distinctions. The majority of the essential fatty acids can be produced by our bodies, which are incredible machines. But it is completely incapable of producing two fatty acids. They are referred to as ALA (alpha linolenic acid) and LA (linoleic acid). This qualifies LA and ALA as "essential," indicating that diet is the only way to obtain them. Fatty acids are essential building blocks of cell membranes in the body and are also transformed into chemical regulators that influence a variety of bodily processes, including blood clotting, blood vessel dilatation, and inflammation. It is uncommon to have clinical deficiencies. People who suffer from severe malabsorption issues are typically found to be lacking in LA. Children that have it experience stunted growth, weakened immune systems, and a scaly, dry rash. The symptoms of ALA deficiency that physicians and researchers are aware of were nerve abnormalities

and vision problems in the few cases.

3. **Fats Carry Fat-Soluble Nutrients:** Fat-soluble nutrients like certain vitamins and phytochemicals that prevent disease, such as lycopene and the carotenoids beta- and alpha-carotene, are dissolved and transported by dietary fats. To give one example, after eating a tossed salad with fat-free salad dressing, participants' blood contained minuscule levels of absorbed carotenoids. The study participants absorbed some carotenoids with reduced-fat dressing, but they absorbed even more with full-fat dressing.
4. **Fats Add to the Texture and Flavor of Foods:** Fat enhances food's flavor, as you already know. Fats dissolve flavorful, erratic compounds, which contributes to this in part. They enhance the mouth feel of food by adding a rich, creamy texture. Think of chocolate without any fat as its texture. Not good, most likely. In conclusion, fats give baked goods a soft, moist texture.

4.3.3. Fats in the Diet

Fatty acid mixtures can be found in fats and oils, together referred to as fats. Olive oil is a type of monounsaturated fat. A lot of people actually do. In actuality, olive oil is a blend of polyunsaturated, saturated, and monounsaturated fatty acids, with a higher concentration of monounsaturated fatty acids. Similarly, lard cannot properly be referred to as a saturated fat. While monounsaturated and polyunsaturated fatty acids are also present, saturated fatty acids make up the majority of its composition.

Except for infants, no population has an adequate intake (AI) or RDA for total fat intake. The AI for infants is 30 or 31 g of fat per day, depending on their age. For men and women 19 years of age and older, the Acceptable Macronutrient Distribution Range (AMDR) is 20–35%. The acceptable daily fat intake for an adult consuming 1600 kcal is therefore between 35 and 62 g. The AMDR for kids is higher and varies according to age; for kids ages 1 to 3, it is 30–40%, and it progressively gets closer to the AMDR for adults. For babies, toddlers, and early children, experts advise against low-fat diets because fat is high in energy and is therefore suitable for their tiny, picky appetites as well as for supporting growth and the developing central nervous system. Adult LA and ALA have AIs ranging from 11–17 g and 1.1 to 1.6 g, respectively.

4.3.4. Saturated Fats

You do not need any saturated fatty acids in your diet because your body can produce all the ones it needs. Increased intakes of the majority of saturated fatty acids are associated with decreased insulin sensitivity and elevated levels of LDL, or bad cholesterol. To lower LDL cholesterol and our risk of heart disease, the Dietary Guidelines for Americans 2010 recommend that we limit our intake of saturated fatty acids to 10% of our total calorie intake (18 g for a person consuming 1600 kcal per day). Only 7% of total calories should be consumed, according to the American Heart Association (12 g for a 1600 kcal diet). But you would quickly discover that you had little to eat if you tried to avoid saturated fatty acids.

After the pan has cooled, what does bacon grease look like? Saturated fat content in bacon can be inferred from its firmness. A large number of saturated fats solidify at room temperature. The tropical oils (coconut, palm, and palm kernel) and dairy fat are also primarily saturated. Pizza, sweets, and full-fat cheese are the main foods in the American diet that are high in saturated fat.

Your experience with cutting back on saturated fats will vary depending on a number of factors, including what you substitute them with. Although it may be tempting to overindulge in fat-free pretzels and gummy candies, diets heavy in highly refined carbohydrates are generally associated with higher triglycerides and lower levels of the good HDL cholesterol, both of which are risk factors for heart disease. A better approach would be to swap out foods high in bad fats with foods high in good fats. Cooking with oils is preferable to cooking with lard or butter. Your heart will benefit from a quick peanut butter sandwich for lunch rather than a slice of pizza. Another wise choice is to replace some of the cheese on your sandwich with a slice or two of avocado. If you consume too many calories, replace whole or 2% reduced-fat milk with 1% low-fat or nonfat milk to reduce your intake of saturated fats and calories.

4.3.5. Trans Fats

Saturated and trans fats are produced when food manufacturers hydrogenate oil to solidify it, a process that extends the shelf life of processed foods like cookies, crackers, and chips. Some unsaturated fatty acids become saturated through partial hydrogenation, but not all of them. Others have their chemical structure altered but still remain unsaturated. These are trans fats that are harmful to health. Like saturated fats, trans fats also raise LDL cholesterol and cause insulin resistance, but there's more bad news, which is why many experts believe trans fats are even worse than saturated fats. They also reduce the good cholesterol, or HDL cholesterol. Less than 1% of total calories, or less than 2 g if we consume 1600 calories a day, is the recommended intake of trans fatty acids by the American Heart Association. Because many foods with labels that claim to have no trans fats actually contain traces of these artery-clogging fats, achieving this may be more difficult than you think. This is so long as a single serving does not contain more than 0 point 49 g of trans fat, which is permitted by law for manufacturers to claim zero trans fats. A few servings of foods like baked goods and margarine crackers, which have trace amounts of trans fat, can easily push you over the advised intake.

Check food labels for traces of trans fats by reading the ingredients lists. An oil that has been partially hydrogenated is transfat. You know that there are at least traces of trans fat present. Trans fats are absent from oil that has been fully hydrogenated (the label will state "fully hydrogenated" or "hydrogenated"). Saturated fatty acids have instead replaced the unsaturated fatty acids.

4.3.6. Unsaturated Fats

When unsaturated fatty acids take the place of saturated and trans fats, blood cholesterol levels and insulin sensitivity improve. Monounsaturated fats and polyunsaturated fats are the two types of unsaturated fatty acids. Sources of monounsaturated fats include olives, almonds, seeds, and avocados. Other sources are canola, olive, and peanut oils.

There are several types of polyunsaturated fats, and they each have different roles in the body:

- Recently, omega-3 fatty acids have gained attention due to their potential to prevent heart disease. Walnuts, ground flaxseed, tofu, soybeans, and common cooking oils like canola, soybean, and walnut oils are good sources of alpha-linoleic acid (ALA), an omega-3 fatty acid. Keep in mind that because your body cannot produce ALA, you must obtain it from your diet. Your body converts ALA into two more vitally important omega-3 fatty acids, EPA and DHA, but the process is quite inefficient. Fish is a better source of EPA and DHA. In addition to their importance for the heart, EPA and DHA also seem to slow down the rate of cognitive decline in the elderly and may lessen the symptoms of arthritis, ulcerative colitis, and other inflammatory diseases. They also support visual acuity and brain development in the fetus, infant, and child. Bluefish, herring, lake trout, mackerel, salmon, sardines, and tuna all contain them.

- Polyunsaturated fats also come in the form of omega-6 fatty acids. LA is an omega-6 fatty acid that can only be obtained by food. Pine nuts, pecans, sunflower seeds, and Brazil nuts are good sources of omega-6 fatty acids. Certain cooking oils, like sesame, corn, sunflower, and safflower oils, are also excellent sources.

Instead of just adding extra calories to your regular diet, make sure to replace solid fats (like butter and bacon grease), whole-milk dairy, and processed foods containing partially hydrogenated oils when you work on cutting them down. If not, you should anticipate slipping into a looser belt as you gain weight.

4.3.7. Digestion and Absorption

Digestion of ingested fats is a complicated process, even though 95% of them are processed. The small intestine is where fats are primarily chemically digested. The mouth does not digest fats. In the stomach, where gastric lipase works on emulsified fats like those in cream and egg yolk, they are only minimally broken down. Before fats reach the small intestine, they must be thoroughly combined with the stomach juices. The fats are emulsified by bile in the small intestine, where they are reduced to fatty acids and glycerol by the enzyme pancreatic lipase. The body then absorbs these substances through villi (Figure 4.9).

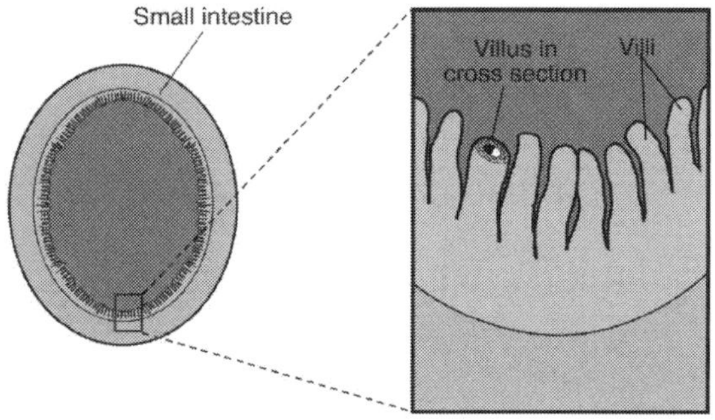

Figure 4.9. *The body absorbs fatty acids and glycerol through the villi of the small intestine.*

Source: https://www.brainkart.com/article/Digestion-and-Absorption-of-Lipids-or-Fats_32698/.

4.3.7.1. Lipoproteins

The primary component of blood is water, which insolublely dissolves fats. For the fats to be absorbed and carried by the blood to the body cells, specific carriers must be made available. Bile combines with the byproducts of fat digestion in the early stages of absorption to transport fat. Later, after fat digestion is complete, protein joins forces with the byproducts to form unique carriers known as lipoproteins. The fats are then transported by the lipoproteins through the blood to the body cells. Based on their density and mobility, lipoproteins are categorized as chylomicrons, LDLs, HDLs, and very-low-density lipoproteins (VLDLs). Following a meal, chylomicrons are the first lipoprotein discovered. They weigh the least and are the biggest lipoproteins. Triglycerides make up between 80 and 90% of their composition. Triglycerides are broken down by lipoprotein lipase into glycerol and free fatty acids. Fat could not enter the cells in the absence of this enzyme. The liver cells are the main source of VLDL, primarily composed of 55–65% triglycerides.

They transport other fats, including triglycerides, to every cell. After the VLDLs lose their triglycerides, they absorb cholesterol from other blood lipoproteins and transform into LDLs. About 45% of LDLs are made up of cholesterol and very little triglycerides. From the liver to the cells, they transport the majority of blood cholesterol. It is believed that elevated blood levels of LDL—more than 130 mg/dl—play a role in atherosclerosis development. Bad cholesterol is another term used to describe LDL.

Lipoproteins with a high-density transport cholesterol from cells to the liver, where it is eventually eliminated. It has been determined that low HDL levels above 40 mg/dl pose a significant risk for heart disease. An HDL level of 60 mg/dl or higher is thought to be protective against heart disease, according to research. One term for HDLs is "good cholesterol." One can raise their HDL by exercising, maintaining a healthy weight, and quitting smoking.

4.3.7.2. Fats and the Consumer

Consumers are still particularly interested in fats. Most people are aware that foods high in fat have high caloric content and are linked to heart disease. However, those outside the medical field might not be aware of the impact fats have on health. As such, they could be readily tricked by deceptive advertisements or salespeople for dietary supplements or novel "health food" items. A health care provider should thoroughly assess any new dietary "supplement" that has a nutrition claim made for it. It is reasonable to presume that medical research has not established the item's necessity if it is not listed in the RDA, DRI, or AI. Ironically, consuming nutritional supplements with questionable benefits might be harmful to one's health.

4.3.7.2.1. Lecithin

A phospholipid is the type of fat that is lecithin. Liver synthesizes this substance, which can be found in both plant and animal foods. Fat is transported through the bloodstream with the aid of this natural emulsifier. Smoothing food products is a commercial use for it. Some salespeople for health food companies have claimed that lecithin supplements can prevent heart disease. This has not been validated by science to date.

4.3.7.2.2. Fat Alternatives

It has taken decades for research on fat substitutes to advance. Fat and carbohydrates are the ingredients of Olestra, the newest product on the market. Only snack foods like tortilla chips, potato chips, and crackers can now use olestra thanks to FDA approval. Olestra "inhibits the absorption of certain vitamins and other nutrients," as required by law to be disclosed on food labels. Foods containing olestra have therefore been supplemented with the fat-soluble vitamins A, D, E, and K. Although Olestra is calorie-free, it can induce diarrhea and cramps. You should use olestra-manufactured products sparingly. One and a third kcal/g of simplesse is derived from either egg white or milk protein. Because it thickens or gels when heated, simple syrup is best used in cold dishes like ice cream. For home use, simplesse is not accessible. A product of oat fiber, oatrim is primarily composed of carbohydrates. Suitable for baking but not frying, oatmeal is heat-stable. For many years, manufacturers have employed thickeners made of carbohydrates. Though far fewer than fat, oatmeal does contain calories.

The possible impacts of these products on human health and nutrition in the long run are uncertain. If consumed in a similar manner to artificial sweeteners by the population in the USA, they may not necessarily lower the overall fat intake in the diet. Instead, they may just become supplements to it. A particular worry among nutrition experts is that these products could be substituted for nutrient-rich foods that offer essential vitamins, minerals, proteins, and carbohydrates in addition to fat.

4.3.7.2.3. Dietary Requirements

The RDA and DRIs do not include a specific dietary requirement for fats; however, failure to meet the daily energy requirement of 10% or more in fats can result in deficiencies. An inflammatory, scaly skin condition known as eczema can arise from a gross deficiency. This has been noted in patients maintained for extended periods on intravenous feedings deficient in linoleic acid as well as in infants fed formulas lacking in this crucial fatty acid. Furthermore, when diets are severely low in fat, weight loss and delayed growth may occur. On the other side, eating a diet high in fat can cause heart disease or obesity. Furthermore, there is evidence linking high-fat diets to cancers of the prostate, uterus, colon, and breast. 30% of total calories should come from fat, according to the Food and Nutrition Board's Committee on Diet and Health's recommendation. Consuming no more than 7% saturated fat, 8% polyunsaturated fat, and 15% monounsaturated fat is the latest advice from the American Heart Association. Right now, 36% of calories in the USA. The foundation of diets is fat.

4.3.7.2.4. Considerations for the Health Care Professional

The medical professional should go over the clients' typical diets with them in order to facilitate dietary change. At that point, changes can be made with the clients' active involvement and presented in a clear, sensitive manner. Clients are unlikely to alter their diets unless they are aware of the need for and desire to make dietary changes.

A Closer Look

Carbs

Carbohydrates provide essential nutrients and are one of the main sources of calories for our bodies. One of the body's primary sources of energy, reveals their multifaceted roles and implications for health. Carbohydrates encompass a broad category of molecules, including sugars, starches, and fibers, found in various foods such as grains, fruits, vegetables, and dairy products. These nutrients serve as the body's main source of glucose, a simple sugar that fuels cellular metabolism and provides energy for physical activity and cognitive function. Carbohydrates are categorized based on their chemical structure into simple carbohydrates (sugars) and complex carbohydrates (starches and fibers). Simple carbohydrates, such as glucose, fructose, and sucrose, are quickly digested and absorbed into the bloodstream, leading to rapid spikes in blood sugar levels. In contrast, complex carbohydrates, found in foods like whole grains, legumes, and vegetables, contain longer chains of sugar molecules that are broken down more slowly, providing a steady release of energy and promoting satiety. Despite their crucial role as a primary energy source, carbohydrates have been the subject of debate and scrutiny in recent years, particularly regarding their impact on health and weight management. Low-carbohydrate diets, such as ketogenic and Atkins diets, advocate for minimizing carbohydrate intake to promote weight loss and improve metabolic health. However, research suggests that the quality and quantity of carbohydrates consumed are more important than simply reducing their intake. Whole food sources of carbohydrates, such as fruits, vegetables, whole grains, and legumes, provide essential nutrients, fiber, and phytochemicals that support overall health and reduce the risk of chronic diseases such as obesity, type 2 diabetes, and cardiovascular disease. Fiber, a type of carbohydrate that cannot be fully digested by the body, plays a crucial role in digestive health, blood sugar regulation, and weight management by promoting satiety, regulating bowel movements, and supporting the growth of beneficial gut bacteria.

Conversely, refined carbohydrates, such as white bread, sugary snacks, and processed foods, are stripped of their fiber and nutrients during processing, leading to rapid spikes in blood sugar levels and contributing to weight gain, insulin resistance, and inflammation when consumed in excess. Added sugars, commonly found in sugary beverages, sweets, and processed foods, provide empty calories and contribute to the development of obesity, metabolic syndrome, and dental caries.

In conclusion, while carbohydrates are a vital source of energy and nutrients, their quality and quantity matter for optimal health. Emphasizing whole, minimally processed carbohydrate sources and incorporating a variety of fruits, vegetables, whole grains, and legumes into the diet can provide essential nutrients, fiber, and health benefits while minimizing the risks associated with excessive consumption of refined carbohydrates and added sugars.

Summary

- Macronutrients (except water) are also called energy-providing nutrients. Energy is measured in calories and is essential for the body to grow, repair and develop new tissues, conduct nerve impulses and regulate life process.
- Carbohydrates are one of the three macronutrients. As such, they are an important energy source for the entire body and are the preferred energy source for nerve cells, including those of the brain.
- Complex carbohydrates, the second major classification of carbohydrate, generally consist of long chains of glucose molecules. Technically, any carbohydrates with three or more monosaccharides are considered complex carbohydrates.
- The glycemic index refers to the potential of foods to raise blood glucose levels. Foods with a high glycemic index cause a sudden surge in blood glucose. This in turn triggers a large increase in insulin, which may be followed by a dramatic drop in blood glucose.
- Monosaccharides—glucose, fructose, and galactose—are simple sugars that may be absorbed from the intestine directly into the bloodstream. They are subsequently carried to the liver, where fructose and galactose are changed to glucose.
- Protein is a macronutrient that is essential to building muscle mass. It is commonly found in animal products, though is also present in other sources, such as nuts and legumes. Proteins are large molecules that our cells need to function properly.
- Proteins are found in both animal and plant foods. The animal food sources provide the highest quality of complete proteins. They include meats, fish, poultry, eggs, milk, and cheese.
- Lipoproteins are classified as chylomicrons, very-low-density lipoproteins (VLDLs), low-density lipoproteins (LDLs), and high-density lipoproteins (HDLs), according to their mobility and density.

References

1. Aranceta, J., & Pérez Rodrigo, C. (2012). Recommended dietary reference intakes, nutritional goals and dietary guidelines for fat and fatty acids: a systematic review. *British Journal of Nutrition, 107*(S2), S8–S22.
2. Brenna, T., Salem, N., Sinclair, A., et al. (2009). ISSFAL official statement number 5 α-linolenic acid supplementation and conversion to n-3 long chain PUFA in humans. *Prostaglandins, Leukotrienes and Essential Fatty Acids, 80*(2/3), 85–91.
3. Djoussé, L., & Gaziano, J. M. (2009). Dietary Cholesterol and Coronary Artery Disease: A Systematic Review. *Current Atherosclerosis Reports, 11*(6), 418–422.
4. Dunford, M. (Ed.). (2006). *Sports Nutrition: A Practice Manual for Professionals*, 4th Edition. American Dietetic Association.
5. EUFIC. (2012). European micronutrient recommendations aligned. EUFIC EU initiatives.
6. European Food Safety Authority (EFSA). (2010). Scientific opinion. *EFSA Journal, 8*(3), 1461.

7. Ferro-Luzi, A., & James, W. P. T. (2001). European diet and public health: The continuing challenge. *Public Health Nutrition, 4*(2a), 275–292.

8. Lecerf, J. M., & De Lorgeril, M. (2011). Dietary cholesterol: from physiology to cardiovascular risk. *British Journal of Nutrition, 106*(1), 6–14.

9. The Fifth Joint Task Force of the European Society of Cardiology and Other Societies on Cardiovascular Disease Prevention in Clinical Practice. (2012). European guidelines on cardiovascular disease (version 2012). *European Heart Journal, 33*, 1635–1701.

10. The Task Force for the management of dyslipidaemias of the European Society of Cardiology (ESC) and the European Atherosclerosis Society (EAS). (2011). ESC/EAS Guidelines for the management of dyslipidaemias. *European Heart Journal, 32*, 1769–1818.

Chapter 5

MICRONUTRIENTS

Contents

Unit Introduction

Micronutrients are present in food sources and help in the synthesis of macronutrients. Even in small doses, they are still vital for overall wellbeing. A micronutrient deficiency can result in major health problems. Micronutrients include both vitamins and minerals. Micronutrients are just as important for healthy nutrition as macronutrients, but in far smaller quantities. Micronutrients only make up 1% to 2% of the dry weight of food, whereas macronutrients make up most of it. Micronutrients can be divided into two groups: inorganic substances called minerals and organic substances called vitamins.

Orientation and Directional Terms

Term	Definition	Illustration
Thiamine	Thiamine is a vitamin, also called vitamin B1. Vitamin B1 is found in many foods including yeast, cereal grains, beans, nuts, and meat. It is often used in combination with other B vitamins, and found in many vitamin B complex products.	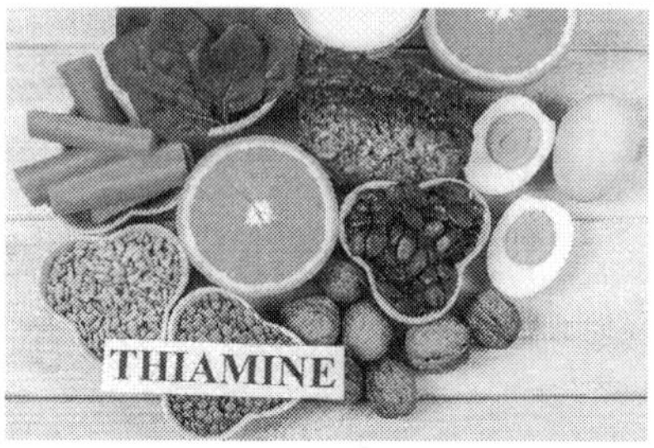
Biotin	Biotin is a water-soluble B-vitamin that helps your body convert food into energy. It is especially important during pregnancy and breastfeeding.	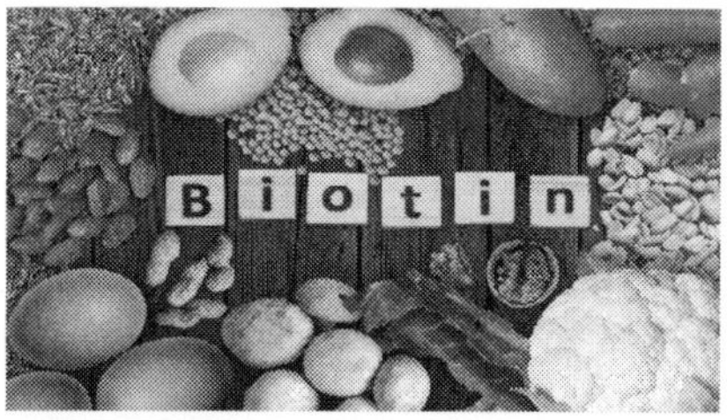
Insulin	Insulin is a peptide hormone produced by beta cells of the pancreatic islets; it is considered to be the main anabolic hormone of the body.	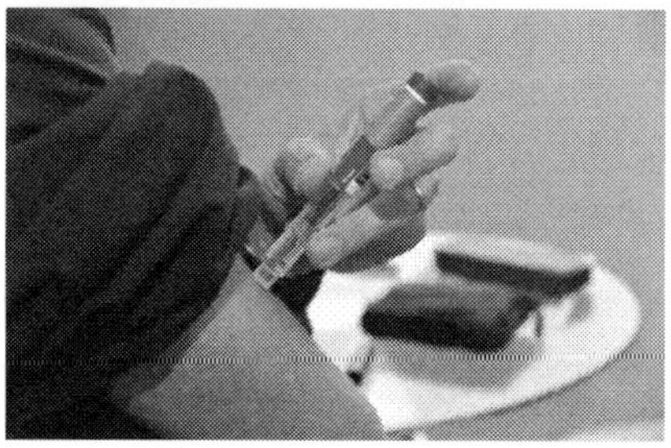
Dietary reference values (DRVs)	Dietary reference values (DRVs) is an umbrella term for a set of nutrient reference values that includes the average requirement (AR), the population reference intake (PRI), the adequate intake (AI) and the reference intake range for macronutrients (RI).	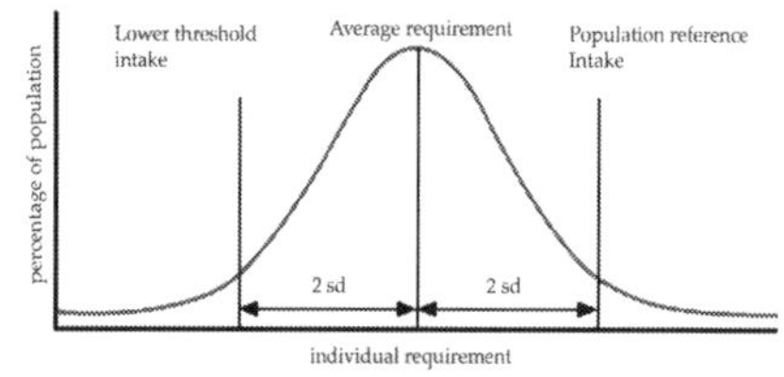
Thyroxine	Thyroxine is a hormone the thyroid gland secretes into the bloodstream. Once in the bloodstream, thyroxine travels to the organs, like the liver and kidneys, where it is converted to its active form of triiodothyronine.	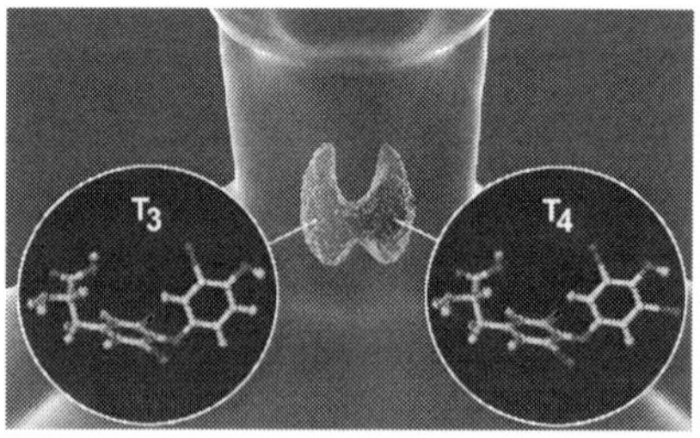

5.1. Vitamins

Vitamins are necessary micronutrients that the body needs in trace amounts to support several critical processes. The two types of vitamins are fat-soluble (A, D, E, and K) and water-soluble (B-complex and C vitamins). Fat-soluble vitamins are stored in the liver and fatty tissues and are removed from the body considerably more slowly than water-soluble vitamins, which the body needs to replace on a regular basis (Figure 5.1).

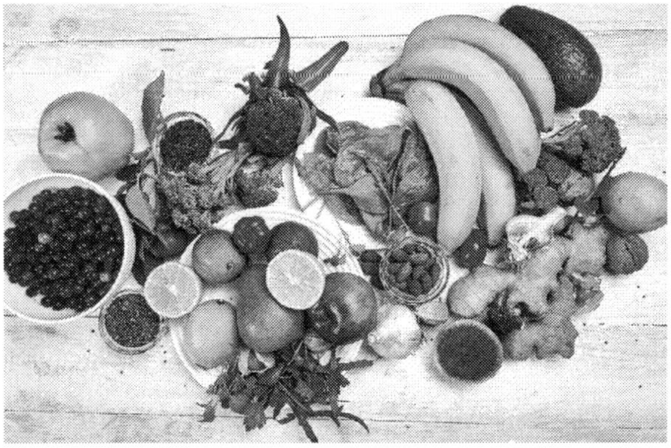

Figure 5.1. *Foods for vitamins and minerals.*

Source: https://content.health.harvard.edu/wp-content/uploads/2021/08/a4591d01-1c90-4211-a11d-ff6815bebac0.jpg.

5.1.1. Water-Soluble Vitamins

Unlike fat-soluble vitamins, which are stored in the body, water-soluble vitamins are absorbed by the body and are typically eliminated through urine. The body requires a constant supply through a consistent daily intake because they cannot be stored. This may come from the meals we consume, the supplements we take, or a mix of the two. Grains, fruits, and vegetables all contain water-soluble vitamins. In contrast to fat-soluble vitamins, they are susceptible to deterioration from heat or air exposure. Additionally, they can be lost in the water used to cook, which implies that when we cook food—especially when it is boiled—we lose a lot of its vitamins. Steaming or grilling food is the best way to retain as much of the water-soluble vitamins as possible.

Nine water-soluble vitamins are found in the human diet:

- Vitamin B1 (thiamine);
- Vitamin B2 (riboflavin);
- Vitamin B3 (niacin);
- Vitamin B5 (pantothenic acid);
- Vitamin B6;
- Vitamin B7 (biotin);
- Vitamin B9;
- Vitamin B12 (cobalamin);
- Vitamin C.

5.1.1.1. Thiamine (Vitamin B1)

The first water-soluble vitamin to be scientifically described was thiamine, sometimes referred to as vitamin B1.

- **Types:** Many forms of thiamine exist, including:
  - **Thiamine Pyrophosphate:** Also known as thiamine diphosphate, thiamine pyrophosphate is the most abundant form of thiamine in your body. It is also the main form found in whole foods.
  - **Thiamine Triphosphate:** This form is found in animal-sourced foods, but is less abundant than thiamine pyrophosphate. It is believed to represent less than 10% of the total thiamine found in animal tissues.
  - **Thiamine Mononitrate:** A synthetic form of thiamine often added to animal feed or processed food.

- **Thiamine Hydrochloride:** The standard, synthetic form of thiamine used in supplements.
- Role and Function:
  - Thiamine functions in the body as a coenzyme, just like the other B vitamins do. This holds true for all of its active forms, the most significant of which is thiamine pyrophosphate.
  - Coenzymes are tiny substances that assist enzymes in starting chemical reactions that they can not initiate on their own.
  - Thiamine participates in a wide range of vital chemical processes. For example, it promotes the formation of sugar and aids in the conversion of nutrients into energy.
- **Dietary Sources:** The highest dietary concentrations of thiamine can be found in whole grains, liver, pig, nuts, and seeds.

The chart in Figure 5.2 shows the thiamine content of some of the best sources.

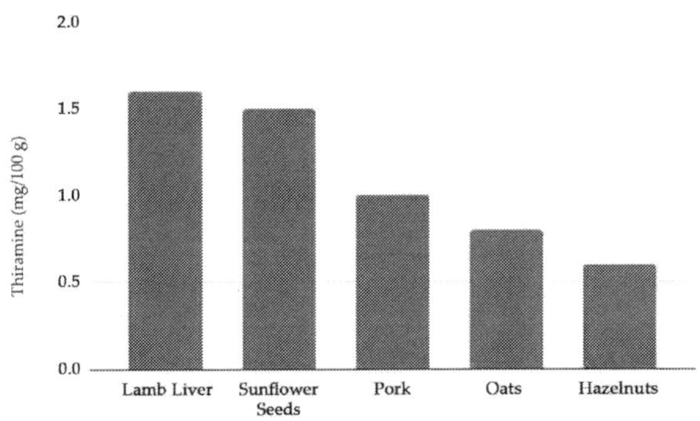

Figure 5.2. *Dietary sources of thiamine.*

Source: https://www.healthline.com/nutrition/water-soluble-vitamins#b1.

- **Recommended Intake:** Table 5.1 shows the recommended dietary allowance (RDA) for thiamine.

  There is no established RDA for infants. Rather, the table displays the appropriate intake, indicated by an asterisk. Like the RDA, the adequate intake (AI) is predicated on less convincing data.

Table 5.1. *The Recommended Dietary Allowance (RDA) for Thiamine*

		RDA (mg/day)
Infants	0–6 months	0.2*
	7–12 months	0.3*
Children	1–3 years	0.5
	4–8 years	0.6
	9–13 years	0.9
Women	14–18 years	1.0
	19+ years	1.1
Men	14+ years	1.2
Pregnancy	–	1.4
Lactation	–	1.4

Source: https://www.healthline.com/nutrition/water-soluble-vitamins#b1.

- **Deficiency:** Although thiamine deficiency is rare, elevated blood sugar levels can enhance the thiamine's excretion through urine, increasing the thiamine's needs and risk. In fact, individuals with type

1 and type 2 diabetes may have 75–76% lower thiamine levels.

Because of their poor diets and impaired absorption of thiamine, people who abuse alcohol also have a higher chance of developing deficiencies.

Conditions like Wernicke-Korsakoff syndrome and beriberi can result from severe deficiencies. Numerous symptoms, such as anorexia, weight loss, impaired neural function, mental health issues, muscle weakness, and heart enlargement, are linked to these disorders.

- **Side Effects and Toxicity:** Thiamine is regarded as secure. When large amounts of thiamine are consumed through food or supplements, no negative effects have been documented. This is partially due to the body's rapid excretion of excess thiamine in urine. Because of this, the upper limit of acceptable thiamine intake has not been determined. This does not, however, rule out the possibility of toxic symptoms at extremely high intakes.
- **Benefits of Supplements:** There is no solid proof that healthy individuals who consume enough thiamine from their diets benefit from taking supplements. However, high-dose supplements may lower blood pressure and blood sugar in people with high blood sugar or low thiamine levels. Low thiamine intake has also been linked to a number of other conditions, including fibromyalgia, depression, and glaucoma. Nevertheless, more investigation is required before firm conclusions can be drawn.

5.1.1.2. Riboflavin (Vitamin B2)

As far as food coloring goes, riboflavin is the only water-soluble vitamin. As the Latin word flavus means "yellow," it is actually named after the color of flesh" (Figure 5.3).

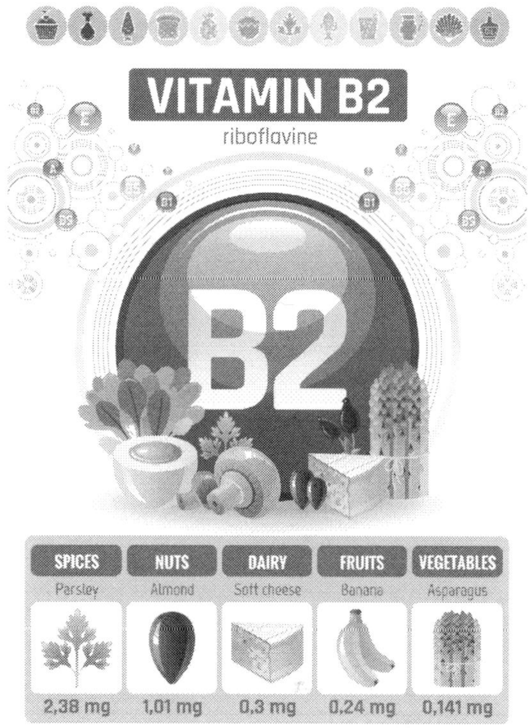

Figure 5.3. *Riboflavin (Vitamin B2).*

Source: https://www.istockphoto.com/vector/riboflavin-vitamin-b2-rich-food-icons-healthy-eating-flat-icon-set-text-icon-gm952360768-259991962.

- Types:
  - In addition to riboflavin, dietary substances known as flavoproteins release riboflavin during digestion.
  - Two of the most common flavoproteins are flavin adenine dinucleotide and flavin mononucleotide. They are found in a wide range of foods.

- **Role and Function:**
  - Riboflavin participates in several chemical reactions as a coenzyme.
  - It participates in the transformation of nutrients into energy, just like thiamine. Additionally, it is necessary for the conversion of tryptophan to niacin (vitamin B3) and for the conversion of vitamin B6 to its active form.
- **Dietary Sources:** The chart in Figure 5.4 shows the riboflavin content of some of its richest dietary sources.

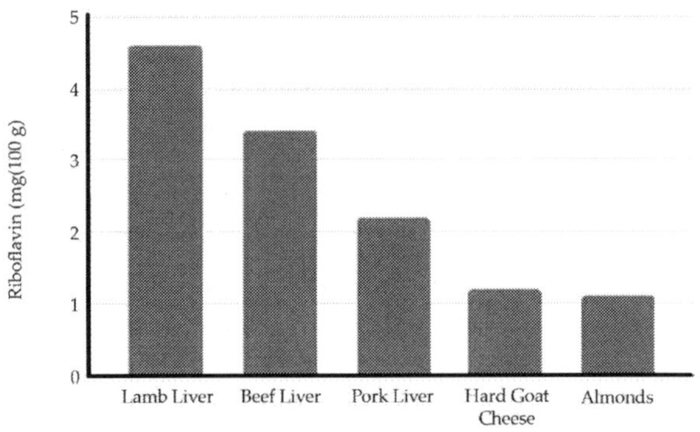

Figure 5.4. *Dietary sources of riboflavin.*

Source: https://www.healthline.com/nutrition/water-soluble-vitamins#b1.

  Spread made from yeast extract is also a particularly high source of riboflavin, with about 18 mg per 100 g. In addition, eggs, broccoli, leafy vegetables, milk, legumes, mushrooms, and meat are excellent providers of riboflavin.

  Furthermore, riboflavin is a yellow-orange food coloring that is frequently added to processed breakfast cereals.

- **Recommended Intake:** Table 5.2 shows the RDA or AI for riboflavin. These values represent the daily intake sufficient to meet the requirements of most people.

Table 5.2. *The Recommended Dietary Allowance (RDA) or Adequate Intake for Riboflavin*

		RDA (mg/day)
Infants	0–6 months	0.3*
	7–12 months	0.4*
Children	1–3 years	0.5
	4–8 years	0.6
	9–13 years	0.9
Women	14–18 years	1.0
	19+ years	1.1
Men	14+ years	1.3
Pregnancy	–	1.4
Lactation	–	1.6

Source: https://www.healthline.com/nutrition/water-soluble-vitamins#b1.

- **Deficiency:** In developed nations, riboflavin deficiency is extremely uncommon. But unhealthy eating habits, advanced age, lung conditions, and alcoholism can raise the risk.

  A condition called ariboflavinosis, which is characterized by anemia, inflammatory tongue, sore throat, and skin and eye issues, is brought on by severe deficiency.

  Additionally, it hinders tryptophan's conversion to niacin and the metabolism of vitamin B6.
- **Side Effects and Toxicity:** There are no known toxic effects from high dietary or supplemental riboflavin intakes.

At higher doses, absorption loses some of its effectiveness. Additionally, the body stores very small amounts in its tissues, and extra riboflavin is eliminated through urine.

As a result, the safe upper intake level of riboflavin has not been established.

- **Benefits of Supplements:** Supplementing with riboflavin is usually not beneficial for individuals who obtain adequate amounts from diet.

Nonetheless, in individuals who are genetically predisposed to heart disease, low-dose riboflavin supplements may potentially lower blood pressure and reduce the risk of heart disease.

It is believed to accomplish this by lowering elevated homocysteine levels in people who carry two copies of the MTHFR 677TT gene.

Higher riboflavin dosages, like 200 mg twice a day, may also lessen migraine symptoms.

5.1.1.3. Niacin (Vitamin B3)

The only other B vitamin your body can make from another nutrient is the amino acid tryptophan, which is referred to as niacin or vitamin B3.

- **Types:** Niacin is a group of related nutrients. The most common forms are:
    - **Nicotinic Acid:** The most common form in supplements. Also found in both plant- and animal-sourced foods. High-dose nicotinic acid supplements may cause a condition called niacin flush.
    - **Nicotinamide (Niacinamide):** Found in supplements and foods.

he compound nicotinamide riboside also has vitamin B3 activity. It is found in trace amounts in whey protein and baker's yeast.

- **Role and Function:** Nicotinamide adenine dinucleotide (NAD+) or nicotinamide adenine dinucleotide phosphate (NADP+), which function as coenzymes, are eventually produced from all dietary forms of niacin.

  It performs the same coenzyme functions as the other B vitamins, supporting vital cellular processes and serving as an antioxidant in the body.

  Driving the metabolic process known as glycolysis, which extracts energy from glucose (sugar), is one of its most significant functions.
- **Dietary Sources:** Animals and plants both contain niacin. The niacin content of some of its best sources is displayed in the chart in Figure 5.5.

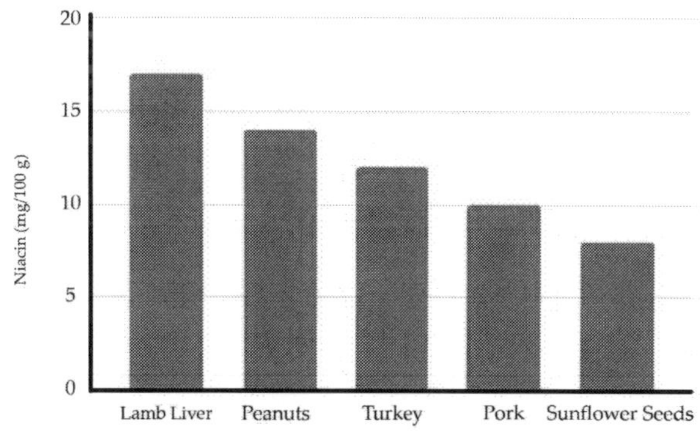

Figure 5.5. *Dietary sources of niacin deficiency.*

Source: https://www.healthline.com/nutrition/water-soluble-vitamins#b1.

Niacin content of yeast extract spread is remarkably high, with approximately 128 mg per 100 g. Additional excellent sources of niacin are fish, chicken, eggs, dairy products, and mushrooms. Niacin is also fortified in breakfast cereals and flour.

Niacin can also be produced by your body from the amino acid tryptophan. According to scientific estimates, 1 mg of niacin can be produced from 60 mg of tryptophan.

- **Recommended Intake:**
  - The RDA, or AI, for niacin is mentioned in Table 5.3. These Figures represent the estimated daily intake of niacin that the majority of people (97.5%) should get from their diets.
  - The tolerable upper intake limit (UL), the maximum daily intake deemed safe for the majority of people, is also displayed.

Table 5.3. *The Recommended Dietary Allowance (RDA) or Upper Intake Limit (UL) for Niacin*

		RDA (mg/day)	UL (mg/day)
Infants	0–6 months	2*	–
	7–12 months	4*	–
Children	1–3 years	6	10
	4–8 years	8	15
	9–13 years	12	20
Women	14+ years	14	30
Men	14+ years	16	30
Pregnancy	–	18	30–35
Lactation	–	17	30–35

Source: https://www.healthline.com/nutrition/water-soluble-vitamins#b1.

- **Deficiency:**
  - In developed nations, pellagra, or a deficiency in niacin, is rare.
  - Inflamed skin, mouth sores, diarrhea, insomnia, and dementia are among the primary signs and symptoms of pellagra. Without treatment, it is lethal, just like all deficiency diseases.
  - Thankfully, a varied diet can easily provide you with the recommended amount of niacin.
  - Deficiency is far more prevalent in developing nations where people typically eat diets low in variety.
  - Cereal grains are especially low in available niacin, since most of it is bound to fiber in the form of niacin.
  - However, your body can synthesize it from the amino acid tryptophan. As a result, severe niacin deficiency can often be avoided on a high-protein diet.
- **Side Effects and Toxicity:**
  - Niacin that occurs naturally in food and does not seem to have any negative effects.
  - On the other hand, excessive niacin supplementation may result in niacin flush, nausea, vomiting, upset stomach, and liver damage.
  - Supplements containing immediate-release nicotinic acid may cause niacin flush as a side effect. A flush in the

face, neck, arms, and chest is one of its characteristics.
- Long-term use of very high doses (3–9 g per day) of sustained-release or slow-release nicotinic acid is linked to liver damage.
- Additionally, taking niacin supplements for a long time may increase insulin resistance and raise blood sugar levels.
- Nicotinic acid may also increase the circulating levels of uric acid, worsening symptoms in people who are predisposed to gout.

- **Benefits of Supplements:**
  - To normalize blood lipid levels, supplements containing 1,300–2,000 mg of nicotinic acid are frequently used.
  - When levels of "bad" low-density lipoprotein (LDL) cholesterol are high, they lower them; when levels of "good" HDL cholesterol are low, they raise them. Supplement users may also experience a decrease in their triglyceride levels.
  - Although the benefits of nicotinic acid are debatable and study results have been mixed, some research has suggested that it lowers the risk of heart disease.
  - Niacin supplementation may also enhance cognition, according to preliminary data, but more research is required before firm conclusions can be drawn.

5.1.1.4. Pantothenic Acid (Vitamin B5)

Almost every food contains pantothenic acid. Its name is appropriately derived from the Greek word pantothen, meaning "from every side."

- **Types:** Pantothenic acid comes in various forms, or there are substances that, when broken down, release the vitamin's active form. In addition to free pantothenic acid, these include:
  - Coenzyme A: A common source of this vitamin in foods. It releases pantothenic acid in the digestive tract.
  - Acyl carrier protein: Like coenzyme A, acyl carrier protein is found in foods and releases pantothenic acid during digestion.
  - Calcium pantothenate: The most common form of pantothenic acid in supplements.
  - Panthenol: Another form of pantothenic acid often used in supplements.
- **Role and Function:**
  - A variety of metabolic processes depend on pantothenic acid.
  - It is needed to make coenzyme A, which is needed to synthesize amino acids, fatty acids, steroid hormones, neurotransmitters, and a host of other vital molecules.
- **Dietary Sources:**
  - Almost every food contains pantothenic acid.
  - Some of its best dietary sources are displayed in the chart in Figure 5.6.

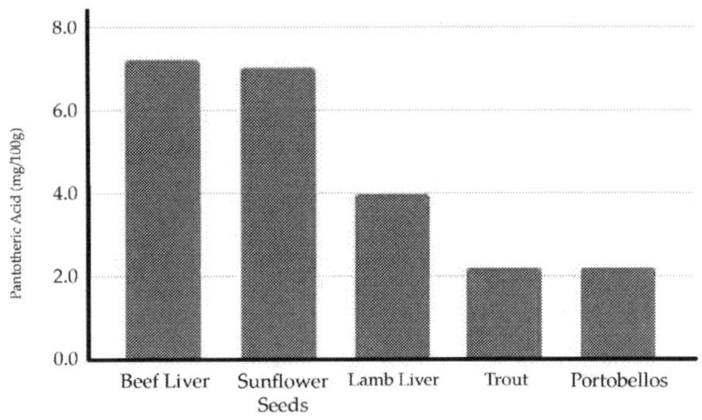

Figure 5.6. *Dietary sources of pantothenic acid.*

Source: https://www.healthline.com/nutrition/water-soluble-vitamins#b1.

- Egg yolks, beef, chicken, shiitake mushrooms, caviar, and yeast extract spread are additional rich sources.
- Many plant-based foods are also excellent providers. These include whole grains, broccoli, tomatoes, and root vegetables in addition to the ones already mentioned.
- Like many other B vitamins, pantothenic acid is often added to breakfast cereals.

- **Recommended Intake:** The majority of people's AI of pantothenic acid is displayed in Table 5.4. There is no established RDA.

Table 5.4. *The Adequate Intake (AI) of Pantothenic Acid*

		AI (mg/day)
Infants	0–6 months	1.7
	7–12 months	1.8
Children	1–3 years	2
	4–8 years	3
	9–13 years	4
Adolescents	14–18 years	5
Adults	19+ years	5
Pregnancy	–	6
Lactation	–	7

Source: https://www.healthline.com/nutrition/water-soluble-vitamins#b1.

- **Deficiency:**
  - Deficiency of pantothenic acid is uncommon in developed nations. Actually, this vitamin is present in so many foods that, outside of extreme malnutrition, deficiencies are practically unheard of.
  - Those who regularly consume excessive amounts of alcohol and those who have diabetes, however, may require more of it.
  - Research conducted on animals demonstrates that a pantothenic acid deficiency negatively affects most organ systems. Many symptoms are linked to it, such as numbness, irritability, restlessness, sleep disturbances, and digestive issues.

- Side Effects and Toxicity:
    - At high doses, pantothenic acid does not seem to have any negative effects. There is no established tolerable upper limit.
    - On the other hand, high dosages, such as 10 g daily, might result in diarrhea and upset stomach.
    - In mice, it was estimated that a lethal dose would be around 4.5 g per pound of body weight (equivalent to 10 g per kg), which translates to 318 g for a human weighing 154 pounds (70 kg).
- **Benefits of Supplements:** Studies have not provided any good evidence of benefits from pantothenic acid supplements in people who get adequate amounts from their diets.

While people take supplements to treat various disorders, including arthritis, dry eyes and skin irritation, there is no strong evidence for its effectiveness in the treatment of any of these disorders.

5.1.1.5. Vitamin B6

Vitamin B6 is a collection of essential nutrients needed for the production of pyridoxal phosphate, which acts as a coenzyme in over 100 various metabolic functions.

- **Types:** Like the other B vitamins, vitamin B6 is a family of related compounds, such as:
    - **Pyridoxine:** This form can be found in supplements, fruits, vegetables, and grains. Pyridoxine additions may also be found in processed foods.
    - **Pyridoxamine:** Utilized in US dietary supplements until recently. But pyridoxamine is now regarded as a pharmaceutical drug by the FDA. Animal-based foods typically contain pyridoxamine phosphate, a common form of vitamin B6.
    - **Pyridoxal:** Pyridoxal phosphate is the main type of vitamin B6 in animal-sourced foods.

In the liver, all dietary forms of vitamin B6 are converted into pyridoxal 5-phosphate, the active form of the vitamin.

- **Role and Function:**
    - Vitamin B6 participates in many chemical reactions as a coenzyme, just like other B vitamins do.
    - It has a role in the synthesis of red blood cells, energy metabolism, and amino acid metabolism. It is also necessary for the body's storage molecule, glycogen, to release glucose, or sugar.
    - In addition, vitamin B6 aids in the body's synthesis of multiple neurotransmitters and promotes the development of white blood cells.
- **Dietary Sources:** Many different foods contain vitamin B6. Some of its richest sources and their contents are displayed in the chart in Figure 5.7.

Potatoes, bananas, chickpeas, turkey, pork, and tuna are additional excellent sources. Additionally, soy-based meat substitutes and breakfast cereals are fortified with vitamin B6. Foods derived from animals typically contain more of this vitamin than foods derived from plants.

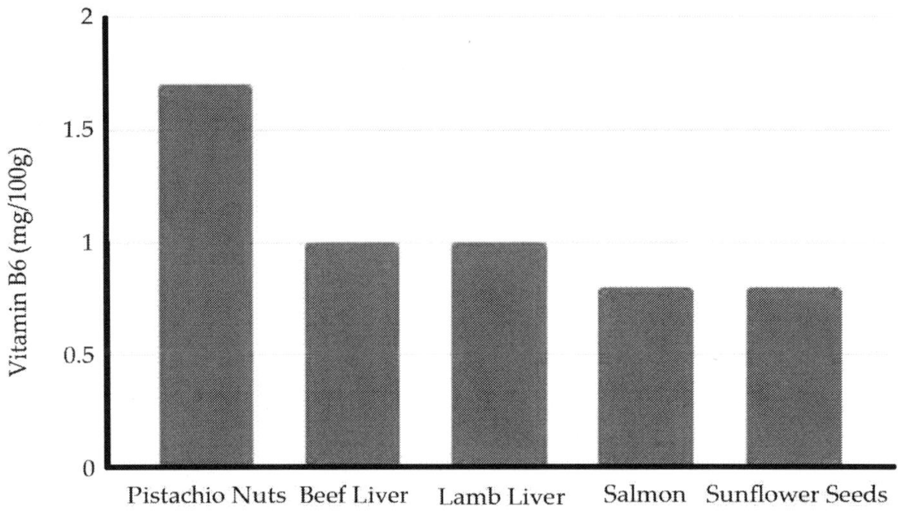

Figure 5.7. *Dietary sources of vitamin B6.*

Source: https://www.healthline.com/nutrition/water-soluble-vitamins#b1.

- **Recommended Intake:** The RDA for vitamin B6 is displayed in Table 5.5. The RDA is the daily intake that most people are expected to find sufficient.

Since the Recommended Dietary Allowance (RDA) has not been determined for infants, the AI is provided instead.

Table 5.5. *The Recommended Dietary Allowance (RDA) for Vitamin B6*

		RDA (mg/day)	UL (mg/day)
Infants	0–6 months	0.1*	–
	7–12 months	0.3*	–
Children	1–3 years	0.5	30
	4–8 years	0.6	40
	9–13 years	1.0	60
Women	14–18 years	1.2	80
	19–50 years	1.3	100
	51+ years	1.5	100
Men	14–18 years	1.3	80
	19–50 years	1.3	100
	51+ years	1.7	100
Pregnancy	–	1.9	80–100
Lactation	–	2.0	80–100

Source: https://www.healthline.com/nutrition/water-soluble-vitamins#b1.

- **Deficiency:**
    - Deficiency of vitamin B6 is uncommon. The most vulnerable group is those who are alcoholics.
    - Anemia, skin rashes, convulsions, disorientation, and depression are among the primary symptoms.
    - A higher risk of cancer has also been linked to deficiencies.
- **Side Effects and Toxicity:**
    - Food-based vitamin B6, which occurs naturally, does not seem to have any negative effects.
    - On the other hand, very high supplemental doses of pyridoxine—2,000 mg or more per day—have been connected to skin lesions and damage to sensory nerves.
    - Breastfeeding mothers may experience decreased milk production if they consume high doses of pyridoxine supplements.
- **Benefits of Supplements:**
    - Pyridoxine in large doses has been used to treat premenstrual syndrome and carpal tunnel syndrome.
    - The benefits are debatable, though. There is insufficient proof to support the efficacy of pyridoxine supplements in treating these ailments.
    - High-dose pyridoxine supplements should only be taken under medical supervision due to their detrimental effects on health.

5.1.1.6. Biotin (Vitamin B7)

Although there is not much proof to support these claims, people frequently take biotin supplements to nourish their skin, hair, and nails. The term "vitamin H" comes from the German word "haut," which means "skin."

- **Types:**
    - There are two types of biotin: unbound and bound to proteins.
    - A substance known as biocytin is released during the digestion of proteins that contain biotin. Next, biocytin is broken down by the digestive enzyme biotinidase into free biotin and the amino acid lysine.
- **Role and Function:**
    - Biotin is a coenzyme, just like all other B vitamins. It is necessary for five carboxylases to function, which are enzymes involved in several essential metabolic processes.
    - For example, biotin is necessary for the synthesis of fatty acids, the production of glucose, and the metabolism of amino acids.
- **Dietary Sources:**
    - There has been less research on the content of biotin in food than there has been on the other B vitamins.
    - Foods derived from animals that are high in biotin include fish, meat, organ meats, egg yolks, and dairy products. Legumes, leafy greens, cauliflower, mushrooms, and nuts are examples of good plant sources.

- Biotin is also produced in small quantities by your gut microbiota.

- **Recommended Intake:** Table 5.6 displays the recommended intake level for biotin, known as the AI. This recommendation is similar to the RDA, but is based on less robust research.

Table 5.6. *The Adequate Intake (AI) for Biotin*

	Age	AI (mcg/day)
Infants	0–6 months	5
	7–12 months	6
Children	1–3 years	8
	4–8 years	12
	9–13 years	20
Adolescents	14–18 years	25
Adults	19+ years	30
Pregnancy	–	30
Lactation	–	35

Source: https://www.healthline.com/nutrition/water-soluble-vitamins#b1.

- **Deficiency:**
  - Deficiency in biotin is not very common.
  - The risk is highest in infants with Leiner's disease, individuals taking antiepileptic medications, individuals genetically predisposed to deficiency, and infants fed formula low in biotin.
  - Untreated biotin deficiency can cause neurological symptoms, such as seizures, mental retardation and loss of muscle coordination.
  - There have also been reports of deficiencies in animals given large quantities of raw egg whites. Avidin, a protein found in egg whites, blocks the absorption of biotin.
- **Side Effects and Toxicity:** Biotin does not have any known adverse effects at high doses and the tolerable upper limit has not been established.
- **Benefits of Supplements:**
  - There is insufficient data to conclude that people who obtain enough biotin from their diets on their own may benefit from taking supplements.
  - For instance, studies suggest biotin may improve symptoms in people with multiple sclerosis (MS).
  - Additionally, observational studies suggest that women with brittle nails may benefit from biotin supplements. Higher caliber research is necessary, though, before any conclusions can be drawn.

5.1.1.7. Vitamin B9

Initially found in yeast, vitamin B9 was subsequently extracted from spinach leaves. Because of this, it was given the names folate or folic acid, which are terms derived from the Latin word folium, which means "leaf" (Figure 5.8).

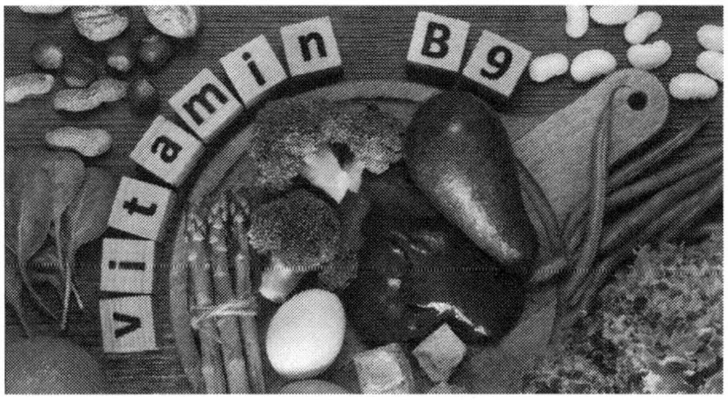

Figure 5.8. *Vitamin B9 sources.*

Source: https://www.healthkart.com/connect/wp-content/uploads/2023/04/900x500_banner_HK-Vitamin-B9-Foods.png.

- **Types:** Vitamin B9 comes in several different forms, including:
  - **Folate:** A family of vitamin B9 compounds that naturally occurs in foods.
  - **Folic Acid:** A synthetic form commonly added to processed foods or sold as a supplement. Some scientists are concerned that high-dose folic acid supplements may cause harm.
  - **L-Methylfolate:** Also known as 5-methyltetrahydrofolate, L-methylfolate is the active form of vitamin B9 in the body. As a supplement, it is thought to be healthier than folic acid.
- **Role and Function:**
  - As a coenzyme, vitamin B9 is necessary for the synthesis of DNA, the growth of cells, and the metabolism of amino acids.
  - During times of rapid cell division and growth, like infancy and pregnancy, it is crucial.
  - It is also necessary for the production of red and white blood cells, so a shortage can result in anemia.
- **Dietary Sources:** A few foods that are excellent sources of vitamin B9 are shown in the chart in Figure 5.9.

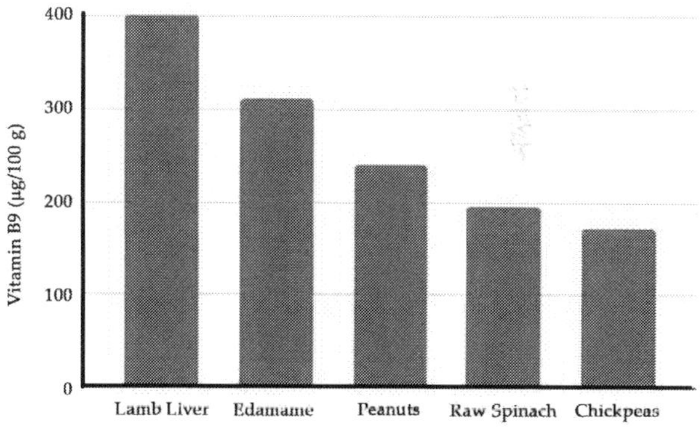

Figure 5.9. *Dietary sources of vitamin B9.*

Source: https://www.healthline.com/nutrition/water-soluble-vitamins#b1.

Asparagus, legumes, sunflower seeds, and leafy greens are additional excellent sources. Spread made with yeast extract has a very high content of vitamin B9—about 3,786 μg per 100 g.

- **Recommended Intake:** The RDA for vitamin B9 is displayed in Table 5.7. Additionally, it displays the daily tolerable upper limit (UL), or the quantity that most people deem safe. For infants, there is currently no established RDA. Alternatively, the table displays the appropriate intake values.

Table 5.7. *The Recommended Dietary Allowance (RDA) for Vitamin B9*

		RDA (mcg/day)	UL (mcg/day)
Infants	0–6 months	65*	–
	7–12 months	80*	–
Children	1–3 years	150	300
	4–8 years	200	400
	9–13 years	300	600
	14–18 years	400	800
Adults	19+ years	400	1,000
Pregnancy	–	600	800–1,000
Lactation	–	500	800–1,000

Source: https://www.healthline.com/nutrition/water-soluble-vitamins#b1.

- **Deficiency:**
  - Deficiency in vitamin B9 seldom happens by itself. It is typically linked to inadequate diet and additional nutrient deficiencies.
  - One of the most common signs of a vitamin B9 deficiency is anemia. It is identical to the anemia brought on by a vitamin B12 shortage.
  - Lack of vitamin B9 may also lead to birth defects of the brain or neural chord, collectively known as neural tube defects.
- **Side Effects and Toxicity:**
  - No serious adverse effects of high vitamin B9 intake have been reported.
  - Yet, studies show that high-dose supplements may mask vitamin B12 deficiency. Some even suggest that they may worsen the neurological damage associated with vitamin B12 deficiency.
  - Additionally, some scientists are concerned that a high intake of folic acid — a synthetic form of vitamin B9 — may cause health problems.
- **Benefits of Supplements:** There isn't much proof that healthy individuals who eat a balanced diet benefit from taking folic acid supplements.

Supplements may improve blood sugar regulation, lower the risk of heart disease, and somewhat lessen depressive symptoms, according to a few studies.

But the advantages of vitamin B9 supplements might only be noticeable to people who were already deficient in the nutrient.

5.1.1.8. Vitamin B12 (Cobalamin)

The only vitamin that has cobalt, a metallic element, in it is vitamin B12. It is frequently referred to as cobalamin because of this.

- **Types:** Adenosylcobalamin, methylcobalamin, hydroxocobalamin, and cyanocobalamin are the four primary forms of vitamin B12.

Supplements contain all of them, with cyanocobalamin being the most widely available. Because of its stability, it is thought to be perfect for supplements, but food only contains trace amounts of it. Hydroxocobalamin is the most common naturally occurring form of vitamin B12, and is widely found in animal-sourced foods.

The other natural forms methylcobalamin and adenosylcobalamin have become popular as supplements in recent years.

- **Role and Function:** As a coenzyme, vitamin B12 functions similarly to all other B vitamins.

Sufficient consumption promotes red blood cell production, neurological development, and brain function.

It is also necessary for DNA synthesis, cell division, and the conversion of protein and fat into energy.

- **Dietary Sources:** Almost the only dietary sources of vitamin B12 are animal-based foods. These consist of eggs, dairy, meat, and seafood. Additional types of liver, heart, octopus, oysters, herring, and tuna are rich sources as well.

However, tempeh and a few algae, such as nori seaweed, may also contain small amounts of vitamin B12. Whether these foods can provide sufficient amounts on their own is a matter of debate.

A class of substances known as pseudovitamin B12, which is comparable to vitamin B12 but not utilised by the body, is present in other algae, such as spirulina.

- **Recommended Intake:** The RDA for vitamin B12 is displayed in Table 5.8. As usual, the AI is given since the RDA has not been determined for infants.

Table 5.8. *The Recommended Dietary Allowance (RDA) for Vitamin B12*

		RDA (mcg/day)
Infants	0–6 months	0.4*
	7–12 months	0.5*
Children	1–3 years	0.9
	4–8 years	1.2
	9–13 years	1.8
Adolescents	14–18 years	2.4
Adults	19+ years	2.4
Pregnancy	–	2.6
Lactation	–	2.8

Source: https://www.healthline.com/nutrition/water-soluble-vitamins#b1.

- **Deficiency:** Even if you aren't getting enough vitamin B12, it may take a while for deficiencies to show symptoms because the vitamin is stored in the liver.

  Those who are at the greatest risk of deficiency are those who never or rarely eat animal-sourced foods. This includes vegetarians and vegans.

  Elderly individuals may also develop deficiencies. In fact, a lot of people need to get regular B12 injections.

  Intrinsic factor is a protein that the stomach produces that is necessary for the absorption of vitamin B12. The production of intrinsic factor may slow down or cease entirely as people get older.

  Those with Crohn's or celiac disease, as well as those who have undergone weight loss surgery, are additional risk groups.

Many health issues, including anemia, loss of appetite, sore tongue, neurological issues, and dementia, can be brought on by deficiencies.

- Ø **Side Effects and Toxicity:** Vitamin B12 can only be absorbed in small amounts through the digestive system. The stomach's synthesis of intrinsic factor determines how much is absorbed.

  Consequently, in healthy individuals, a high intake of vitamin B12 has not been associated with any negative effects. There is no established upper intake level that is tolerable.

- Ø **Benefits of Supplements:** Although vitamin B12 supplements are beneficial for those who are at risk of deficiency, their effects on people whose diets provide adequate amounts are less well understood.

  More research is necessary, but a small study suggests that giving patients recovering from strokes 1,000 mcg daily may help with verbal learning.

  In addition, hydroxocobalamin injections are used, typically in conjunction with sodium thiosulfate, to treat cyanide poisoning.

5.1.1.9. Vitamin C

The only water-soluble vitamin that is not a member of the vitamin B family is vitamin C. It is essential for the synthesis of collagen and one of the body's primary antioxidants.

Types: There are two forms of vitamin C; ascorbic acid is the most widely used form. Dehydroascorbic acid, an oxidized form of ascorbic acid, also possesses vitamin C activity.

- **Role and Function:** Vitamin C supports many essential body functions, including:
  - Antioxidant defenses: Your body uses antioxidants to protect itself against oxidative stress. Vitamin C is one of its most important antioxidants.
  - Collagen formation: Without vitamin C, the body is unable to synthesize collagen, the main protein in connective tissue. As a result, deficiency affects your skin, tendons, ligaments and bones.
  - Immune function: Immune cells contain high levels of vitamin C. During an infection, its levels are quickly depleted.

Vitamin C, in contrast to the B vitamins, is not a coenzyme; however, it is a cofactor for prolyl hydroxylase, an enzyme that is critical to the production of collagen.

- **Dietary Sources:** Fruits and vegetables are the primary dietary sources of vitamin C. Vitamin C is almost nonexistent in cooked foods derived from animals, although it is present in trace amounts in raw liver, eggs, fish roe, meat, and fish.
- **Recommended Intake:** The estimated daily requirement of vitamin C for the majority of people is known as the RDA.

Additionally, the tolerable UL, or maximum intake level deemed entirely safe for the majority of people, is displayed in Table 5.9.

For newborns, no RDA has been set. Rather than using the RDA, scientists have estimated their AI, which is based on less reliable data.

Table 5.9. *The Recommended Dietary Allowance (RDA) for Vitamin C*

		RDA (mg/day)	Upper Limit (UL, mg/day)
Infants	0–6 months	40*	–
	7–12 months	50*	–
Children	1–3 years	15	400
	4–8 years	25	650
	9–13 years	45	1,200
Women	14–18 years	65	1,800
	19+ years	75	2,000
Men	14–18 years	75	1,800
	19+ years	90	2,000
Pregnancy	–	80–85	1,800–2,000
Lactation	–	115–120	1,800–2,000

Source: https://www.healthline.com/nutrition/water-soluble-vitamins#b1.

- **Deficiency:** While deficiency is uncommon in Western nations, it can occur in those who consume very little fruit or vegetable in their diet or who follow restrictive eating plans. Individuals who suffer from alcoholism or drug addiction are also more vulnerable.

It results in scurvy, a disease characterized by the degeneration of connective tissue. Weakness and exhaustion are the initial signs of deficiency.

Spotted skin and inflamed gums are possible symptoms of scurvy progression.

In addition to bleeding gums and skin, advanced scurvy can also result in joint issues, dry eyes, swelling, and slowed wound healing. Scurvy is lethal without treatment, just like all vitamin deficiencies.

- **Side Effects and Toxicity:** High vitamin C dosages are generally tolerated by most people without any negative effects.

But extremely high doses—more than 3 g daily—cause nausea, cramping in the abdomen, and diarrhea. This is because a single dosage of vitamin C can only absorb so much.

In individuals who are predisposed, taking high-dose supplements exceeding 1,000 mg daily may also raise the risk of kidney stones.

- **Benefits of Supplements:** There is conflicting data regarding the health benefits of vitamin C supplements for those who consume enough of it through diet.

On the other hand, vitamin C can help people who are low or deficient in iron absorb iron better from meals.

Furthermore, a comprehensive review of 29 studies found that taking supplements containing a minimum of 200 mg of vitamin C daily could potentially aid in the recovery from the common cold.

There is no proof that vitamin C supplements lower the risk of heart disease, even though they might help lower blood pressure.

Research indicates that vitamin C could potentially lower the risk of cognitive decline, enhance blood vessel function, and decrease blood sugar levels. However, more rigorous studies are necessary in order to draw solid conclusions.

5.1.2. Fat-Soluble Vitamins

The majority dissolve in water when it comes to water solubility. The fat-soluble vitamins, on the other hand, behave like oil and are water-soluble. The majority of fat-soluble vitamins can be found in foods high in fat, and eating fat improves their absorption into the bloodstream.

There are four fat-soluble vitamins in the human diet:

- Vitamin A;
- Vitamin D;
- Vitamin E;
- Vitamin K.

5.1.2.1. Vitamin A

Vitamin A is essential for keeping your vision intact. You would go blind without it.

- **Types:** A single vitamin is not what vitamin A is. Instead, it is a class of fat-soluble substances called retinoids.

Retinol is the most widely consumed dietary form of vitamin A. The body contains other forms of retinoic acid and retinal, which are either rare or nonexistent in food.

Vitamin A2 (3,4-dehydroretinal) is an alternative, less active form found in freshwater fish.

- **Role and Function of Vitamin A:** Vitamin A supports many critical aspects of body function, including:
    - **Vision Maintenance:** Vitamin A is essential for maintaining the light-sensing cells in the eyes and for the formation of tear fluid.
    - **Immune Function:** Vitamin A deficiency impairs immune function, increasing susceptibility to infections.
    - Body Growth: Vitamin A is necessary for cell growth. Deficiency may slow or prevent growth in children.
    - **Hair Growth:** It is also vital for hair growth. Deficiency leads to alopecia, or hair loss.
    - **Reproductive Function:** Vitamin A maintains fertility and is vital for fetal development.
- **Dietary Sources:** Animal products are the only source of vitamin A in food. Liver, butter, and fish liver oil are the primary naturally occurring food sources.

The vitamin A content of 3.5 ounces (100 g) of some of the highest-quality food sources (Figure 5.10).

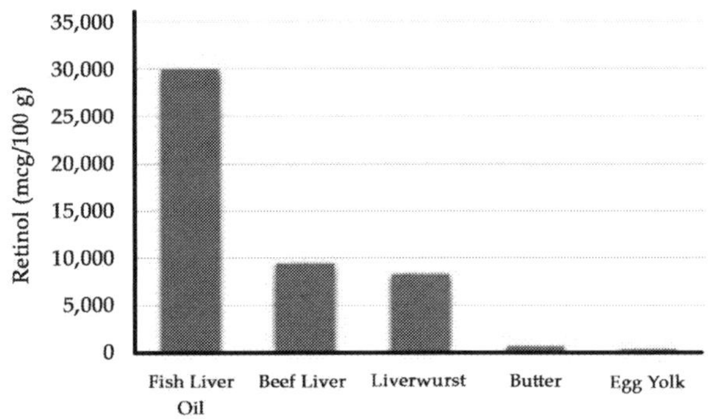

Figure 5.10. *Dietary sources in animal-sourced foods.*

Source: https://www.healthline.com/nutrition/fat-soluble-vitamins#vitamin-a.

Certain carotenoid antioxidants that are present in plants can also be used to make vitamin A. They are referred to as pro-vitamin A collectively.

The most effective of these is beta-carotene, found in large amounts in a variety of vegetables, including spinach, kale, and carrots.

- **Recommended Intake:** The RDA for vitamin A is displayed in Table 5.10. The RDA represents the estimated amount of vitamin A that the majority of people (roughly 97.5%) require to meet their daily requirements. The tolerable UL, the highest daily intake level that 97.5%

of healthy individuals deem safe, is also displayed in Table 5.10.

Table 5.10. *Dietary Sources in Animal-Sourced Foods*

		RDA (IU/ mcg)	Upper Limit (UL, IU / mcg)
Infants	0–6 months	1,333 / 400	2,000 / 600
	7–12 months	1,667 / 500	2,000 / 600
Children	1–3 years	1,000 / 300	2,000 / 600
	4–8 years	1,333 / 400	3,000 / 900
	9–13 years	2,000 / 600	5,667 / 1700
Women	14–18 years	2,333 / 700	9,333 / 2800
	19–70 years	2,333 / 700	10,000 / 3000
Men	14–18 years	3,000 / 900	9,333 / 2800
	19–70 years	3,000 / 900	10,000 / 3000

Source: https://www.healthline.com/nutrition/fat-soluble-vitamins#vitamin-a.

- **Vitamin A Deficiency:** Deficiency of vitamin A is uncommon in developed nations. But since pre-formed vitamin A can only be found in foods derived from animals, vegans might be in danger. Provitamin A is found in large quantities in many fruits and vegetables, but it is not always effectively converted into retinol, which is vitamin A's active form. Genetics determines how well this conversion occurs.

Deficiency is also common in some developing nations with limited food variety. It is prevalent in populations whose diets are low in meat, fat, and vegetables and high in refined rice, white potatoes, or cassava. A common symptom of early deficiency includes night blindness. As it progresses, it may lead to more serious conditions, such as:

- **Dry Eyes:** Severe deficiency may cause xerophthalmia, a condition characterized by dry eyes caused by reduced tear fluid formation.
- **Blindness:** Serious vitamin A deficiency may lead to total blindness. In fact, it is among the most common preventable causes of blindness in the world.
- **Hair Loss:** If you are vitamin A deficient, you may start to lose your hair.
- **Skin Problems:** Deficiency leads to a skin condition known as hyperkeratosis or goose flesh.
- **Poor Immune Function:** Poor vitamin A status or deficiency makes people prone to infections.

- **Vitamin A Toxicity:** Taking too much vitamin A can result in a condition called hypervitaminosis A, which can have serious health effects. This most commonly occurs when individuals consume excessive amounts of vitamin A from supplements, liver, or fish liver oil. Consuming high levels of provitamin A, however, does not typically lead to hypervitaminosis. Symptoms of vitamin A toxicity may include fatigue, headaches, irritability, stomach pain, joint pain, decreased appetite, vomiting, blurry vision, skin issues, and inflammation in the mouth and eyes. In severe cases, overdosing on vitamin A can result in liver damage, bone loss, and hair loss, and may even be fatal. To prevent hypervitaminosis A, it is recommended that adults do not exceed the daily upper limit of 10,000 IU (900 mcg) of vitamin A.

Adults who consume higher doses, up to 300,000 IU (900 mg), may develop acute hypervitaminosis A. Children are susceptible to negative effects in far smaller doses. Tolerance varies greatly amongst individuals. Extra caution is necessary because children and those suffering from liver diseases such as cirrhosis and hepatitis are more vulnerable.

- **Benefits of Vitamin A Supplements:** Although those who are deficient can benefit from supplements, most people get enough vitamin A from their diet and do not require supplements.

However, even if a person's diet satisfies the essential requirements, controlled studies indicate that vitamin A supplements may be beneficial for some individuals.

For example, vitamin A supplements can aid in the treatment of pediatric measles. They can prevent pneumonia linked to measles and lower mortality rates by 50–80%. Research indicates that vitamin A functions by inhibiting the measles virus.

5.1.2.2. Vitamin D

The human body naturally produces vitamin D when it is exposed to sunlight. Bone health and development are aided by vitamin D.

- **Types:** The term "vitamin D" refers to a group of related fat-soluble substances.

Also known as calciferol, vitamin D comes in two main dietary forms:

  - **Vitamin D2 (Ergocalciferol):** Found in mushrooms and some plants.
  - **Vitamin D3 (Cholecalciferol):** Found in animal-sourced foods, such as eggs and fish oil, and produced by your skin when exposed to sunlight.

- **Role and Function of Vitamin D:** Although vitamin D has many uses, only a small number of them have been thoroughly studied. These include the following:
  - **Bone Maintenance:** Vitamin D regulates the circulating levels of calcium and phosphorus, which are the most important minerals for bone growth and maintenance. It promotes the absorption of these minerals from the diet.
  - **Immune System Regulation:** It also regulates and strengthens immune system function.

The biologically active form of vitamin D, calcitriol, is produced by the liver and kidneys after calciferol is absorbed into the bloodstream. Calciferol can also be stored for later use as calcidiol. Compared to vitamin D2, vitamin D3 is converted into calcitriol more effectively.

- **Sources of Vitamin D:** If you expose a significant portion of your skin to sunlight on a regular basis, your body can generate all the vitamin D it needs.

But a lot of people either avoid the sun altogether or only spend a short while there. Some people, understandably enough, use sunscreen to protect their skin from sunburns. Although wearing sunscreen is strongly advised, it actually reduces the amount of vitamin D your skin produces.

Since few foods naturally contain vitamin D, most people must rely on their diets to get enough of it. The best dietary sources are fatty fish and fish oil, but mushrooms that have been exposed to UV light may also contain significant amounts of the vitamin. The following chart displays how much vitamin D is found in 30.5 ounces (100 g) of some of the highest-quality food sources (Figure 5.11):

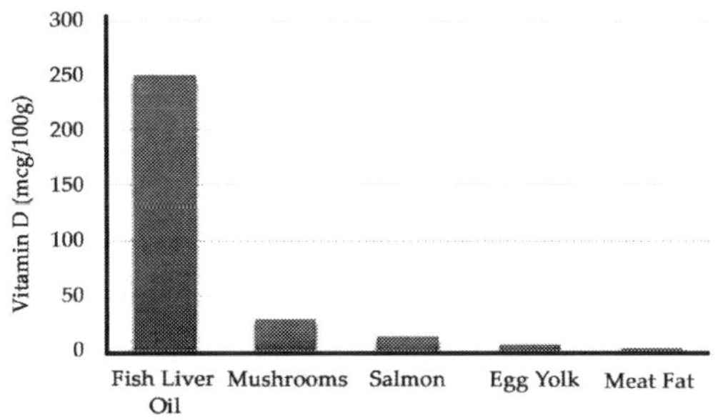

Figure 5.11. *Dietary sources of vitamin D.*

Source: https://www.healthline.com/nutrition/fat-soluble-vitamins#vitamin-a.

- **Recommended Intake:** The UI and RDA for vitamin D are displayed in Table 5.11.

The values indicated with an asterisk represent the AI for infants, as there is no established RDA for them. Though it is supported by less evidence, the AI and RDA are comparable.

Table 5.11. *The Recommended Dietary Allowance (RDA) and Upper Limit (UI) for Vitamin D*

Age Group	RDA (IU / mcg)	UL (IU / mcg)
0–6 months	400 / 10*	1,000 / 25
7–12 months	400 / 10*	1,500 / 38
1–3 years	600 / 15	2,500 / 63
4–8 years	600 / 15	3,000 / 75
9–70 years	600 / 15	4,000 / 100
70+ years	800 / 20	4,000 / 100

Source: https://www.healthline.com/nutrition/fat-soluble-vitamins#vitamin-a.

- **Vitamin D Deficiency:** Although severe vitamin D deficiency is uncommon, hospitalized patients and the elderly frequently have mild forms of the deficiency or insufficiency. Dark skin tone, advanced age, obesity, limited sun exposure, and illnesses that hinder the absorption of fat are risk factors for deficiencies.

The most well-known effects of low vitamin D include weakened muscles, brittle bones, and a higher chance of bone fractures. In adults, this is known as osteomalacia; in children, it is known as rickets. Inadequate levels of vitamin D are also linked to weakened immune systems, heightened vulnerability to infections, and autoimmune disorders. Additional indicators of inadequacy or inadequacy could be lethargy, despondency, baldness, and slowed wound healing. Additionally, observational studies have connected low vitamin D levels or deficiencies to a higher risk of heart attacks and cancer-related mortality.

- **Vitamin D Toxicity:** It is extremely rare to be vitamin D toxic. Although excessive sun exposure does not result in vitamin D toxicity, taking large doses of supplements can be harmful.

The primary effect of toxicity is hypercalcemia, which is a disorder marked by elevated blood calcium levels.

A few symptoms include high blood pressure, kidney and heart damage, fatigue, headaches, nausea, lack of appetite, weight loss, and abnormalities in the fetus.

The general consensus is that individuals should refrain from consuming more vitamin D than what is recommended, which for adults is 4,000 IU per day.

When taken daily for one or two months, higher amounts, ranging from 40,000–100,000 IU (1,000–2,500 mcg) per day, may cause toxic symptoms in adults. Remember that much lower doses can be harmful to small children.

- **Benefits of Vitamin D Supplements:** Supplements can prove to be highly advantageous for individuals who eat little liver or fatty fish and spend little time in the sun.

People's lives appear to be prolonged by taking supplements on a regular basis, particularly those of elderly patients in hospitals or institutions. Supplements may also reduce the risk of respiratory tract infections. They may also have many other benefits in people with vitamin D deficiency, but more studies need to examine their effects in people with sufficient vitamin D levels.

5.1.2.3. Vitamin E

Antioxidant vitamin E can assist the body in eliminating free radicals. Unstable atoms known as free radicals have the potential to initiate the growth of cancer cells. As a result, vitamin E may be crucial in preventing cancer.

- **Types:** Vitamin E is a family of eight structurally similar antioxidants that are divided into two groups:
    - **Tocopherols:** Alpha-tocopherol, beta-tocopherol, gamma-tocopherol, and delta-tocopherol.
    - **Tocotrienols:** Alpha-tocotrienol, beta-tocotrienol, gamma-tocotrienol, and delta-tocotrienol.

Alpha-tocopherol is the most common form of vitamin E. It makes up around 90% of the vitamin E in the blood.

- **Role and Function of Vitamin E:** Vitamin E's main role is to act as an antioxidant, preventing oxidative stress and protecting fatty acids in your cell membranes from free radicals.

These antioxidant properties are enhanced by other nutrients, such as vitamin C, vitamin B3 and selenium.

In high amounts, vitamin E also acts as a blood thinner, reducing the blood's ability to clot.

- **Dietary Sources:** The highest dietary concentrations of vitamin E can be found in nuts, seeds, and certain vegetable oils. The following chart lists some of the highest-quality sources of vitamin E along with how much of each food is contained in 3 point five ounces (100 g) (Figure 5.12).

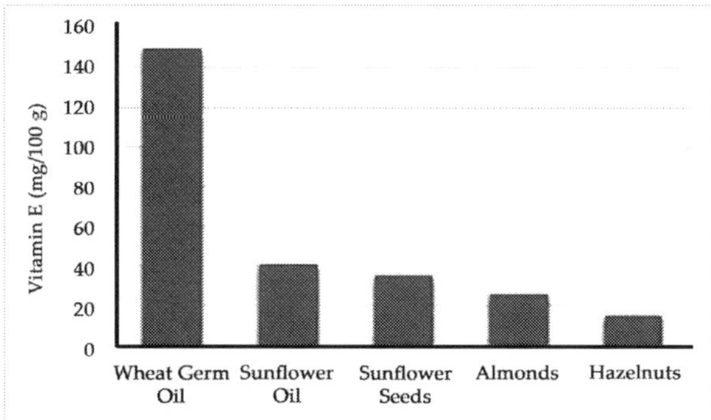

Figure 5.12. *Dietary sources of vitamin E.*

Source: https://www.healthline.com/nutrition/fat-soluble-vitamins#vitamin-a.

- **Recommended Intake:** The RDA and acceptable upper limit for vitamin E intake are displayed in Table 5.12. Since there are no RDA values available for infants, the values indicated with an asterisk represent the AI.

Table 5.12. *The Recommended Dietary Allowance (RDA) and Tolerable Upper Limit for Vitamin E Intake*

		RDA (IU / mg)	UL (IU / mg)
Infants	0–6 months	6 / 4*	Not known
	7–12 months	8 / 5*	Not known
Children	1–3 years	9 / 6	300 / 200
	4–8 years	11 / 7	450 / 300
	9–13 years	17 / 11	900 / 600
Adolescents	14–18 years	23 / 15	1,200 / 800
Adults	19–50 years	23 / 15	1,500 / 1,000
	51+	18 / 12	1,500 / 1,000

Source: https://www.healthline.com/nutrition/fat-soluble-vitamins#vitamin-a.

- **Vitamin E Deficiency:** It is rare and never found in otherwise healthy individuals to have a vitamin E deficiency. It occurs most frequently in conditions like cystic fibrosis and liver disease that hinder the body's ability to absorb fat or vitamin E from food.

Symptoms of vitamin E deficiency include muscle weakness, walking difficulties, tremors, vision problems, poor immune function and numbness. Severe, long-term deficiency may lead to anemia, heart disease, serious neurological problems, blindness, dementia, poor reflexes and the inability to fully control body movements

- **Vitamin E Toxicity:** It is difficult to consume too much vitamin E when it comes from natural food sources. Toxicological cases have only been documented following extremely high supplement dosages. Still, taking too much vitamin E seems safe when compared to vitamin A and D. It might thin the blood, negating the benefits of vitamin K and leading to excessive bleeding. Therefore, high vitamin E dosages should be avoided by those who use blood thinners. Additionally, vitamin E may have pro-oxidant effects at high doses exceeding 1,000 mg daily. In other words, it may turn into the antithesis of an antioxidant and cause oxidative stress.
- **Benefits and Risks of High Vitamin E Intake or Supplements:** Several advantages have been associated with high consumption of vitamin E, either from food or supplements. Gamma-tocopherol, one type of vitamin E, has been shown to promote blood vessel dilatation, which increases blood flow and may lower blood pressure and the risk of heart disease.

Gamma-tocopherol supplements may also have a blood-thinning effect as well as reducing levels of "bad" LDL cholesterol. On the other hand, some research indicates that taking high doses of vitamin E supplements could be harmful, even without any noticeable signs of toxicity. For example, observational studies have found a connection between taking vitamin E supplements and a higher risk of developing prostate cancer and overall mortality. Due to the potential negative impacts of vitamin E supplements, it is not advisable to use them currently. More rigorous studies are necessary to determine the long-term safety of these supplements before definitive conclusions can be drawn.

5.1.2.4. Vitamin K

An essential component of blood clotting is vitamin K. You would be in danger of dying from bleeding to death without it.

- **Types:** Vitamin K is actually a group of fat-soluble compounds divided into two main groups:
    - Vitamin K1 (phylloquinone): Found in plant-sourced foods, phylloquinone is the main form of vitamin K in the diet (49Trusted Source).
    - Vitamin K2 (menaquinone): This variety of vitamin K is found in animal-sourced foods and fermented soy products, like natto. Vitamin K2 is also produced by gut bacteria in the colon (50Trusted Source, 51Trusted Source).

Additionally, there are at least three synthetic forms of vitamin K. These are known as vitamin K3 (menadione), vitamin K4 (menadiol diacetate) and vitamin K5.

- **Role and Function of Vitamin K:** Vitamin K plays an essential role in blood clotting. In fact, the "K" stands for "koagulation," the Danish word for coagulation, which means clotting.

However, vitamin K serves additional purposes as well, such as promoting bone health and assisting in the prevention of blood vessel calcification, which may lower the risk of heart disease.

- **Dietary Sources:** While vitamin K2 (menaquinone) is primarily found in foods derived from animals and fermented soy products, vitamin K1 (phylloquinone) is best obtained through diet. Some of the primary sources of vitamin K1 are listed in Figure 5.13, along with how much of each food type makes up 3 point five ounces (100 g).

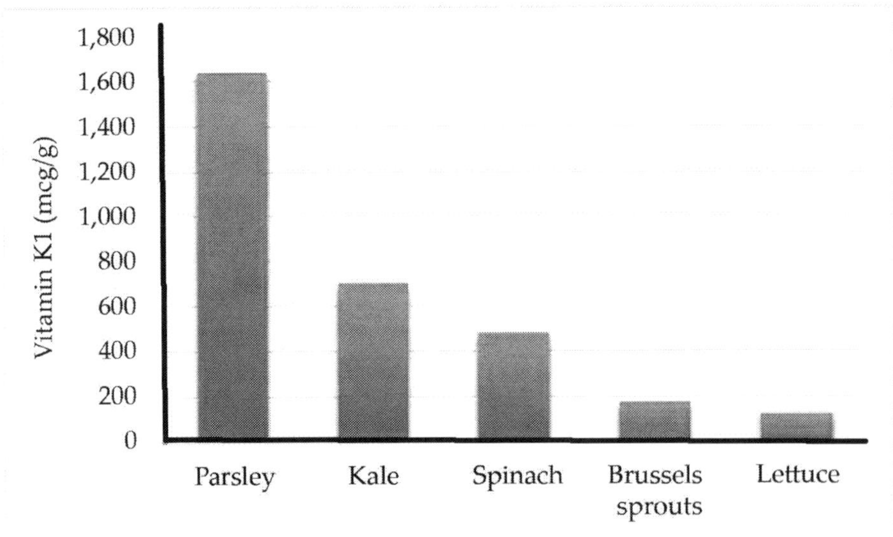

Figure 5.13. *Dietary sources of vitamin K1.*

Source: https://www.healthline.com/nutrition/fat-soluble-vitamins#vitamin-a.

In contrast to phylloquinone, menaquinone is only found in small amounts in certain high-fat, animal-sourced foods, such as egg yolks, butter and liver.

- **Recommended Intake:** Table 5.13 displays the recommended vitamin K intake values known as AI. AI is comparable to the RDA, as it represents the daily intake level believed to satisfy the needs of 97.5% of individuals. However, AI is derived from less robust evidence compared to RDA.

Table 5.13. *The Adequate Intake (AI) Values for Vitamin K*

		AI (mcg)
Infants	0–6 months	2
	7–12 month	2.5
Children	1–3 years	30
	4–8 years	55
	9–13 years	60
Adolescents	14–18 years	75
Women	18+ years	90
Men	18+ years	120

Source: https://www.healthline.com/nutrition/fat-soluble-vitamins#vitamin-a.

- **Vitamin K Deficiency:** Vitamin K is not significantly stored in the body like vitamins A and D are. Because of this, eating a diet low in vitamin K could cause you to become deficient in the vitamin in as little as one week. Individuals who have poor fat digestion and absorption capacities are most vulnerable to vitamin K deficiency. This covers people with cystic fibrosis, inflammatory bowel disease, and celiac disease.

The risk of deficiency may also be increased by the use of broad-spectrum antibiotics and very high doses of vitamin A, which appear to decrease the absorption of vitamin K. Excessive dosages of vitamin E have the potential to mitigate the clotting effects of vitamin K. Your blood wouldn't clot without vitamin K, and even a small cut could start a chain reaction of bleeding. Fortunately, because the body only requires trace amounts of vitamin K to maintain blood clotting, vitamin K deficiency is uncommon. In women, low vitamin K levels have also been associated with decreased bone density and a higher risk of fractures.

- **Vitamin K Toxicity:** There are no known toxic symptoms associated with natural forms of vitamin K, in contrast to other fat-soluble vitamins. Consequently, researchers have been unable to determine an upper limit of vitamin K intake that is considered tolerable. Additional research is required.

In contrast, a synthetic form of vitamin K, known as menadione or vitamin K3, may have some adverse effects when consumed in high amounts.

- **Benefits of Vitamin K Supplements:** Numerous well-controlled studies have investigated the impact of vitamin K supplements on humans. The findings suggest that both vitamin K1 and vitamin K2 supplements may be effective in reducing bone loss and lowering the likelihood of bone fractures.

Additionally, taking vitamin K2 supplements at 45–90 mg per day slightly increased the survival of patients with liver cancer.

An increased consumption of vitamin K2 may also reduce the risk of heart disease, according to observational studies. The data from controlled trials, however, is scant and equivocal. Lastly, older men's development of insulin resistance was slowed by vitamin K1 supplements administered at 0.5 mg daily for three years, as opposed to a placebo. For women, no discernible differences were found.

5.2. Major Minerals and Trace Elements

Minerals and vitamins are essential micronutrients that humans need for overall health and development. Along with macronutrients like fats, carbohydrates, and proteins, they play a crucial role in maintaining metabolic and developmental processes. Deficiency in micronutrients can lead to chronic metabolic issues, as seen in the potentially harmful consequences of not having enough vitamins. While many processed foods are now enriched with vitamins to prevent deficiencies, minerals are not as commonly supplemented. Minerals, such as calcium, play important roles in nerve transmission, muscle activation, and enzyme function. Trace minerals, needed in small amounts, act as cofactors for various enzymes. Their importance lies in their ability to regulate essential biochemical reactions at a cellular level.

5.2.1. What Are Minerals?

The body needs minerals, which are inorganic substances, in trace amounts for a number of purposes. These include the development of teeth and bones, their role as vital components of bodily tissues and fluids, their role as parts of enzyme systems, and their role in maintaining normal nerve function. More of some minerals are required than of others, e.g. Chloride, sodium, potassium, magnesium, calcium, and phosphorus. Some are referred to as trace minerals and are needed in smaller amounts, such as e. g. copper, zinc, iodine, fluoride, and selenium. Trace minerals are just as important as other minerals even though they are needed in smaller quantities. When minerals are consumed in food as opposed to supplements, the body is able to absorb them more effectively. Additionally, a diet lacking in one mineral may also be lacking in others, so the first line of action in addressing this is to evaluate and enhance the diet overall. For healthy individuals, eating a varied diet will help guarantee an adequate supply of most minerals.

According to data from the National Diet and Nutrition Surveys (NDNS), certain population subgroups consume inadequate amounts of other minerals, such as potassium, magnesium, and zinc in men and iron, calcium, copper, and iodine in women. Young adults in Britain, particularly women, tend to eat particularly poorly, which could jeopardize their long-term health if changes aren't made. The majority of people do not exhibit deficiencies, but this does not imply that their intakes or nutritional status are sufficient. For instance, because their dietary intake may not meet their needs, some vegans and vegetarians, women of childbearing age, and adolescent girls are more prone to low iron status and iron deficiency anemia. Concerns have also been raised concerning some teenagers' and young and older women's calcium intake and its potential effects on bone health in the future.

5.2.2. Requirements and Recommended Dietary Intakes

Due to the various functions that each mineral performs, the body needs varying amounts of each mineral. Conditions differ based on age, gender, and physical condition (e.g., pregnancy). Their health status might also have an impact. Dietary Reference Values (DRVs) for minerals have been published by the Department of Health for various categories of healthy individuals. The amount of a nutrient that will meet the needs of almost the entire population is known as the

Reference Nutrient Intake (RNI) (i.e. 97.5%); in other words, surpassing the RNI is typically not required. Additionally, Lower Reference Nutrient Intakes (LRNI) have been determined. Only 2.5% of the population is thought to be served by these levels; the remaining individuals will need more. Therefore, it is very likely that the majority of a population group will not be getting enough of a nutrient if, say, 10% of them consume it at levels below the LRNI.

The mean intakes of mineral and trace elements from food sources as a percentage of LRNI, by age and sex. These tables give an indicator of where intakes of minerals and trace elements are of concern. But certain groups of people may have higher requirements for specific minerals, e.g. women with particularly heavy periods may need extra iron, and extra calcium (and vitamin D) is sometimes recommended by doctors for women at high risk of osteoporosis. In such cases, supplements may be useful but should not replace a varied and healthy diet.

5.2.3. The Bioavailability and Absorption of Minerals

The bioavailability of a mineral (i.e., how readily it can be absorbed and used by the body) may be influenced by a variety of factors. Bioavailability is contingent on the chemical form of the mineral, other compounds in the diet, and (for nutrients like iron) the specific requirements of the individual based on the amount of the nutrient stored in the body. This is due to the body's sensitive mechanisms that guard against the storage of nutrients that, in excess, can be harmful (such as iron).

A few food ingredients lower bioavailability. For instance, the presence of phytates in wholegrain cereal-based products (particularly in unleavened breads like chapattis) can bind and thereby decrease the absorption of calcium, iron, and zinc. Nitrates may get in the way of iodine absorption. In a similar vein, any calcium present is bound by the oxalate found in spinach and rhubarb, preventing absorption. Also, an excess of one mineral may hinder the absorption of another by competing for the same transport systems in the gut, e.g., excess iron reduces zinc absorption. This generally only becomes a problem when zinc intakes are already marginal. Unlike some vitamins, minerals are fairly stable in normal food processing and storage conditions.

5.2.4. Calcium

The most prevalent mineral in the body and one that is necessary for many essential processes is calcium (Ca). For the development and maintenance of strong bones and teeth, the body requires enough calcium from the diet in addition to vitamin D and a number of other nutrients like vitamin K. In addition, calcium is essential for many other systems, such as intracellular signaling, which permits the integration and control of metabolic processes, nervous system information transmission, control of heart and muscle contraction, and blood clotting. Additionally, it has been proposed that consuming enough calcium (from, say, reduced-fat dairy products) may help prevent colon cancer and lower high blood pressure, though more research is required to fully support these claims.

The majority of calcium in the body, around 99%, is found in the skeleton, totaling approximately 1 kg in adult bones. The main components of bone are calcium and phosphate, which combine to form hydroxyapatite. This mineral structure is intertwined with collagen fibers, creating a strong and rigid framework. The body's need for calcium varies depending on the rate of bone growth. Additionally, the skeleton serves as a reserve of minerals, such as calcium and phosphorus, which can be accessed or stored as needed to support bodily functions and development. Blood calcium levels are meticulously controlled, and blood plasma levels are kept within strict bounds. Calcium balance can be maintained at a range of different levels of calcium intake because calcium absorption is well regulated to match the needs of the body. There is evidence, for instance, from Gambia, that calcium balance can be reached even at low intake levels. The maintenance of calcium status involves the regulation of calcium absorption from the gastrointestinal tract, kidney excretion, and bone mobilization and deposition. These sites are regulated by feedback mechanisms that are governed by a number of hormones, such as parathyroid hormone and activated vitamin D. Abnormal calcium plasma levels only arise when this homeostatic mechanism breaks down, usually not as a result of variations in calcium intake from food. The reason the body makes this effort is that even slight changes in plasma calcium concentrations can have detrimental effects on the general health of the body as well as the operation of essential organs. Hypocalcaemia refers to low blood calcium levels, and hypercalcaemia refers to high blood calcium levels.

5.2.4.1. Deficiency

Low blood levels of certain nutrients indicate a nutritional deficiency; however, low blood levels of some nutrients, like calcium, are uncommon for the reasons mentioned above. Since bone serves as a reservoir in times of need, the effects of a low calcium supply are typically reflected in bone density due to the requirement to maintain blood levels. For instance, low vitamin D levels can lead to insufficient calcium in the bones, as calcium absorption depends on vitamin D. A vitamin D deficiency causes rickets in children and osteomalacia (weak bones due to calcium deficiency) in adults.

A notable number of young women, including 8% aged 19–24 years and 6% aged 25–34 years, have calcium intakes below the LRNIs, suggesting their intake may be insufficient. Adequate calcium intake is crucial for overall health, especially during periods of growth such as childhood, adolescence, pregnancy, and lactation when peak bone mass is established. In some cases, supplements are advised for individuals at risk of osteoporosis.

5.2.4.2. Adverse Effects

It is unlikely to have any negative effects from getting calcium from a varied diet, but taking high-dose supplements can occasionally result in diarrhea and stomach pain.

5.2.4.3. Food Sources

Approximately half of the calcium in the UK diet comes from milk, cheese, and other dairy products. Since most bread flour in the UK is required by law to be fortified with calcium (though not whole meal), bread is another important source. Some green leafy vegetables, like broccoli and cabbage (but not spinach), fortified soy products, and fish that is eaten with the bones, like sardines, canned salmon, and whitebait, are also good sources of calcium.

5.2.4.4. Calcium Absorption

There are several promoting and inhibiting factors that affect calcium absorption. Lactose, vitamin D, non-digestible oligosaccharides, dietary protein, and an acidic environment in the small intestine are all considered promoting factors. Calcium is most readily absorbed from milk and dairy products. Inhibitory factors include phytates (e.g. in wholegrain cereals, pulses), oxalate (e.g. from spinach, rhubarb, beetroot), use of antacids, unabsorbed dietary fats, excessive intakes of dietary fibre and large intakes of phosphoric acid (e.g. from carbonated drinks). Phytates and oxalates in plant foods can bind calcium, making it difficult for the body to absorb the mineral into the bloodstream from the intestine. This is why calcium from plant foods is frequently less available. However, absorption from some plant foods is good e.g. broccoli, although the amount present is usually lower than in milk.

5.2.5. Phosphorus

The primary role of phosphorus is in the synthesis of hydroxyapatite, the component of bone, in conjunction with calcium. As calcium salts found in the skeleton contain 80% of the phosphorous in the body, they are vital for strong bones and teeth. The adult's ongoing bone remodeling is characterized by a dynamic equilibrium between calcium and phosphate. Every cell in the body contains the remaining phosphorus. Intercellular phosphorus is involved in several energy metabolism-related processes and is necessary for the structure of cell membranes (in phospholipids).

5.2.5.1. Deficiency

Phosphorus is unlikely to be in short supply in UK diets because it is available in many foods.

5.2.5.2. Adverse Effects

Phosphorus has very low toxicity.

5.2.5.3. Food Sources

Phosphorus is abundant in red meat, dairy products, fish, poultry, bread, rice and oats and is usually found in foods that also contain calcium.

5.2.6. Magnesium

All human tissues contain the necessary mineral magnesium, but bone contains the most of it. It functions both physiologically and biochemically, and it has significant interactions with sodium, potassium, and calcium. It is required for the release of parathyroid hormone, which is involved in bone metabolism, as well as the activation of numerous enzymes, including those involved in DNA replication and RNA synthesis. Additionally, it's necessary for nerve and muscle function.

5.2.6.1. Deficiency

Neuromuscular dysfunction and progressive muscle weakness are the hallmarks of a rare nutritional deficiency. Individuals with malabsorption disorders, alcoholism, and critically ill patients frequently experience mild hypomagnesaemia, or low blood magnesium levels.

On the other hand, excessively low magnesium intakes are fairly common in the United Kingdom. Despite the fact that a wide variety of foods contain magnesium, one in five women between the ages of 19 and 34, as well as over half of teenage girls (51% of those in the 11–14 age group and 53% of those in the 15–18 age group) and over 20% of boys in the same age group are at risk of having low intakes.

5.2.6.2. Adverse Effects

Large dietary intakes have not been shown to be harmful to people with normal kidney function. On the other hand, taking high dose supplements on a regular basis may cause diarrhea as well as elevated blood levels of magnesium and related side effects.

5.2.6.3. Food Sources

Due to its widespread availability and presence in both plant and animal cells, magnesium is a mineral that is found in chlorophyll, the green pigment found in plants. Green leafy vegetables, bread, nuts, fish, meat, and dairy products are examples of sources.

5.2.7. Sodium

Sodium is in charge of controlling the electrolyte balance and body water content. Nerves and hormones work together to maintain a balance between sodium excretion and absorption by the kidneys, which controls blood sodium levels. Additionally, the gut's ability to absorb certain nutrients and water depends on sodium. Sodium chloride (NaCl) is a common salt that contains sodium.

5.2.7.1. Deficiency

The homeostatic regulation of sodium levels in blood and tissues is similar to that of certain other minerals. The kidneys closely control the amount of sodium in urine, and when the supply is too high, they can excrete sodium in the urine or make it nearly salt-free. Sodium intakes in the UK are considered to be too high and so deficiency of sodium is unlikely but under some circumstances losses can occur:

- Excess sweating, e.g. due to exercise in a hot environment, may cause some sodium depletion.
- Diarrhea can cause fluid loss and dehydration leading to some sodium depletion.
- The kidneys normally act to protect the body's stores of sodium, but in Addison's disease failure to produce aldosterone (hormone that allows the kidneys to retain sodium and water) leads to the kidneys inability to conserve sodium.
- Renal failure: The kidneys may also lose sodium in some types of renal failure.
- Drugs: Diuretic drugs may remove large amounts of sodium in the urine.

5.2.7.2. Adverse Effects

Excessive consumption of sodium, obesity, and alcohol are thought to be among the risk factors for hypertension, or elevated blood pressure, which raises the possibility of heart disease and stroke. Hypertension may be treated with a low-sodium diet.

5.2.8. Potassium

Potassium is necessary for the equilibrium of water and electrolytes as well as the proper operation of all cells, including nerve cells. Because potassium encourages the excretion of sodium in the urine, higher dietary intakes of. this mineral have been linked to a drop in blood pressure. It has been proposed that increasing potassium intakes could mitigate the effects of some dietary sodium and safeguard cardiovascular health.

5.2.8.1. Deficiency

Low blood potassium levels (hypokalemia) can result from severe diarrhea. Symptoms include weakness, mental confusion and, if extreme, heart failure.

Low dietary potassium intakes have been observed in the UK: in the NDNS of adults about 1 in 5 women had intakes below the LRNI and in common with some other minerals, potassium intakes were lower among younger women. In the NDNS of young people, 10–15% of boys had intakes below the LRNI but among girls, about 1 in 5 11–14 year olds and about 2 in 5 15–18 year olds had intakes below the LRNI.

5.2.8.2. Adverse Effects

High additional potassium dosages can be dangerous, particularly if the kidneys aren't working well.

5.2.8.3. Food Sources

While practically everything contains potassium, some good sources include fruit (especially bananas), vegetables, meat, fish, shellfish, nuts, seeds, pulses, and milk. Generally speaking, processed foods have less than raw foods.

5.2.9. Iron

Red blood cells require iron in order to produce hemoglobin, which carries oxygen throughout the body by binding to it. Iron plays a crucial role in the immune system and is a necessary component of many enzyme reactions. It is also necessary for the regular metabolism of energy, medications, and foreign materials that the body must eliminate.

5.2.9.1. Deficiency

Iron deficiency anemia can develop as a result of the body's iron stores being depleted by a diet low in iron. Due to their higher needs than those of men of the same age, teenage girls and women who are childbearing in particular must make sure they get enough iron from their diet. Additionally, significant menstrual losses or blood loss from injuries raise the short-term need for iron. The average daily iron intake for women in all age groups—with the exception of older women (over 54 years old)—is found to be below the recommended daily iron intake (RNI), according to data from the NDNS. A very significant proportion of younger women (2 out of 5) have intakes below the LRNI i.e. intakes that are likely to be inadequate.

As the extra demand should be countered by pre-existing body stores, absence of menstrual blood loss, and the mother's increased intestinal absorptive capacity during the second and third trimesters of pregnancy, there are currently no recommendations for increasing iron intake during pregnancy. The most prevalent nutritional deficiency condition, iron deficiency anemia affects over 2 billion people globally.

5.2.9.2. Adverse Effects

As with some other minerals, under normal circumstances absorption of iron is tightly controlled as iron can have adverse effects owing to its ability to generate oxygen free radicals. However, 1 person in 200 of northern European descent is genetically predisposed to the iron loading disease hemchromatosis.

5.2.9.3. Food Sources

There are two main forms of dietary iron. Either as non-haem iron (derived from plants) or as haem iron (derived from animal sources). The most bioavailable form of iron is hem iron. Non-haem iron, which can be found in cereals, vegetables, pulses, beans, nuts, and fruit, is the main type of iron in all diets.

A number of food-related factors influence the absorption of non-hem iron. In the intestine, non-haem iron can be bound by phytate (found in cereals and pulses), fiber, tannins (found in tea), and calcium, which decreases absorption. However, when consumed concurrently with other foods, such as meat, vitamin C, which is found in fruit and vegetables, helps the body absorb non-hem iron.

5.2.10. Trace Elements

5.2.10.1. Zinc

As a cofactor for many different enzymes, zinc plays a major role in human metabolism. In a variety of reactions, zinc plays a crucial role as a catalyst. It is also necessary for cell division, which is necessary for growth, tissue repair, and normal reproductive development. It is directly or indirectly involved in the major metabolic pathways that deal with the metabolism of proteins, lipids, carbohydrates, and energy. Zinc also plays a critical role in wound healing because it is necessary for the immune system to function as well as for the structure and function of the skin.

- **Deficiency:** Although it is not certain that zinc deficiency is the only cause, delayed puberty and small stature have been related to zinc deficiency in some countries.

- **Adverse Effects:** Excess zinc in the body from very high doses can interfere with copper metabolism.
- **Food Sources:** A third of the zinc consumed in the UK comes from meat, although zinc is found in a wide variety of foods and is best absorbed from this source. Additionally, milk, cheese, eggs, seafood, wholegrain cereals, nuts, and pulses contain it. Phytates restrict the availability of zinc in cereals and pulses.

5.2.10.2. Iodine

Thyroxine and triiodothyronine, the thyroid hormones that regulate metabolic rate and both physical and mental development, require iodine as a necessary component.

- **Deficiency:** A lack of iodine causes sluggishness and swelling of the thyroid gland in the neck, which can lead to a goiter. In the UK, iodine deficiency is comparatively uncommon, but it is still a major nutritional public health concern in many other parts of the world. Children born to mothers with severe iodine deficiency may experience cretinism, or mental retardation. When it comes to low dietary intakes in the UK, the NDNS data show that 1 in 8 young women, or 12%, have intakes that are below the LRNI. This could be linked to insufficient consumption of milk and milk derivatives.
- **Adverse Effects:** Excess iodine is not absorbed so toxicity is unlikely in healthy individuals.
- **Food Sources:** The amount of iodine present in the growing plant's surroundings, which can vary greatly in the soil or water, determines the amount of iodine in plant foods like vegetables and cereal grains. Seafoods (sea fish, shellfish, and seaweed) are the only foods high in iodine, though milk is also a good source. In certain nations, specific foods, like. g. Iodine is used to fortify salt and bread.

5.2.10.3. Fluoride

The primary role of fluoride in the body is to help teeth and bones mineralize. In addition to preventing dental caries, or tooth decay, fluoride is now frequently added to the majority of toothpastes. Fluorosis can occasionally be brought on by extremely high levels of (non-dietary) fluoride. The symptoms can range from minor ones like tooth mottling and crumbling to more serious ones that cause skeletal changes like calcification of ligaments and tendons, which results in issues with the muscles, joints, and bones. Fish, tea, and fluoridated water all contain fluoride. The diet accounts for only about 25% of the total required amount. In places where the fluoride content of the water supply is low, toothpaste containing fluoride is crucial.

5.2.10.4. Copper

After iron and zinc, copper is the third most common trace metal in food. It is required for the synthesis of red and white blood cells and is a component of numerous enzymes. In addition to being necessary for the body's effective use of iron, copper is also believed to be critical for healthy bone development, immunological function, brain development, and newborn growth. Due to the abundance of copper in food and its excellent absorption efficiency, dietary-induced copper deficiency is exceedingly uncommon. However, Menke's disease, a rare genetic condition that causes the inability to absorb copper, results in skeletal and vascular issues, failure to keratinize hair, and severely impaired mental development.

Similar to certain other minerals, absorption of copper is normally strictly regulated, making copper overload extremely uncommon. Wilson's disease, a different genetic disorder, on the other hand, causes an accumulation of copper in the body, particularly in the liver and brain, and results in pathological damage because it prevents the body from excreting excess copper in bile.

5.2.10.5. Selenium

The primary role of selenium is as an ingredient in several significant antioxidant enzymes, such as e. g. glutathione peroxidase), and as a result, to shield the organism from oxidative harm. It is also required for the production of thyroid hormone, immune system function, and reproductive system function, among other uses of iodine.

The most well-known example of a selenium deficiency condition is Keshan disease, a cardiac condition that afflicts children and women who are fertile in rural China. Low levels of selenium in the soil cause the condition to persist throughout the food chain. Because there are few trustworthy biomarkers for selenium status and requirements, the implications of lower-than-DRV selenium intakes in the UK, remain unclear.

Selenium in excess is highly toxic. Brittle hair and nails, skin lesions, and a garlic-like odor on the breath are signs of selenosis, or an excess of sulfur in the body. Many foods contain selenium, but bread, eggs, meat, fish, and Brazil nuts are particularly high in the mineral. The amount of selenium in cereals is directly correlated with the amount of selenium in the soil.

5.2.10.6. Manganese

Energy metabolism and bone formation both depend on manganese. Moreover, it is a component of an antioxidant enzyme that guards against cell damage caused by free radicals.

Manganese deficiency is rarely seen. Manganese toxicity is not a problem because blood levels are carefully controlled. It is present in plant foods such as vegetables, cereals and nuts. Tea is also a rich source. In the UK, 50% of manganese intake is derived from cereals and cereal products.

5.2.10.7. Chromium

The active form of this nutrient is chromium (III), and it appears that metabolism of fats and carbohydrates is one of its primary functions. It is believed that this type of chromium helps the hormone insulin, which regulates blood glucose levels, function better. Individuals who consume enough dietary chromium have better blood lipid profiles and better blood glucose regulation. Impaired glucose tolerance is a notable feature of chromium deficiency that can be remedied with chromium supplementation. For those who were not initially deficient, chromium supplementation does not, however, improve insulin action. Chromium is not known to show toxicity. Sources of chromium include meat, nuts, cereal grains, brewer's yeast and molasses.

A Closer Look

Dietary Sources

Dietary sources reveal the wide variety of foods that provide essential nutrients necessary for optimal health and well-being. A balanced diet should include a diverse array of nutrient-rich foods from all food groups to ensure adequate intake of vitamins, minerals, protein, carbohydrates, and fats.

Fruits and vegetables are rich sources of vitamins, minerals, fiber, and phytochemicals that support overall health and reduce the risk of chronic diseases. Dark leafy greens such as spinach and kale are excellent sources of vitamin K, folate, and antioxidants, while citrus fruits like oranges and strawberries provide vitamin C and fiber. Additionally, colorful vegetables such as carrots, bell peppers, and sweet potatoes are packed with vitamins A and C, potassium, and other beneficial nutrients.

Whole grains such as oats, quinoa, brown rice, and whole wheat are important sources of complex carbohydrates, fiber, B vitamins, and minerals such as iron and magnesium. Including whole grains in the diet can help regulate blood sugar levels, promote digestive health, and reduce the risk of heart disease and type 2 diabetes.

Lean protein sources such as poultry, fish, eggs, tofu, legumes, and nuts are essential for building and repairing tissues, synthesizing hormones and enzymes, and supporting immune function. Fish, particularly fatty fish like salmon and mackerel, are rich in omega-3 fatty acids, which have anti-inflammatory properties and are beneficial for heart health and cognitive function.

Dairy products such as milk, yogurt, and cheese are excellent sources of calcium, protein, vitamin D, and other nutrients important for bone health, muscle function, and overall growth and development. For those who are lactose intolerant or prefer non-dairy options, fortified plant-based milk alternatives like soy, almond, or oat milk can provide similar nutrients.

Healthy fats found in foods such as avocados, olive oil, nuts, seeds, and fatty fish are essential for absorbing fat-soluble vitamins, supporting brain function, and reducing inflammation. Including these sources of unsaturated fats in the diet can help improve cholesterol levels and reduce the risk of heart disease. While whole, minimally processed foods should form the foundation of a healthy diet, it's also important to enjoy foods in moderation that may be higher in added sugars, saturated fats, and sodium. These include sugary snacks, processed meats, fried foods, and sweetened beverages, which should be consumed sparingly as part of an overall balanced eating pattern. In conclusion, a diverse and balanced diet that includes a variety of nutrient-rich foods from all food groups is essential for meeting the body's nutritional needs and supporting optimal health. By focusing on whole foods and minimizing intake of processed and refined products, individuals can ensure they are getting the vitamins, minerals, and other nutrients necessary for overall well-being.

Summary

- Micronutrients aid in the synthesis of macronutrients and can be found in food sources. They are necessary in small amounts although still essential for good health. A deficiency in a micronutrient can cause serious health issues.
- Water-soluble vitamins (as oppose to fat-soluble vitamins) are not stored in the body, it absorbs what it needs and then it usually excretes the excess in your urine. Due to the fact that they cannot be stored, the body needs a continuous supply through a steady daily intake.
- Riboflavin is the only water-soluble vitamin used as a food coloring. In fact, it is named for its color — the Latin word *flavus* means "yellow."
- Most are water-soluble, meaning they dissolve in water. In contrast, the fat-soluble vitamins are similar to oil and do not dissolve in water. Fat-soluble vitamins are most abundant in high-fat foods and are much better absorbed into your bloodstream when you eat them with fat.
- Vitamin D is produced naturally in the human body when the skin is exposed to the sun. Vitamin D aids in bone health and development.
- Vitamin E is an antioxidant that can help the body destroy free radicals. Free radicals are unstable atoms that may cause the formation of cancer cells. As such, vitamin E could play an important part in preventing cancer.
- Vitamin K plays a key role in blood clotting. Without it, you would run the risk of bleeding to death.
- Minerals constitute one of two major classes of biologically critical micronutrients required for normal health and development of humans. The other class are the vitamins. Humans must consume both macronutrients (the major sources of calories: fats, carbohydrates, proteins) and micronutrients in order to maintain virtually all metabolic and developmental processes.

References

1. Berdanier, C., Berdanier, L., & Zempleni, J. (2009). *Advanced Nutrition: Macronutrients, Micronutrients, and Metabolism.* Boca Raton, FL: CRC Press, Taylor & Francis Group.
2. National Academy Press. (2000). *Dietary Reference Intakes for Vitamin C, Vitamin E, Selenium, and Carotenoids.* Washington, DC.
3. Duyff, A.D.A. (2006). *American Dietetic Association: Complete Food and Nutrition Guide.* Hoboken, NJ: John Wiley & Sons, Inc.
4. Duyff, R. (2012). *American Dietetic Association: Complete Food and Nutrition Guide.* Hoboken, NJ: John Wiley & Sons, Inc.
5. Gropper, S., & Smith, J. (2009). *Advanced Nutrition and Human Metabolism.* Belmont, CA: Wadsworth, Cengage Learning.
6. Holick, M., & Chen, T. (2008). Vitamin D deficiency: a worldwide problem with health consequences. *American Journal of Clinical Nutrition, 87*(4), 1080–1086.

7. Institute of Medicine (US). (2000). *Dietary Reference Intakes for Vitamin C, Vitamin E, Selenium, and Carotenoids.* Washington, DC: National Academy Press.

8. Institute of Medicine (US). (2002). *Dietary Reference Intakes for Vitamin A, Vitamin K, Arsenic, Boron, Chromium, Copper, Iodine, Iron, Manganese, Molybdenum, Nickel, Silicon, Vanadium, and Zinc.* Washington, DC: National Academy Press.

9. Wessells, K. R., & Brown, K. H. (2013). Estimating the global prevalence of zinc deficiency: Results based on zinc availability in national food supplies and the prevalence of stunting. *PLoS ONE, 7*(11), e50568.

10. Zimmermann, M. B. (2009). Iodine deficiency. *Endocrine Reviews, 30*(4), 376–408.

11. Zimmermann, M. B., & Andersson, M. (2012). Assessment of iodine nutrition in populations: past, present, and future. *Nutrition Reviews, 70*(10), 553–570.

12. Adrogue, H. J., & Madias, N. E. (2000). Hypernatremia. *The New England Journal of Medicine, 342*, 1493–1499.

13. Alexander, M. F., Fawcett, J. N., & Runciman, P. J. (2006). *Nursing Practice: Hospital and Home: The Adult* (3rd ed.). Edinburgh: Elsevier Churchill Livingstone.

14. Atkinson, M., & McHanwell, S. (2002). *Basic Medical Science for Speech and Language Therapy Students.* London: Whurr.

15. Institute of Medicine. (2004). *Dietary reference intakes for water, potassium, sodium, chloride, and sulfate.* Washington: The National Academies Press.

16. Maughan, R. J., & Griffin, J. (2003). Caffeine ingestion and fluid balance: a review. *Journal of Human Nutrition and Dietetics, 16*, 411–420.

17. Metheny, N. (2000). *Fluid and electrolyte balance.* Philadelphia: Lippincott Williams & Wilkins.

18. Metheny, N. (2012). *Fluid and Electrolyte Balance* (5th ed.). Sudbury, MA: Jones & Bartlett Learning.

19. Shirreffs, S. M. (2005). The importance of good hydration for work and exercise performance. *Nutrition Reviews, 63*, S14–S21.

20. Shirreffs, S. M., Cheuvront, S., et al. (2004). Fluid and electrolyte needs for the preparation and recovery from training and competition. *Journal of Sports Sciences, 22*, 57–63.

21. Ganong, W. F. (2005). *Review of medical physiology* (22nd ed.). Lange Medical Books/McGraw-Hill.

22. Giebisch, G., Klose, R. M., & Windhager, E. E. (2003). *Kidney physiology and pathophysiology.* Lippincott Williams & Wilkins.

23. Huang, C. L., & Kuo, E. (2007). Mechanism of hypokalemia in magnesium deficiency. *Journal of the American Society of Nephrology, 18*(10), 2649–2652.

24. Kurtz, I. (2010). Regulation of electrolyte balance. In Seldin and Giebisch's *The Kidney* (4th ed., pp. 305–342). Academic Press.

25. Lang, F., & Vallon, V. (2012). Potassium homeostasis and renal potassium transport: implications for pathogenesis and treatment of potassium depletion and hypokalemia. *Journal of the American Society of Nephrology, 23*(5), 595–605.

26. Nijenhuis, T., Vallon, V., & van der Kemp, A. W. (2005). Enhanced passive Ca2+ reabsorption and reduced Mg2+ channel abundance explains thiazide-induced hypocalciuria and hypomagnesemia. *Journal of Clinical Investigation, 115*(6), 1651–1658.

27. Palmer, B. F., & Clegg, D. J. (2014). Electrolyte and acid–base disturbances in patients with Diabetes Mellitus. *New England Journal of Medicine, 2015*(373), 548–559.

28. Pham, P. C., Pham, P. A., Pham, S. V., Pham, P. T., Pham, P. M., & Pham, P. T. (2017). Hypomagnesemia: a clinical perspective. *International Journal of Nephrology and Renovascular Disease, 10*, 219–230.

29. Sebastian, A., & Morris, R. C. (2007). Hypomagnesemia and potassium depletion. *New England Journal of Medicine, 357*(17), 1736–1737.

30. Sica, D. A. (2006). Diuretic use in renal disease. *Nature Reviews Nephrology, 2*(12), 632–644.

31. Skou, J. C. (2003). The identification of the sodium pump. *Biochimica et Biophysica Acta (BBA)-Biomembranes, 1617*(1–2), 6–11.

32. Verbalis, J. G. (2007). Disorders of body water homeostasis. *Best Practice & Research Clinical Endocrinology & Metabolism, 21*(1), 27–41.

33. Voets, T., Nilius, B., & Hoefs, S. (2004). TRPM6 forms the Mg2+ influx channel involved in intestinal and renal Mg2+ absorption. *Journal of Biological Chemistry, 279*(1), 19–25.

34. Weiner, I. D., & Verlander, J. W. (2011). Renal ammonia metabolism and transport. *Comprehensive Physiology, 3*(1), 201–220.

35. Wingo, C. S., & Smolka, A. J. (2005). Renal regulation of potassium homeostasis. *Comprehensive Physiology, 5*(1), 237–283.

Chapter 6

WATER AND ELECTROLYTES

Contents

Unit Introduction

The most prevalent material in the body is water, which is the main constituent of bodily fluids. Numerous physiological functions, including digestion, nutrient absorption and utilization, distribution, waste excretion, perfusion, and hemodynamic maintenance, depend on water. Fluid and electrolyte homeostasis is maintained by intricate systems that guarantee optimal operation. From birth to adulthood, pediatric patients experience rapid growth and development that is linked to altered pharmacokinetics. In order to prevent fluid and electrolyte imbalances, maintain a patient's fluid balance, and maximize pharmacotherapy, it is imperative to comprehend these continuous dynamic changes. For instance, by changing the volume of distribution, total body water (TBW) and hydration state impact the pharmacokinetics of drugs. For some drugs, electrolytes can also have an impact on drug therapy, or vice versa. This chapter covers specific electrolyte abnormalities in pediatric patients as well as the homeostasis and therapeutic management of fluids and electrolytes in a variety of pediatric populations.

Orientation and Directional Terms

Term	Definition	Illustration
Water conservation	Water conservation is the practice of using water efficiently to reduce unnecessary water usage. According to Fresh Water Watch, water conservation is important because fresh clean water is a limited resource, as well as a costly one.	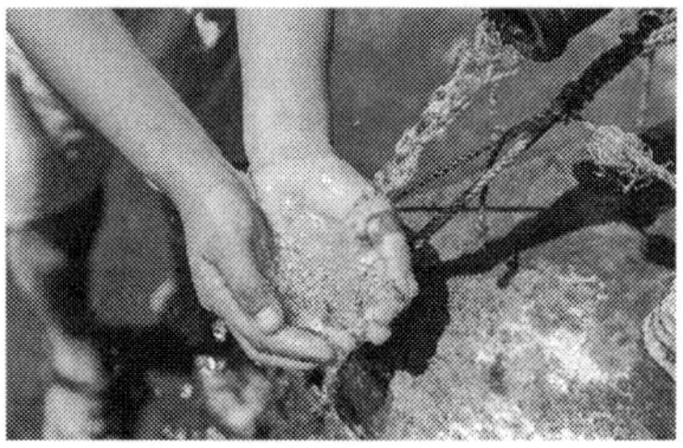
Plasma osmolality	Plasma osmolality measures the body's electrolyte-water balance. There are several methods for arriving at this quantity through measurement or calculation.	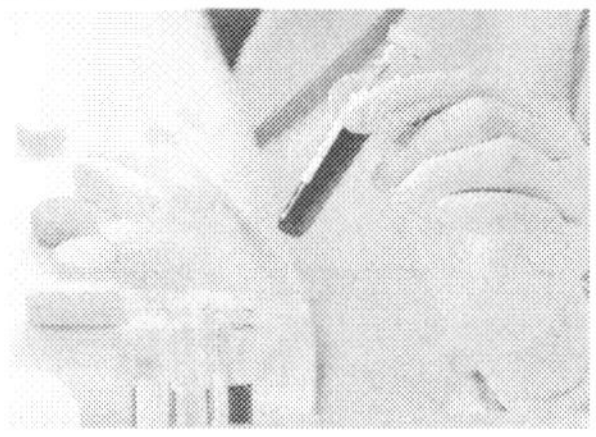
Sodium ions	Sodium ions are necessary for regulation of blood and body fluids, transmission of nerve impulses, heart activity, and certain metabolic functions.	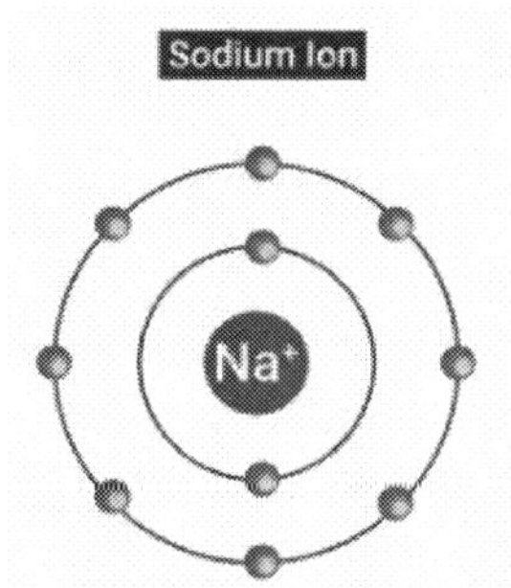
Osmosis	Osmosis is the spontaneous net movement or diffusion of solvent molecules through a selectively-permeable membrane from a region of high water potential to a region of low water potential, in the direction that tends to equalize the solute concentrations on the two sides.	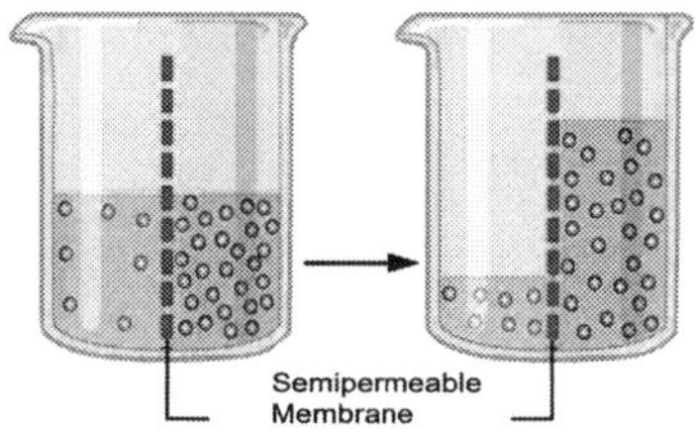

6.1. Body Fluids and Fluid Compartments

Living things undergo chemical reactions in aqueous solutions. Solutes are the materials that dissolve in a solution.

Solutes in the human body can vary depending on the area of the body, but they can include proteins, which are involved in the transportation of lipids, carbohydrates, and—most importantly—electrolytes.

An electrolyte is a term used frequently in medicine to describe a mineral that has separated from a salt and contains an ion, or electrical charge. Electrolytes, for example, include sodium ions (Na^+) and chloride ions (Cl^-).

Osmosis is the process by which water travels throughout the body's compartments and through semi-permeable cell membranes. Osmosis is essentially the diffusion of water through a semi-permeable membrane along an osmotic gradient from areas of higher concentration to regions of lower concentration.

Depending on the relative concentrations of water and solutes present, water will enter and exit cells and tissues. To guarantee proper function, the solutes inside and outside of cells must be kept in the proper balance.

6.1.1. Body Water Content

The majority of human body mass is made up of water, which ranges from roughly 75% in newborns to between 50% and 60% in adults for both sexes, and as low as 45% in old age.

Because the percentage of the body devoted to each organ, as well as to muscles, fat, bone, and other tissues, varies from infancy to adulthood, the percentage of body water also varies with development (Figure 6.1). Nearly 80 to 85% of the mass of your kidneys and brain is made up of water. Teeth, on the other hand, contain the least amount of water—between 8 and 10%.

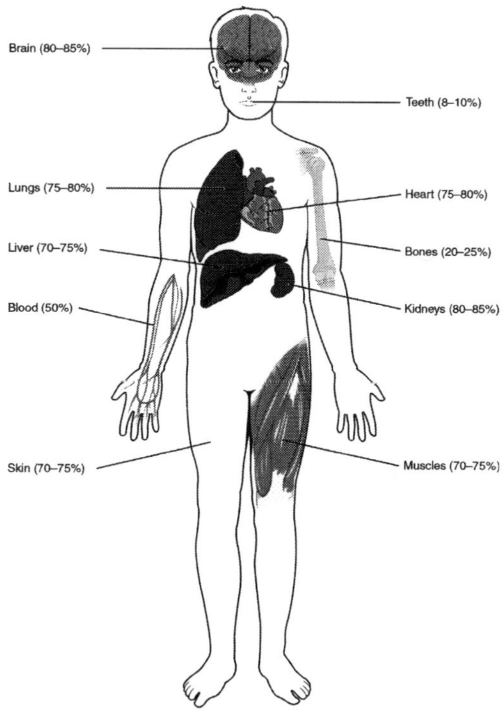

Figure 6.1. *Water content of the body's organs and tissues. Water content varies in different body organs and tissues, from as little as 8% in the teeth to as much as 85% in the brain.*

Source: https://encrypted-tbn0.gstatic.com/images?q=tbn:ANd9GcT1OTDDxbHLA_C4EQP7ch5AEjIbaK9VclxJl7Z2fIX0xw&s.

6.1.2. Fluid Compartments

Body fluids are referred to in terms of their own fluid compartment, which is primarily isolated from other compartments by a physical barrier. All fluid that is encased in cells by their plasma membranes is part of the ICF compartment. Every cell in the body is surrounded by ECF. The two main components of ECF are the ISF, which envelops all cells not in the bloodstream, and the fluid component of blood called plasma (Figure 6.2).

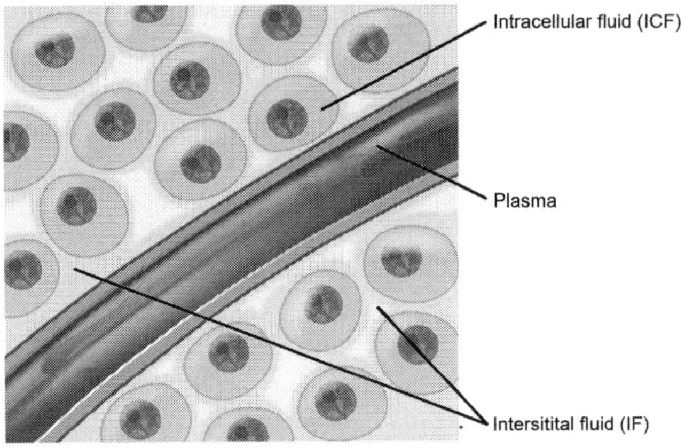

Figure 6.2. Fluid compartments in the human body. The intracellular fluid (ICF) is the fluid within cells. The interstitial fluid (IF) is part of the extracellular fluid (ECF) between the cells. Blood plasma is the second part of the ECF. Materials travel between cells and the plasma in capillaries through the IF.

Source: https://courses.lumenlearning.com/suny-ap2/chapter/body-fluids-and-fluid-compartments-no-content/.

6.1.2.1. Intracellular Fluid

The ICF is the main part of the cytosol and cytoplasm and is found inside cells. An adult male of average size has an ICF that holds approximately 25 L (seven gallons) of fluid, or roughly 60% of the total water in the human body (Figure 6.3).

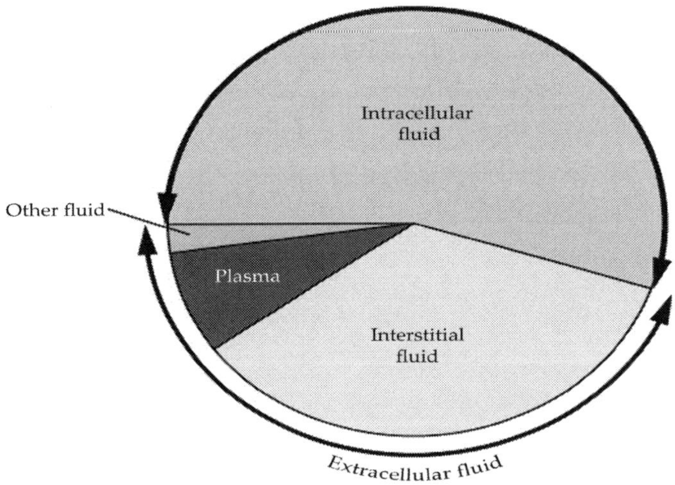

Figure 6.3. A pie graph showing the proportion of total body fluid in each of the body's fluid compartments. Most of the water in the body is intracellular fluid. The second largest volume is the interstitial fluid, which surrounds cells that are not blood cells.

Source: https://textimgs.s3.amazonaws.com/osanp/m46411/2703_Distribution_of_Water_in_the_Human_Body_in_Terms_of_ICF_and_ECF_Pie_Chart.jpg.

The fluid volume in living cells is usually highly stable due to the tight regulation of water content. A cytosol becomes too concentrated with solutes to support regular cellular functions when the volume of water inside the cell drops too low; conversely, when a cell absorbs too much water, it may burst and perish.

6.1.2.2. Extracellular Fluid

The remaining one-third of the body's water content is made up of the ECF. The plasma contains about 20% of the ECF. A variety of substances, including blood cells, proteins (such as clotting factors and antibodies), electrolytes, nutrients, gases, and waste products, are transported by plasma as it passes through blood vessels in the body.

Through the IF, gases, nutrients, and waste products move between capillaries and cells. A selectively permeable cell membrane that keeps materials from passing through between the IF and the inside of the cell divides cells from the IF. There are more water-based ECF in the body. These consist of the aqueous humor of the eye, lymph, pleural fluid in the pleural cavities, pericardial fluid in the cardiac sac, lymph, the cerebrospinal fluid that surrounds the brain and spinal cord, and synovial fluid in joints. These fluids are also regarded as elements of the ECF compartment because they are not contained within cells.

6.1.3. Composition of Body Fluids

The two ECF components—the IF and the plasma—have compositions that are more similar to one another than they are to the ICF (Figure 6.4). High levels of sodium, chloride, bicarbonate, and protein are found in blood plasma.

The IF has comparatively low protein concentrations but high sodium, chloride, and bicarbonate concentrations. On the other hand, the ICF has higher than normal levels of magnesium, potassium, phosphate, and protein. All things considered, the ICF has high potassium and phosphate (HPO_4^{2-}) concentrations, while the plasma and the ECF both have high sodium and chloride concentrations.

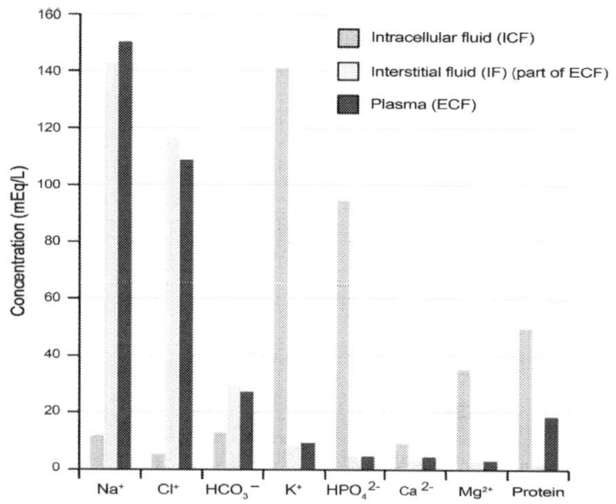

Figure 6.4. *The concentrations of different elements in key bodily fluids. The graph shows the composition of the ICF, IF, and plasma. The compositions of plasma and IF are similar to one another but are quite different from the composition of the ICF.*

Source: https://courses.lumenlearning.com/suny-ap2/chapter/body-fluids-and-fluid-compartments-no-content/.

The majority of bodily fluids have no charge. As a result, the balance of positively charged ions, or cations, and negatively charged ions, or anions, exists in fluids. Potassium (K^+) ions are concentrated inside cells, while sodium (Na^+) and chloride (Cl^-) ions are concentrated in the body's ECF. The high potassium and low sodium levels in the ICF are sustained by sodium-potassium pumps in the cell membranes, despite the fact that both potassium and sodium can "leak" through "pores" into and out of cells, respectively. These pumps move potassium into the cell and sodium out of the cell using the energy provided by ATP (Figure 6.5).

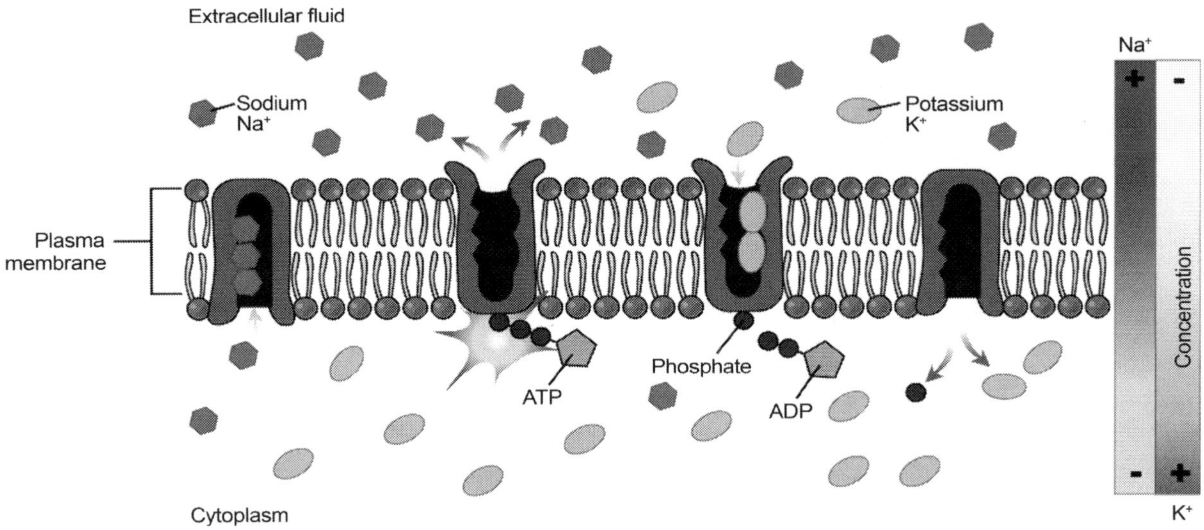

Figure 6.5. *The sodium-potassium pump. The sodium-potassium pump is powered by ATP to transfer sodium out of the cytoplasm and into the ECF. The pump also transfers potassium out of the ECF and into the cytoplasm.*

Source: https://courses.lumenlearning.com/suny-ap2/chapter/body-fluids-and-fluid-compartments-no-content/.

6.1.4. The Importance of Water in Vitality

When you wake up in the morning, you drink coffee, drive, clean the dirt off your windshield, flush wastes down the toilet, take a shower, and brush your teeth. You drive home, make dinner, use the restroom numerous times, eat lunch and wash it down with a glass of water, all while standing next to a fountain. The countless uses that water has in the human body are far greater than the sum of all the ways you use it on a daily basis. Water is the most important nutrient since it can be fatally absent in a matter of days. Numerous mechanisms have been adapted by organisms to conserve water.

The four basic roles that water plays in the human body are as a transportation medium, a lubricant/shock absorber, a medium for chemical reactions, and a temperature regulator.

6.1.4.1. Water as a Transportation Vehicle

Water is referred to as the "universal solvent" due to the fact that it dissolves more substances than any other fluid. Because hydrogen and oxygen molecules can form slack bonds with other molecules, molecules can dissolve in water. Substances are encircled by water molecules (H_2O), which suspend them in a sea of water molecules. Water acts as a solvent, making it easier to move materials around. It would be difficult to move a glob of fat, a bubble of gas, or a pile of undissolved salt through tissues. Approximately 78% of blood, the body's main transport fluid, is made of water. Proteins, lipoproteins, glucose, electrolytes, and metabolic waste products like urea and carbon dioxide are among the materials dissolved in blood. These materials are either taken up by the blood's aqueous environment and transported to cells for essential functions, or they are eliminated from cells to avoid waste accumulation and toxicity. In addition to serving as the body's principal means of transportation, blood serves as the structural support for blood vessels that would burst without it. In a similar vein, the brain is composed of 75% water, which gives it structure.

6.1.4.2. Water as a Medium for Chemical Reactions

Even the simplest chemical reactions require water. Enzymes need a medium to carry out their unique chemical reactions after they are formed, and in all organisms, that medium is water. Because it is electrically neutral, has a pH of 7.0, which means it is neither acidic nor basic, and can store a lot of heat, water is a perfect medium for chemical reactions. Water also functions as an agent to break or form bonds in many enzymatic reactions by being taken out of molecules.

6.1.4.3. Water as a Lubricant/Shock Absorber

Although many people find sneezing's slimy byproducts repulsive, sneezing is a necessary respiratory function that requires water to occur. More than 90% of mucus is made up of water, which is necessary for breathing, the movement of nutrients through the digestive tract, and the evacuation of waste products through the rectum in addition to being necessary for the discharge of nasal irritants. The first line of defense against harm and outside invaders is mucus. It has immune system cells that eliminate pathogens, traps pathogens, and shields tissues from irritants. The primary ingredient in the lubricating fluid that coats joints and facilitates the movement of articulated bones is water.

The fluids that surround the brain and spinal cord and the extra space in the eyes, known as the aqueous and vitreous humors, and cerebrospinal fluid, are mostly composed of water and act as a cushion for these organs against abrupt changes in their surroundings. The watery fluids that envelop the organs offer mechanical and chemical defense. Water fills the amniotic sac of a pregnant woman just two weeks after fertilization, protecting the developing embryo.

6.1.4.4. Water as a Temperature Regulator

Body water is essential for maintaining homeostasis in the body's thermoregulation, which is the process of balancing heat intake and heat output. The body's set temperature is 98.6°F (37°C), which is the narrow range of temperatures within which human life is supported. Enzymes become inactive in extremes of temperature, which slows down metabolism. Muscle failure and hypothermia occur at 82.4%F (28°C). The central nervous system fails and death ensues at the opposite extreme of 111.2°F (44.4°C). Because water has a high heat capacity, it can retain heat well and helps the body's temperature stabilize even in the face of environmental changes.

The body uses a number of mechanisms to transfer body water from one location to another in order to distribute heat and maintain a consistent body temperature (Figure 6.6). The thermoregulatory center of the brain is the hypothalamus. Blood temperature is detected by unique protein sensors found in the hypothalamus. Additionally, temperature sensors in the skin react fast to changes in the immediate environment. A neural signal is transmitted to the hypothalamus in response to cold sensors in the skin. The hypothalamus then transmits a signal to the smooth muscle tissue surrounding blood vessels, causing the blood vessels to constrict and decrease blood flow. As a result, less heat is lost to the surroundings. The hypothalamus also triggers the endocrine glands, such as the thyroid, to release hormones that can speed up metabolism, and it instructs muscles to tense their muscles and tremble. By doing these things, you promote heat conservation and encourage the body to produce more heat when the temperature drops.

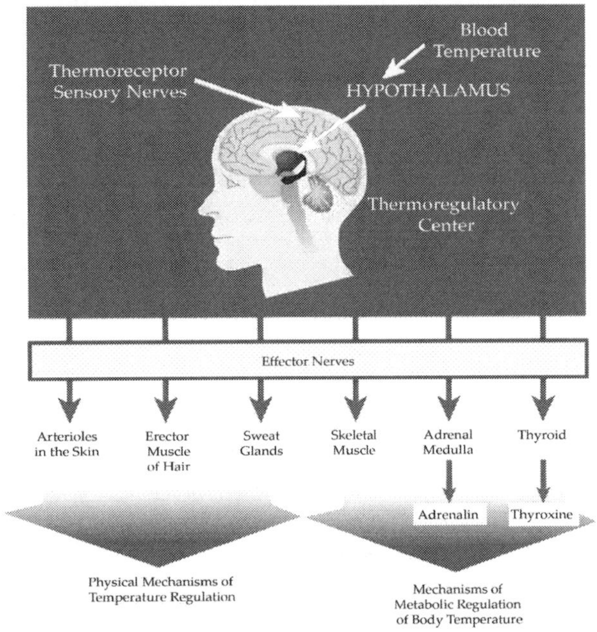

Figure 6.6. *Thermoregulation is the ability of an organism to maintain body temperature despite changing environmental temperatures.*

Source: https://pressbooks.oer.hawaii.edu/humannutrition/chapter/waters-importance-to-vitality/.

The hypothalamus senses an increase in blood temperature when body temperature rises, as it does during exercise. The smooth muscle in blood vessels dilates as a result of a signal sent by the hypothalamus to this effect, increasing blood flow to the body's periphery.

Extra heat is expelled from the body through perspiration, or sweat, which is made up of 98–99% water once it reaches the skin.

The body cools as a result of the energy-intensive process of water on the skin's surface evaporating and losing heat. Perspiration is a process that combines fluid and electrolyte homeostasis with temperature homeostasis. Maintaining fluid and electrolyte balance requires replacing lost water and electrolytes through perspiration.

6.1.5. Composition of Body Fluids

6.1.5.1. Fluid Distribution/Total Body Water

The proportion of TBW to body weight varies from childhood to adulthood and is influenced by age, weight, sex, and body fat percentage (Table 6.1).

TBW is separated into three compartments: TCF (e.g., synovial, pleural, CSFs), ECF, and intracellular fluid (ICF). Because the percentage of TCF is low (e.g., 1.5%–2.5% of TBW) and does not significantly contribute to fluid losses, this compartment will not be a focus of further discussion.

Throughout life, the ECF/ICF ratio fluctuates, with an earlier ECF/ICF ratio during development. Age-related changes in muscle mass, cellular growth, hydration status, nutritional status, and renal function/urinary output are secondary to variations in the ECF/ICF ratio.

The ECF/ICF ratio can also change due to clinical status and disease states like protein-losing enteropathy, liver failure, and nephrotic syndrome.

Approximately two thirds of TBW by adolescence/adulthood go to the ICF, with the remaining portion going to the ECF.

75% of the fluid in the ECF is located in the interstitial fluid compartment (i.e. 25% circulating intravascularly, and the remaining 25% passing between cells in the extravascular space (Figure 6.7). Born Wet, Human Babies Are 75% Water was an NPR segment that highlighted the shifting composition of TBW.

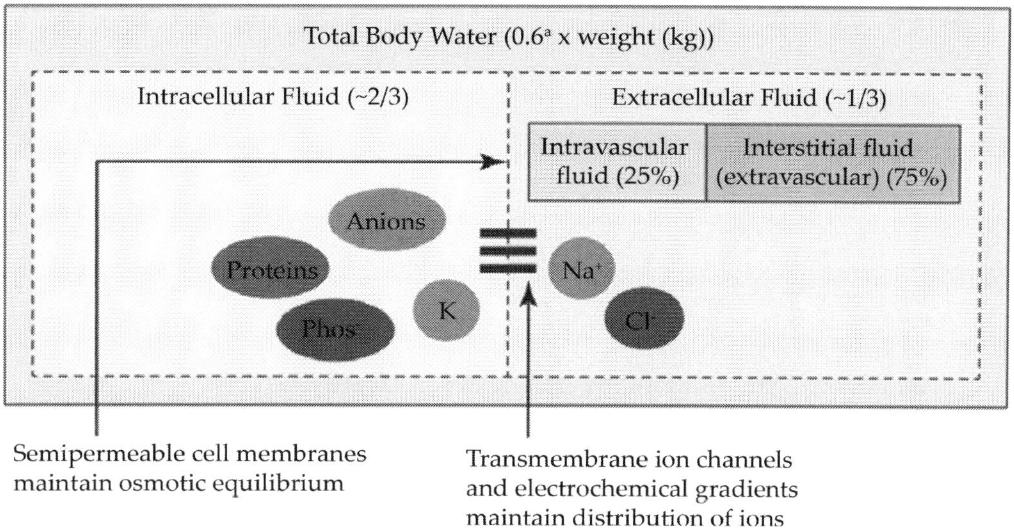

Figure 6.7. *Body distribution of fluid and solutes in adolescents/adults.*

Source: https://courses.minia.edu.eg/Attach/8429Med%20Post%20Pharma%20(1).pdf.

6.1.5.2. Osmotic Equilibrium

The body uses three main principles to maintain osmotic equilibrium: capillary permeability, oncotic pressure, and hydrostatic pressure.

The main extracellular cation, potassium, and the sodium-potassium-adenosine triphosphatase (Na^+-K^+-ATPase) pump, which uses cellular energy to maintain sodium and potassium concentrations, outweigh variations in the composition of solutes. Osmotic pressure controls the flow of water between the ECF and ICF. Semipermeable membranes that preserve osmotic equilibrium and transmembrane ion channels and electrochemical gradients are two factors influencing this distribution. Large anions and proteins pass through cellular membranes relatively easily, but water passes through them freely.

Osmolality is the concentration of all solutes in a given weight of water. Sodium, glucose, and urea are the primary osmoles in blood, leading to the following equation for calculating osmolality:

calculated serum osmolality

$$= 2\ Na^+\ \frac{mmol}{L} + \frac{glucose\ \frac{mg}{dL}}{18} + \frac{BUN\ \frac{mg}{dL}}{2.8}$$

The normal range for serum osmolality is 275–295 mOsm/kg. Hyperosmolality occurs when there is not enough water compared to solute in the ECF, resulting in a serum osmolality greater than 295 mOsm/kg. This can be caused by reduced water intake or increased water excretion and may be related to conditions such as diabetes insipidus, osmoreceptor dysregulation, acute tubular necrosis, burns, GI illness, or iatrogenic factors. Hypoosmolality, on the other hand, occurs when there is an excess of water compared to solute in the ECF, leading to a serum osmolality < 275 mOsm/kg. This can be due to increased TBW, depletion of body solutes, or a combination of the two. Common causes of hypoosmolality include a syndrome of inappropriate antidiuretic hormone (ADH) secretion, salt-losing nephropathy, diuretic use, mineralocorticoid deficiencies, GI illnesses, nephrotic syndrome, heart failure, and cirrhosis.

Table 6.1. *Age-Related Changes in TBW*

	Neonate (% body weight)	Infant (% body weight)	1 Yr (% body weight)	Adolescent/ Adult (% body weight)
TBW	23–27 wk GA: 85–90 28–32 wk GA: 82–85 36–40 wk GA: 71–76	~70	~60	~60 (male) ~55 (female)
Extracellular fluid	23–27 wk GA: 60–70 28–32 wk GA: 50–60 36–40 wk GA: ~40	~70	~55	~30
Intracellular fluid	23–27 wk GA: 30–40 28–32 wk GA: 40–50 36–40 wk GA: 60	~30	~45	~70
Transcellular fluid	~2.5	~2	~1.8	~1.7

GA = gestational age; TBW = total body water.

Source: https://courses.minia.edu.eg/Attach/8429Med%20Post%20Pharma%20(1).pdf.

6.1.5.3. Fluid Regulation (Hypervolemia/Hypovolemia)

The metabolism of water is equilibrium between intake and output. Water produced by the oxidation of consumed macronutrients is one type of intake; other factors include ingested water from foods and beverages and regulated factors like drinking water when thirsty. A rise in serum tonicity, the release of angiotensin II, the activation of osmoreceptors in the anterior hypothalamus, and baroreceptor activation all contribute to the feeling of thirst. The primary control mechanism for the metabolism of water is excretion. Water is lost through sensible losses like urine excretion as well as insensible losses through the skin, respiratory system, and gastrointestinal tract. Hydraulic feedback from the renin-angiotensin-aldosterone system (RAAS), ADH/arginine vasopressin (AVP), and other substances like prostaglandins and natriuretic peptides is the primary driver of water output.

Hypovolemia, defined as a decrease in TBW, causes an increased serum osmolarity, which results in the release of two hormones: AVP and aldosterone. Arginine vasopressin is synthesized in the hypothalamus and stored in the pituitary. Arginine vasopressin is superbly sensitive, with small alterations in serum osmolality (e.g., 1%) leading to large, minute-to-minute changes in AVP release and physiologic responses.

The AVP V2 receptors on the kidneys interact with the AVP that is secreted by the posterior pituitary. Increased free water reabsorption results from this interaction's stimulation of aquaporin 2 channel insertion on the collecting tubules' luminal surface. The RAAS also facilitates the release of aldosterone. Renin is released in response to a low ECF, and this process changes angiotensin I into angiotensin II. In the distal convoluted tubules of the kidneys, angiotensin II causes vasoconstriction and the release of aldosterone, which results in the reabsorption of salt and water. Hypovolemia can arise from various clinical scenarios, such as hemorrhaging or losing blood, gastrointestinal disorders like vomiting and/or diarrhea, burns, excessive perspiration or diuresis, and diabetes insipidus. In these situations, the disease state outweighs the body's natural capacity to control volume.

Decreased serum osmolality and decreased AVP concentrations are the results of hypervolemia, characterized by an increase in TBW. Under normal conditions, hypervolemia causes the kidneys to excrete more water and reduce thirst. However, hypervolemia does not prevent AVP in some clinical circumstances, such as heart failure, which leads to hyponatremia and further volume expansion. Additional conditions that can lead to hypervolemia include sepsis, kidney or liver failure, and syndrome of inappropriate ADH secretion.

6.1.6. Fluid Considerations: Historical Perspective and Maintenance Requirements

All patients must receive maintenance fluid therapy in order to maintain fluid homeostasis. The primary goal of maintenance fluid therapy is to replenish normal, continuous physiological losses with an appropriate amount of fluid. Maintenance fluid therapy does not offer nutritional support or makes up for losses that have already occurred or are still occurring. Children have higher maintenance fluid requirements (ml/kg/day) than adult patients due to higher respiratory rates, higher body surface area-to-weight ratios, and higher metabolic rates. The amount of maintenance fluid needed can be estimated using a variety of techniques. In actuality, though, the Holliday-Segar and 4-2-1 approaches (*see* Table 6.2) are the most often applied ones nowadays. The patient's underlying clinical condition must be considered in individualized and tailored therapy for overall fluid requirements, even though these calculations are reasonable for providing estimates of fluid requirements. Fluid requirements are increased by a few conditions, including hypermetabolic states, burn injuries, and gastroschisis. Certain illnesses, like heart or respiratory problems, reduce the need for fluids. To start with, estimates of maintenance fluid needs are used, and then fluid therapy is closely monitored (e.g. laboratory results, vital signs, clinical indicators, and volume status symptoms), as well as adjustments based on each patient's response to treatment.

Table 6.2. *Common Methods to Estimate Maintenance Fluid Requirements in Pediatric Patients*

Method to Estimate Maintenance Fluid Needs	Details	Pros	Cons
Holliday-Segar (daily requirement)	0–10 kg: 100 mL/kg/day > 10 kg to ≤ 20 kg: [1000 mL + (50 mL x each kg > 10 kg)]/day > 20 kg: [1500 mL + (20 mL x each kg > 20 kg)]/day	Simple calculation	Does not account for abnormal clinical circumstances
4-2-1 (hourly requirement)	0–10 kg: 4 mL/kg/hr > 10 kg to ≤ 20 kg: 40 mL/hr + (2 mL/hr x each kg > 10 kg) > 20 kg: 60 mL/hr + (1 mL/hr x each kg > 20 kg)		

Source: https://courses.minia.edu.eg/Attach/8429Med%20Post%20Pharma%20(1).pdf.

6.1.6.1. Special Population Consideration: Neonates

In a neonatal patient, fluid homeostasis needs to consider both the demands of fast growth and development as well as the shift from intrauterine to extrauterine existence. The placenta controls the fluid and electrolyte balance during fetal development; the neonate is responsible for maintaining this balance after birth. To adjust to this shift, premature neonates rely on developing organ and hormone systems. During the early neonatal period, challenges that need to be taken into consideration include maintaining nutrition and hydration, preventing dehydration, and avoiding fluid overload.

Both gestational age and intrauterine growth affect postnatal adaptation. Under normal physiological conditions, the kidneys excrete water and sodium through natriuresis and diuresis during the first 24 to 48 hours of the early postnatal period. Body weight is reduced by 5–15% as a result of the contraction of the ECF due to water loss. Along with immature skin barriers and a higher body surface area/weight ratio, premature neonates and/or small for gestational age have a higher percentage of TBW. As a result, the birth weight and gestational age have an inverse relationship with the percentage of weight loss. The reduced incidence rates of prematurity-related complications like patent ductus arteriosus, necrotizing enterocolitis, bronchopulmonary dysplasia, and intracranial hemorrhage—all of which are linked to poor neurodevelopmental outcomes—are a result of the processes of natriuresis and diuresis. Therefore, one of the objectives of fluid and electrolyte therapy in the neonatal period is to permit these processes to take place in order to prevent fluid retention and related problems. With careful volume and electrolyte provision, complications related to fluid retention can be avoided.

Delivery volume must consider neonatal renal function, which is dependent on their degree of prematurity. Nephrogenesis starts at 4–5 weeks gestation during fetal development, but nephron development does not start until 20–22 weeks gestation and ends at 34–35 weeks gestation. Along with their low response to aldosterone, high ECF volume, and tubular immaturity, newborns are also unable to expel excess fluid and electrolytes. During the neonatal stage, volume provision is also influenced by outside variables. For the premature neonate, incubators and radiant warmers offer a thermoregulated environment; nevertheless, they may also result in higher insensible water losses. Additionally, phototherapy impacts insensible water loss. These difficulties can be solved by changing the environment's humidity level or the fluid therapy to compensate for the extra losses.

It is best to delay giving electrolytes until after renal function has been established. For the previously mentioned reasons, early sodium administration should be avoided until renal function is established as it can cause fluid retention. There are some exceptions, such as gastroschisis, where fetal fluid loss causes infants to be born deficient in sodium. Potassium shouldn't be added to newborn fluids until the urinary output is established in order to prevent hyperkalemia and the problems that come with it. Moreover, hypoglycemia in newborn patients can be dangerous. One of the most dangerous consequences of hypoglycemia is neurodevelopmental impairment, which can happen if the condition is not treated. Thus, to maintain euglycemia during the neonatal period, a higher dextrose content is needed. Within the first 24 to 48 hours, restricted volumes (60–100 mL/kg/day) of 10% dextrose without additional electrolytes are usually administered as a fluid. Fluid volume can be liberalized and sodium, potassium, and other electrolytes can be carefully added once renal function and diuresis have occurred.

6.2. Water Balance

An adult will typically consume about 2500 mL, or nearly 3 quarts, of aqueous fluid in a single day. About 230 mL (8 ounces) are produced metabolically each day during the final stages of aerobic respiration, even though the majority of intake passes through the digestive tract.

Furthermore, the body loses roughly the same amount of water (2,500 mL) every day through a variety of pathways; the majority of this water is eliminated as urine. The kidneys' mechanisms for removing water from the filtrate and urine allow them to also regulate blood volume. The kidneys have the ability to control the body's water balance. If you are dehydrated, they can help you retain water by diluting your urine, which can help you eliminate extra water when needed. Water is lost through the skin as a result of air being exhaled from the lungs and evaporating from the skin's surface without obvious sweating. Because a person is typically unaware of this type of water loss, it is referred to as insensible water loss.

6.2.1. Regulation of Water Intake

The ratio of solutes to solvent volume in a solution is known as osmolality. Thus, the ratio of solutes to water in blood plasma is known as plasma osmolality. A person's level of hydration is indicated by their plasma osmolality value. A healthy body uses a number of processes to control the intake and output of water in order to keep plasma osmolality within a specific range. It is thought that drinking water is optional. Now that we know how the body controls water intake, let us look at an example of someone who is dehydrated—a person who has lost a net amount of water, leaving their blood and other tissues with inadequate levels of water. Blood plasma contains the water expelled from the body, such as sweat, urine, or exhaled air. A series of physiological processes known as the thirst response are set off when the blood becomes more concentrated (Figure 6.8). Osmoreceptors are sensory receptors in the hypothalamic thirst center that track the blood's solute concentration, or osmolality. Sensation of thirst is brought on by signals sent by the hypothalamus when blood osmolality rises above optimal levels. Drinking water is the appropriate (and typical) response for the individual. ADH is also released by the hypothalamus of a dehydrated individual through the posterior pituitary gland. By instructing the kidneys to extract water from urine, ADH essentially dilutes blood plasma. A dehydrated person's hypothalamus also signals their salivary glands in the mouth to conserve water through the sympathetic nervous system. Stickier, thicker mucus output increases and watery, serous output decreases as a result of the signals. A "dry mouth" and a feeling of thirst are brought on by these modifications in secretions.

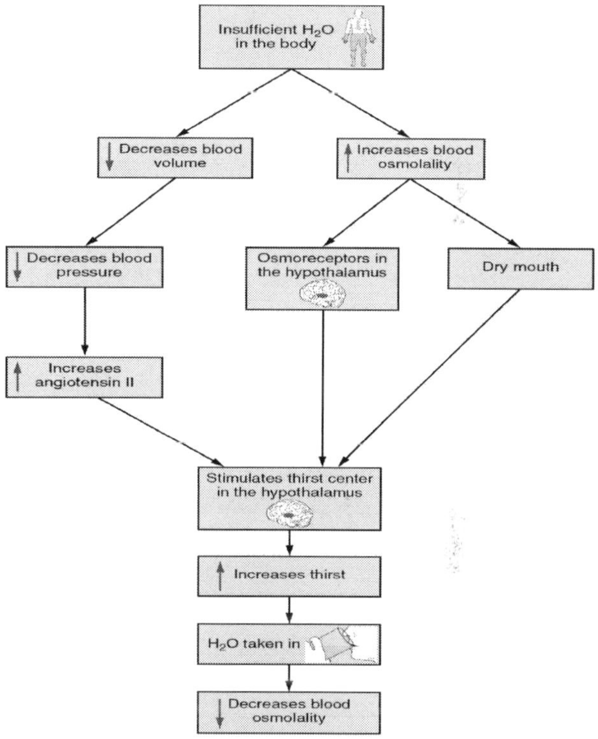

Figure 6.8. *A flowchart showing the thirst response. The thirst response begins when osmoreceptors detect a decrease in water levels in the blood.*

Source: https://commons.wikimedia.org/wiki/File:2708_Flowchart_of_Thirst_Response-01.jpg.

Two more effects result from decreased blood volume caused by water loss. First, a drop in blood volume causes a decrease in blood pressure, which is detected by baroreceptors, blood-pressure receptors in the carotid arteries in the neck and the arch of the aorta. Eventually, a signal is sent to the heart to accelerate and/or deepen its contractions in order to make up for the dropped blood pressure. Second, the kidneys' renin-angiotensin hormonal system raises the body's production of angiotensin II's active form, which not only helps to increase thirst but also causes the adrenal glands to release more aldosterone. In the kidneys, aldosterone promotes the reabsorption of sodium in the distal tubules of the nephrons, and water is subsequently reabsorbed and returned to the bloodstream.

Dehydration occurs when a person does not drink enough fluids, leaving their body with insufficient water to perform as intended. Infants, whose body mass is so low, can quickly become dangerously dehydrated. A person who vomits or has diarrhea on a regular basis may also become dehydrated. Distance runners and other endurance athletes frequently experience dehydration during lengthy races. If the body is not quickly rehydrated, a dehydrated person may lose consciousness, go into a comatose state, or even pass away. Dehydration can be a medical emergency.

6.2.2. Regulation of Water Output

The kidneys are the main organ through which the body loses water. Urine production is approximately 10.5 liters (10.6 quarts) per day on average for an individual. There is a minimum volume of urine production necessary for normal body functions, even though the volume of urine changes in response to hydration levels. To get rid of various excess salts and other water-soluble chemical wastes, the kidney excretes 100 to 1200 milliosmoles of solutes daily, the most common ones being creatinine, urea, and uric acid. Insufficient urine production can lead to ineffective removal of metabolic wastes from the body, potentially compromising organ function. About 0:47 liters (0:5 quarts) of urine production per day is the minimal amount required to sustain normal function.

6.2.3. Role of Antidiuretic Hormone

Vasopressin, another name for ADH, regulates the volume of water that the kidney's tubules and collecting ducts reabsorb. The posterior pituitary receives this hormone, which is made in the hypothalamus, and stores and releases it (Figure 6.9). The hypothalamus signals the posterior pituitary's release of ADH into the blood when its osmoreceptors identify an increase in blood plasma concentration.

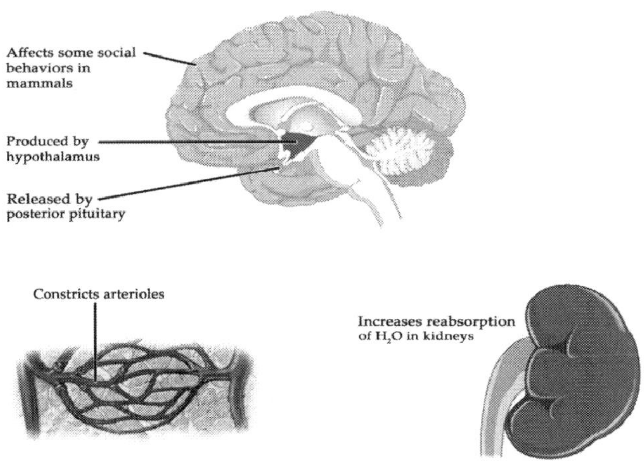

Figure 6.9. *Antidiuretic hormone (ADH) is produced in the hypothalamus and released by the posterior pituitary gland. It causes the kidneys to retain water, constricts arterioles in the peripheral circulation, and affects some social behaviors in mammals.*

Source: https://commons.wikimedia.org/wiki/File:2709_ADH.jpg.

ADH primarily affects two things. By narrowing the peripheral circulation's arterioles, it increases blood flow to the body's core while decreasing blood flow to the extremities. Aquaporins are water channel proteins that are moved from the inside of the cell to the apical surface of the cell, where they are inserted into the cell membrane, by the epithelial cells that line the renal collecting tubules as a result of ADH (Figure 6.10).

The end effect is an increase in these cells' water permeability, which increases the amount of water that passes from the urine through the collecting tubule walls and back into the circulation. The removal of aquaporins from collecting tubule cell membranes and a decrease in the amount of water that passes from urine into the blood occur when blood plasma concentration falls and ADH levels drop.

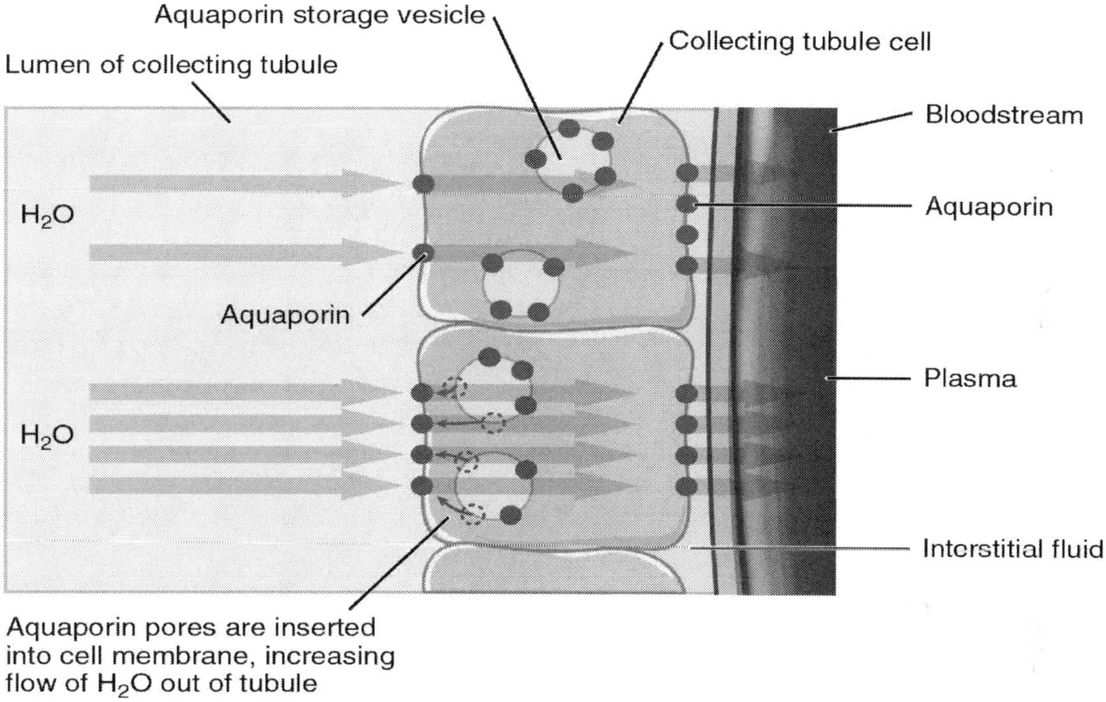

Figure 6.10. *Aquaporins. The binding of antidiuretic hormone to receptors on the cells of the collecting tubule results in aquaporins being inserted into the plasma membrane, shown in the lower cell. This dramatically increases the flow of water out of the tubule and into the bloodstream.*

Source: https://open.oregonstate.education/app/uploads/sites/157/2021/02/2710_Aquaporins-01.jpg.

A diuretic is a substance that causes the body to produce more urine, which reduces its ability to conserve water. Diuretics are prescribed to treat menstrual-related fluid retention, hypertension, and congestive heart failure. Because alcohol prevents the release of ADH, it has a diuretic effect. Moreover, caffeine has a diuretic effect when taken in large quantities.

6.3. Electrolytes

Minerals called electrolytes help the body perform a variety of tasks, such as preserving water balance, facilitating the contraction and relaxation of muscles, including the heart, and facilitating the transmission of nerve impulses. Along with water, the most common electrolytes lost through sweat are sodium, potassium, and chloride. "Electrolyte" is the umbrella term for particles that carry a positive or negative electric charge. In nutrition, the term refers to essential minerals found in your blood, sweat and urine.

These minerals dissolve in a liquid to form electrolytes, which are either positive or negative ions that are used in metabolism.

Electrolytes found in your body include:

- Sodium;
- Potassium;
- Chloride;
- Calcium;
- Magnesium;
- Phosphate;
- Bicarbonate.

6.3.1. Sodium

Sodium is necessary for many other vital functions as well as for preserving fluid balance. Sodium is absorbed very efficiently in the small intestine, unlike many other minerals, and in a healthy person, the kidneys eliminate any excess sodium. Because the kidneys actively reabsorb sodium, only 200 mg of sodium per day are actually needed in the diet. The hormonal regulation of kidney reabsorption of sodium maintains a relatively constant concentration of sodium in the blood.

6.3.1.1. Other Functions of Sodium in the Body

The transmission of nerve impulses is sodium's second important role. The entry of sodium cations into a nerve cell produces a charge difference, or voltage, between the nerve cell and its extracellular environment, which is what causes nerve impulse transmission. A sodium current flows through a nerve cell in a manner akin to that of a current flowing through a wire. Together with other ion movements, sodium ion movement plays a role in inducing a muscle contraction. A nerve impulse must reach a muscle in order for it to contract. Acetylcholine is a neurotransmitter that is released by the movement of sodium current in the nerve and communicates with the muscle. Acetylcholine causes the muscle's sodium channels to open, allowing sodium to flood in and create a second current that eventually causes the muscle to contract. The sodium-potassium pump is now required to remove the sodium that was absorbed during a stimulus in both muscle and nerve cells.

Both the small intestine's and the kidney's processes of reabsorbing nutrients depend on sodium. Water, glucose, and amino acids have to travel through the small intestine to reach the blood. They travel through intestinal cells to reach the blood in order to accomplish this. The sodium-potassium pump, which raises the concentration of sodium outside the cell by removing sodium, facilitates the movement of nutrients through intestinal cells (requiring ATP).

6.3.1.2. Sodium Imbalances

Sweating affects fluid and electrolyte balance and is a homeostatic mechanism for regulating body temperature. Though mostly composed of water, sweat also contains certain electrolytes, primarily sodium and chloride. In typical environmental circumstances (i.e. not hot, muggy days), sweating causes very little loss of water and sodium but varies greatly from person to person. One liter of sweat is thought to be produced during 60 min of vigorous exercise, such as a game of tennis; however, the quantity of sweat produced is greatly influenced by the surrounding circumstances. One liter of sweat has 1–2 g of sodium, so for some people, working out for several hours can result in a significant loss of sodium. Furthermore, sweating profusely during hard labor can result in significant sodium loss. Either way, the next meal or snack will easily make up for the lost sodium. Athletes may develop hyponatremia, a condition characterized by low blood-sodium levels, not primarily due to excessive sodium loss through sweat, but rather from consuming too much water. When excess water is consumed, it dilutes the sodium levels in the blood. Additionally, illnesses that result in vomiting, sweating, and diarrhea can also lead to hyponatremia. Common symptoms of hyponatremia, also known as water intoxication, include nausea, muscle cramps, confusion, dizziness, and in severe cases, coma or even death.

The physiological events that occur in water intoxication are the following:

1. Excessive sodium loss and/or water intake.
2. Sodium levels fall in blood and in the fluid between cells.
3. Water moves to where solutes are more concentrated (i.e. into cells).
4. Cells swell.
5. Symptoms, including nausea, muscle cramps, confusion, dizziness, and in severe cases, coma and death result.

Table 6.3. *Dietary Reference Intakes for Sodium*

Age Group	**Adequate Intake (mg/day)**	**Chronic Disease Risk Reduction Intake (mg/day)**
Infants (0–6 months)	110	Not determined
Infants (7–12 months)	370	Not determined
Children (1–3 years)	800	Reduce intake if above 1,200
Children (4–8 years)	1,000	Reduce intake if above 1,500
Children (9–13 years)	1,200	Reduce intake if above 1,800
Adolescents (14–18 years)	1,500	Reduce intake if above 2,300
Adults (>19 years)	1,500	Reduce intake if above 2,300
Pregnancy and lactation	1,500	Reduce intake if above 2,300

Source: https://spscc.pressbooks.pub/principlesofnutrition/chapter/13-5-sodium/.

6.3.1.3. Needs and Dietary Sources of Sodium

For healthy adults between the ages of 19 and 50, the IOM has established an AI level for sodium at 1,500 mg, or 1.5 g. Approximately 40% of table salt is sodium and 60% is chloride. To put this into perspective, the diet needs to contain just ⅔ teaspoon of salt to meet the AI for sodium. In addition to accounting for the appropriate intake of other nutrients, like chloride, the AI also considers the amount of sodium lost through perspiration during recommended physical activity levels. This means that in order to obtain all the other nutrients in our diet, we must permit a higher intake of sodium.

For adults, the Tolerable Upper Intake Level (UL) for sodium is 2.3 g per day. (A little more than one teaspoon of salt has the recommended 2 g of sodium). The UL is regarded as suitable for people in good health, but not for people who have high blood pressure, or hypertension. According to IOM estimates, in America, over 95% of men and 75% of women consume more salt than is recommended.

Reducing salt intake lowers blood pressure after hypertension is diagnosed, lowers the risk of cardiovascular disease, and prevents hypertension, according to numerous scientific studies. The Institute of Medicine (IOM) suggests that individuals over 50, African Americans, diabetics, and those suffering from chronic kidney disease should limit their daily sodium intake to 12.5 g. According to the American Heart Association (AHA), consuming less than 1.5 grams of sodium daily is recommended for all Americans, not just those on the list, to prevent cardiovascular disease. The American Heart Association (AHA) suggests doing this because lower-sodium diets are scientifically shown to be a preventive measure against hypertension, and millions of people have risk factors for the condition (Table 6.3).

6.3.1.4. Food Sources for Sodium

The majority of sodium in the average American diet is found in prepared and processed foods. Foods are salted by manufacturers for two reasons: as a preservative and to enhance flavor and texture. The salt content of comparable food items varies greatly. Certain foods, like poultry, meat, and dairy products, naturally contain sodium. For example, one cup of low-fat milk contains 107 mg of sodium. Naturally occurring sodium accounts for less than 12% of dietary intake in a typical diet. For the sodium contents of various foods see Table 6.4.

Table 6.4. *Sodium Contents of Selected Foods*

Food Group	**Serving Size**	**Sodium (mg)**
Breads, all types	1 oz.	95–210
Rice Chex cereal	1 ¼ c.	292
Raisin bran cereal	1 c.	362
Frozen pizza, plain, cheese	4 oz.	450–1200
Frozen vegetables, all types	½ c.	2–160
Salad dressing, regular fat, all types	2 Tbsp.	110–505
Salsa	2 Tbsp.	150–240
Soup (tomato), reconstituted	8 oz.	700–1260
Potato chips	1 oz. (28.4 g)	120–180
Tortilla chips	1 oz. (28.4 g)	105–160
Pork	3 oz.	59
Chicken	(½ breast)	69
Chicken fast food dinner	–	2243
Chicken noodle soup	1 c.	1107
Dill pickle	1	928
Soy sauce	1 Tbsp.	1029
Canned corn	1 c.	384
Baked beans, canned	1 c.	856
Hot dog	1	639
Burger, fast-food	1	990
Steak	3 oz.	55
Canned tuna	3 oz.	384
Fresh tuna	3 oz.	50
Dry-roasted peanuts	1 c.	986
American cheese	1 oz.	406
Tap water	8 oz.	12

Source: https://spscc.pressbooks.pub/principlesofnutrition/chapter/13-5-sodium/.

6.3.1.5. Sodium on the Nutrition Facts Panel

The amount of sodium (measured in mg) in each serving of the food in question is shown on the Nutrition Facts panel (Figure 6.11). Food additives frequently have high sodium contents; monosodium glutamate (MSG) has 12% of sodium, for instance. A considerable amount of sodium can also be found in baking soda, baking powder, disodium phosphate, sodium alginate, and sodium nitrate or nitrite. You can find out where the extra sodium is coming from by looking at the ingredients list on the Nutrition Facts label of a food.

Various claims about the sodium content in foods must be in accordance with Food and Drug Administration (FDA) regulations (Table 6.5).

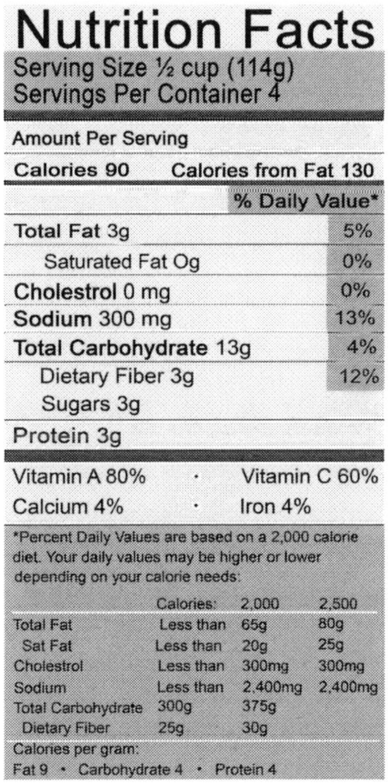

Nutrition Facts
Serving Size ½ cup (114g)
Servings Per Container 4

Amount Per Serving	
Calories 90	Calories from Fat 130
	% Daily Value*
Total Fat 3g	5%
Saturated Fat Og	0%
Cholestrol 0 mg	0%
Sodium 300 mg	13%
Total Carbohydrate 13g	4%
Dietary Fiber 3g	12%
Sugars 3g	
Protein 3g	

Vitamin A 80% • Vitamin C 60%
Calcium 4% • Iron 4%

*Percent Daily Values are based on a 2,000 calorie diet. Your daily values may be higher or lower depending on your calorie needs:

	Calories:	2,000	2,500
Total Fat	Less than	65g	80g
Sat Fat	Less than	20g	25g
Cholestrol	Less than	300mg	300mg
Sodium	Less than	2,400mg	2,400mg
Total Carbohydrate	300g	375g	
Dietary Fiber	25g	30g	

Calories per gram:
Fat 9 • Carbohydrate 4 • Protein 4

Figure 6.11. *Sodium levels in milligrams is a required listing on a Nutrition Facts label.*

Source: https://spscc.pressbooks.pub/principlesofnutrition/chapter/13-5-sodium/.

Table 6.5. *Food Packaging Claims Regarding Sodium*

Claim	Meaning
"Light in sodium" or "low in sodium"	Sodium is reduced by at least 50%
"No Salt added" or "unsalted"	No salt added during preparation and processing*
"Lightly salted"	50% less sodium than that added to similar food
"Sodium free" or "salt free"	Contains less than 5 mg sodium per serving
"Very low salt"	Contains less than 35 mg sodium per serving
"Low salt"	Contains less than 140 mg sodium per serving

Source: https://spscc.pressbooks.pub/principlesofnutrition/chapter/13-5-sodium/.

*Must also declare on package "This is not a sodium-free food" if food is not sodium-free.

6.3.1.6. Salt Substitutes

Using a salt substitute when preparing food is one option for people who have hypertension or are trying to cut back on their salt consumption.

Even so, the sodium content of many salt substitutes is still lower than that of table salt. Potassium is frequently used in place of sodium in salt substitutes. It is advised that people with kidney disorders stay away from potassium-containing salt substitutes because they frequently have trouble eliminating excess potassium from their diets.

People with liver disorders should also avoid salt substitutes containing potassium because their treatment is often accompanied by potassium dysregulation. Table 6.6 "Salt Substitutes" displays the sodium and potassium amounts in some salt substitutes.

Table 6.6. *Salt Substitutes*

Product	Serving Size	Sodium (mg)	Potassium (mg)
Salt	1 tsp.	2,300	0
Mrs. Dash	1 tsp.	0	40
Spike (Salt-Free)	1 tsp.	0	96
Veg-It	1 tsp.	<65	<65
Accent low-sodium seasoning	1 tsp.	600	0
Salt sense	1 tsp.	1,560	0
Pleasoning mini-mini salt	1 tsp.	440	0
Morton lite salt	1 tsp.	1,100	1,500
Estee salt-it	1 tsp.	0	3,520
Morton nature's seasons	1 tsp.	1,300	2,800
Morton salt substitute	1 tsp.	0	2,730
No salt	1 tsp.	5	2,500
Nu-salt	1 tsp.	0	529

Source: https://spscc.pressbooks.pub/principlesofnutrition/chapter/13-5-sodium/.

6.3.1.7. Alternative Seasonings

There are other ingredients that give your food a different flavor and zest besides table salt, which may seem like a necessary component of delicious food (Table 6.7).

Table 6.7. *"Salt Alternatives" for an AHA List of Alternative Food Seasonings*

Seasoning	Foods
Allspice	Lean ground meats, stews, tomatoes, peaches, applesauce, cranberry sauce, gravies, lean meat
Almond extract	Puddings, fruits
Caraway seeds	Lean meats, stews, soups, salads, breads, cabbage, asparagus, noodles
Chives	Salads, sauces, soups, lean-meat dishes, vegetables
Cider vinegar	Salads, vegetables, sauces
Cinnamon	Fruits, breads, pie crusts
Curry powder	Lean meats (especially lamb), veal, chicken, fish, tomatoes, tomato soup, mayonnaise,

Dill	fish sauces, soups, tomatoes, cabbages, carrots, cauliflower, green beans, cucumbers, potatoes, salads, macaroni, lamb
Garlic (not garlic salt)	Lean meats, fish, soups, salads, vegetables, tomatoes, potatoes
Ginger	Chicken, fruits
Lemon juice	Lean meats, fish, poultry, salads, vegetables
Mace	Hot breads, apples, fruit salads, carrots, cauliflower, squash, potatoes, veal, lamb
Mustard (dry)	lean ground meats, lean meats, chicken, fish, salads, asparagus, broccoli, Brussels sprouts, cabbage, mayonnaise, sauces
Nutmeg	Fruits, pie crust, lemonade, potatoes, chicken, fish, lean meatloaf, toast, veal, pudding
Onion powder	Lean meats, stews, vegetables, salads, soups
Paprika	Lean meats, fish, soups, salads, sauces, vegetables
Parsley	Lean meats, fish, soups, salads, sauces, vegetables
Peppermint extract	Puddings, fruits
Pimiento	Salads, vegetables, casserole dishes
Rosemary	Chicken, veal, lean meatloaf, lean beef, lean pork, sauces, stuffings, potatoes, peas, lima beans
Sage	Lean meats, stews, biscuits, tomatoes, green beans, fish, lima beans, onions, lean pork
Savory	Salads, lean pork, lean ground meats, soups, green beans, squash, tomatoes, lima beans, peas
Thyme	Lean meats (especially veal and lean pork), sauces, soups, onions, peas, tomatoes, salads
Turmeric	Lean meats, fish, sauces, rice

Source: https://spscc.pressbooks.pub/principlesofnutrition/chapter/13-5-sodium/.

6.3.2. Chloride

The main anion in ECF is chloride. Apart from its passive uptake of sodium, chloride also resides in cell membranes through its own protein channels. The pancreas, lungs, and digestive system have a disproportionately high concentration of these protein channels.

6.3.2.1. Chloride's Role in Fluid Balance

The primary reason chloride helps with fluid balance is that it follows sodium to preserve charge neutrality. Chloride channels are also involved in controlling the secretion of fluids, including pancreatic juice into the small intestine and water into mucus. Mucus and fluid secretion are essential for numerous biological processes. The indications and symptoms of the genetic illness cystic fibrosis serve as an excellent example of their significance.

6.3.2.2. Cystic Fibrosis

Among those of European descent, one of the most common inherited diseases is cystic fibrosis, or CF. A mutation in a protein that moves chloride ions out of the cell is the cause. Salty skin, poor growth due to poor digestion and absorption, sticky mucus buildup in the lungs (which increases susceptibility to respiratory infections), liver damage, and infertility are some of the signs and symptoms of cystic fibrosis (CF).

When chloride channels do not transport chloride out of cells, the following signs and symptoms of CF become apparent:

1. **Salty Skin:** Defective chloride channels in the sweat glands cause excess release of chloride, which sodium then follows into the sweat.
2. **Poor Digestion and Growth:** Defective chloride channels in the pancreas cause pancreatic juices to thicken. As a result of the thickening, the release of pancreatic juices is slowed and nutrient digestion is compromised.
3. **Respiratory Infection:** Defective chloride channels in the lungs cause thickened mucus. The mucus then traps bacteria.
4. **Liver Damage:** Defective chloride channels in the gall bladder cause thickened gall-bladder secretions. The gall-bladder ducts then become blocked, leading to liver damage.
5. **Infertility:** Defective chloride channels in male and female reproductive organs can result in impaired sperm transport and viscous mucus in the cervix, respectively.

6.3.2.3. Other Functions of Chloride

The balance of acid and base is one of the many additional roles that chloride plays in the body. Blood pH is kept within a specific range, and the quantity of positively and negatively charged substances is the same.

Blood pH is maintained by negatively charged proteins like albumin as well as bicarbonate and chloride ions.

A gastric acid that is a combination of hydrogen and chlorine, hydrochloric acid facilitates digestion and inhibits the growth of undesirable bacteria in the stomach.

The body needs chloride for immune system cells, and red blood cells use chloride anions to expel carbon dioxide.

6.3.2.4. Chloride Imbalances

Low blood levels of chloride can be caused by a low dietary intake of the mineral and, more frequently, diarrhea.

Typically, the symptoms resemble those of hyponatremia and include headache, nausea, and weakness. It is uncommon to have too much chloride in the blood, and there are no obvious symptoms.

6.3.2.5. Needs and Dietary Sources of Chloride

The majority of chloride in food comes from salt. 60% of salt is chloride. 5.6 g is equal to one teaspoon of salt, and each teaspoon has 2.2 g of sodium and 3.4 grams of chloride.

The IOM has set an adult chloride AI of 2.3 g. For both sodium and chloride, therefore, a mere ⅔ teaspoon of table salt each day is adequate. The AIs for other age groups are listed in Table 6.8 "Adequate Intakes for Chloride."

Table 6.8. *Adequate Intakes for Chloride*

Age Group	mg/day
Infants (0–6 months)	180
Infants (6–12 months)	570
Children (1–3 years)	1,500
Children (4–8 years)	1,900
Children (9–13 years)	2,300
Adolescents (14–18 years)	2,300
Adults (19–50 years)	2,300
Adults (51–70 years)	2,000
Adults (> 70 years)	1,800

Source: https://courses.lumenlearning.com/sunyltnutrition/chapter/chloride/#:~:text=A%20teaspoon%20of%20salt%20equals,chloride%20as%20well%20as%20sodium.

6.3.2.6. Other Dietary Sources of Chloride

In the diet, chloride can also be found in potassium chloride, which is a different type of salt.

Chloride can be found in food items such as seafood, whole-grain foods, tomatoes, lettuce, olives, celery, and rye. Salt alternatives can still contain chloride even though many of them are sodium-free.

6.3.2.7. Bioavailability

The components of sodium chloride separate into sodium cations and chloride anions in the small intestine. Chloride is passively absorbed by intestinal cells after the sodium ion, which makes chloride absorption highly effective. Chloride is also readily absorbed when it is present as a potassium salt. Although some mineral salts, like magnesium chloride, are not as well absorbed, their bioavailability is still quite high.

6.3.3. Potassium

The most prevalent positively charged ion within cells is potassium. Just 1% of potassium is found in blood plasma, compared to 90% in intracellular fluid, 10% in ECF, and 10% in both.

The blood's potassium levels are strictly regulated, just like sodium's. Although insulin and other hormones (such as aldosterone) also have an impact, aldosterone is the main hormone that regulates potassium levels. The adrenal glands release aldosterone in response to elevated blood potassium levels.

Through its action on the kidney's collecting ducts, aldosterone causes a rise in the quantity of sodium-potassium pumps. More potassium is then expelled and sodium is reabsorbed. Approximately 200 mg of potassium are lost from the body each day because it is necessary to maintain sodium levels and, consequently, fluid balance.

6.3.3.1. Other Functions of Potassium in the Body

Nerve impulse involves potassium in addition to sodium. When sodium ions enter a cell, a nerve impulse travels along the nerve.

Potassium ions shoot out of the nerve cell to stop the impulse, which lowers the positive charge within the nerve cell. In turn, this lessens the stimulus.

The sodium-potassium pump exchanges potassium ions for sodium ions to return the intracellular and ECF to their initial ion concentrations.

A nerve cell is prepared to receive the subsequent impulse once the restored ion concentrations are complete.

Similar to this, potassium plays a role in muscle cells to stop a contraction and return the membrane potential to normal. In addition to its roles in energy metabolism, platelet function, and protein synthesis, potassium also functions as a buffer in blood, contributing to the maintenance of acid-base balance.

6.3.3.2. Imbalances of Potassium

Hypokalemia, or low potassium in the body, can be brought on by eating too little potassium-rich food or too much sodium, but diuretics, in particular, are the main medications that cause this condition.

The effects of potassium on nerve cells and, subsequently, the contraction of smooth and skeletal muscles, are linked to the indications and symptoms of hypokalemia.

Constipation, respiratory distress, and muscle weakness and cramps are some of the warning signs and symptoms.

Severe potassium deficiency can even be lethal, resulting in irregular heartbeats. Hyperkalemia, or elevated potassium in the blood, has an impact on the heart as well.

Since it frequently shows no symptoms or indicators, it is a silent condition.

Overly elevated potassium levels in the blood can stop the heart by interfering with the electrical impulses that stimulate it. Kidney dysfunction is typically the cause of hyperkalemia.

6.3.3.3. Needs and Dietary Sources of Potassium

The levels of potassium linked to a drop in blood pressure, a reduction in sensitivity to salt, and a low risk of kidney stones served as the foundation for the IOM's artificial intelligence calculations.

The recommended daily intake of potassium for adults over the age of 19 is 4.7 g for both males and females. The AIs for other age groups are listed in Table 6.9.

Table 6.9. *Adequate Intakes for Potassium*

Age Group	mg/day
Infants (0–6 months)	400
Infants (6–12 months)	700
Children (1–3 years)	3,000
Children (4–8 years)	3,800
Children (9–13 years)	4,500
Adolescents (14–18 years)	4,700
Adults (> 19 years)	4,700

Source: https://courses.lumenlearning.com/sunyltnutrition/chapter/potassium-3/.

6.3.3.4. Food Sources for Potassium

High-potassium fruits and vegetables include spinach, lettuce, broccoli, peas, tomatoes, potatoes, bananas, apples, and apricots. High in potassium are meats, whole grains, seeds, and some fish (like flounder, cod, and salmon).

6.3.3.5. Bioavailability

The small intestine absorbs more than 90% of the potassium that is consumed through diet. Potassium is a very soluble mineral that is easily lost during food processing and cooking, despite being highly bioavailable. Foods that are fresh or frozen provide more potassium than those that are canned.

6.3.4. Calcium

Over 99% of the calcium that is present in the body is found in bone tissue, making it the most abundant mineral in the body. The blood and soft tissues contain only 1% of the calcium in the human body, but this is where it serves the majority of its vital purposes. Blood calcium levels are closely monitored, and in the event that they fall, the body quickly reacts by inducing bone resorption, which releases calcium that has been stored in the body into the blood. To keep blood calcium levels stable, bone tissue thus gives up its calcium reserves. This explains why dietary calcium intake is essential for maintaining healthy bones as well as the reason that blood calcium levels do not always match dietary intake. The body uses calcium for many purposes, including the development of teeth and bones. The most well-known benefit of calcium is that it helps to strengthen and develop teeth and bones. Remember that osteoid tissue, which is rich in proteins and not hardened, is what forms the first part of bone during the modeling or remodeling process. The protein matrix is covered in calcium phosphates (salts) during the osteoblast-directed process of bone mineralization. Bone tissue normally consists of approximately 65% calcium salts. A diet low in calcium causes the mineral content of bone to decrease, making the bone weak and brittle. Therefore, consuming more calcium aids in raising the mineralized content of bone tissue. Increased BMD and bone strength are correlated with higher mineralized bone tissue. The residual calcium helps electrical impulses travel from one nerve cell to another, which is how it contributes to nerve impulse transmission. Because the movement of calcium ions is necessary for the interaction of the muscle proteins (actin and myosin), calcium in muscle cells is critical for muscular contraction. Additionally, calcium is necessary for blood clotting because it activates clotting factors that repair damaged tissue. Apart from its four principal functions, calcium also performs several minor functions that are equally important for preserving normal physiology. For instance, the release of the hormone insulin from pancreatic cells and the breakdown of glycogen in muscle cells to provide energy for muscular contraction would not be possible in the absence of calcium.

6.3.4.1. Maintaining Calcium Levels

Because calcium is involved in so many essential bodily processes, parathyroid hormone (PTH), calcitriol, and calcitonin all play a major role in controlling blood calcium levels. PTH is secreted to raise blood calcium levels through three distinct mechanisms when blood calcium levels are low. PTH first causes the calcium that has been stored in the bone to be released. Second, PTH stimulates calcium reabsorption and reduces calcium excretion in the urine by acting on kidney cells. Third, PTH activates kidney enzymes that convert vitamin D into calcitriol. The hormone that stimulates intestinal cells to absorb more calcium from food is called calcitriol. Certain thyroid gland cells release the hormone calcitonin when blood calcium levels rise too high, which also causes PTH secretion to cease. At higher nonphysiological concentrations, calcitonin inhibits bone resorption directly, increases calcium excretion in the urine, and stops further absorption of calcium in the gut (Figure 6.12).

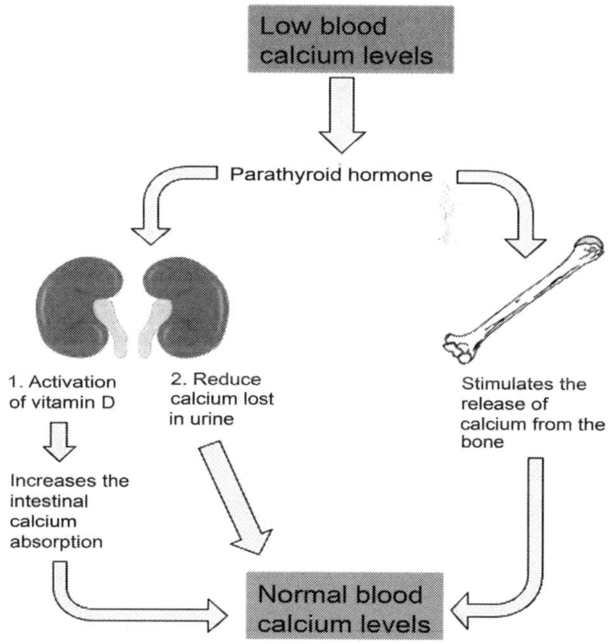

Figure 6.12. *Maintaining blood calcium levels.*

Source: https://courses.lumenlearning.com/sunyltnutrition/chapter/major-minerals-2/.

6.3.4.2. Other Health Benefits of Calcium in the Body

It has been demonstrated that calcium has additional health benefits for the body besides helping to form and maintain strong bones and teeth, such as:

- **Cancer:** According to the National Cancer Institute, there is sufficient scientific data to draw the conclusion that increased calcium intake lowers the risk of colon cancer and may inhibit the growth of polyps, which frequently cause cancer. While consuming more calcium prevents colon cancer, some research has examined the link between calcium and prostate cancer and found that higher intakes may raise the risk for prostate cancer. Nevertheless, the evidence is conflicting, and additional research is required to validate any negative association.
- **Blood Pressure:** Multiple studies provide clear evidence that higher calcium consumption reduces blood pressure. A review of 23 observational studies concluded that for every 100 mg of calcium consumed daily, systolic blood pressure is reduced 0.34 millimeters of mercury (mmHg) and diastolic blood pressure is decreased by 0.15 mmHg.
- **Cardiovascular Health:** There is emerging evidence that higher calcium intakes prevent against other risk factors for cardiovascular disease, such as high cholesterol and obesity, but the scientific evidence is weak or inconclusive.
- **Kidney Stones:** Another health benefit of a high-calcium diet is that it blocks kidney stone formation. Calcium inhibits the absorption of oxalate, a chemical in plants such as parsley and spinach, which is associated with an increased risk for developing kidney stones. Calcium's protective effects on kidney stone formation occur only when you obtain calcium from dietary sources. Calcium supplements may actually increase the risk for kidney stones in susceptible people.

The elderly and teenage girls are the groups most likely to suffer from calcium insufficiency. A healthy diet rich in calcium is essential for strong bones. The typical American diet does not provide the recommended amounts of calcium in the diet, despite the abundance of evidence demonstrating the many health benefits of calcium, especially for bone health. In actuality, the average daily intake of calcium in females over the age of nine is only roughly 70% of the recommended intake. Here, we'll focus on specific demographics that might need to consume more calcium.

- **Adolescent Teens:** A calcium-deficient diet is common in teenage girls as their dairy consumption often considerably drops during adolescence.
- **Amenorrheic Women and the "Female Athlete Triad:"** The term "amenorrhea" describes the lack of a menstrual cycle. Less estrogen is produced in women who do not menstruate, which can upset and negatively affect the calcium balance in their bodies. Amenorrhea, irregular eating habits, and osteoporosis are the three

conditions collectively referred to as the "female athlete triad." Bone mass can be lowered by amenorrhea brought on by exercise or amenorrhea associated with anorexia nervosa. Low bone mineral density, irregular menstruation, personal food preferences, and a history of stress-related illnesses are associated with a higher risk of stress fractures in female athletes and active military personnel.

- **The Elderly:** Age-related changes in dietary habits, decreased calcium bioavailability, decreased kidney function in converting vitamin D into its most active form, decreased skin vitamin D synthesis, and decreased exposure to sunlight are all factors that contribute to the kidneys' inefficiency in retaining calcium. This increases the risk of calcium insufficiency.
- **Postmenopausal Women:** Absorption of calcium is improved by estrogen. Particularly at risk for calcium deficiency are postmenopausal women due to the reduction in this hormone during and after menopause. Both a decrease in calcium absorption and an increase in bone resorption are caused by decreases in estrogen production. Annual drops in bone mass during the first few years of menopause range from 3 to 5%. Decreases are usually less than 1% after 65 years of age.
- **Lactose-Intolerant People:** Groups of people, such as those who are lactose intolerant, or who adhere to diets that avoid dairy products, may not have an adequate calcium intake.
- **Vegans:** These typically absorb reduced amounts of calcium because their diets favor plant-based foods that contain oxalates and phytates.

Furthermore, vegans may eat fewer foods overall that are high in calcium because they abstain from dairy. Remember that there are plenty of plant-based foods that are high in calcium and that there are dairy products that are low in lactose or lactose-free available if you are lactose intolerant, allergic to milk, vegan, or just don't like dairy products.

6.3.4.3. Calcium Supplements: Which One to Buy?

Many individuals opt to meet their daily calcium needs by using calcium supplements. These supplements are available in various forms such as calcium carbonate, calcium citrate, calcium lactate, and calcium phosphate, each containing around 200 mg of elemental calcium per pill. It is important to remember that calcium carbonate requires an acidic stomach environment to be effectively utilized. While this is not an issue for most individuals, it may pose a problem for those taking medication to reduce stomach acid or for elderly individuals with a decreased ability to produce stomach acid. In such cases, calcium citrate may be a better option. However, calcium carbonate is the most cost-effective choice for others. The body can absorb approximately 30% of calcium from these supplement forms.

6.3.4.3.1. Beware of Lead

Since supplements made from natural sources like oyster shell, bone meal, and dolomite (a type of rock containing calcium magnesium carbonate) are known to contain high amounts of lead, there is concern regarding the lead content of some brands of calcium supplements regarding public health. In a study involving 22 calcium supplement brands, it was established that the acceptable limit for lead content was exceeded by eight of the brands. This was discovered to be the case with supplements made of refined calcium carbonate and oyster shell. Additionally, brands that purported to be lead-free had extremely low levels of lead, according to the same study. It is vital to understand that supplements that aren't made from oyster shell or other naturally occurring materials typically have low lead contents because the lead content of these products isn't stated on the labels. Furthermore, it was discovered that one brand only contained 77% of the claimed calcium content and that another brand did not dissolve as required for absorption.

6.3.4.3.2. Diet, Supplements, and Chelated Supplements

Generally speaking, calcium supplements don't offer as many of the health advantages associated with increased calcium intake as dietary calcium sources do. This is partially explained by the fact that dietary calcium sources provide extra nutrients that have health-promoting properties. Because the chelation process shields the calcium from oxalates and phytates that could bind with the calcium in the intestines, it is said that chelated forms of calcium supplements are easier to absorb. These more costly supplements, however, only slightly improve calcium absorption—by 10%. When combined with a vitamin D supplement, calcium supplements have little effect on bone health in individuals with low calcium intakes. However, there are numerous advantages to bone health when calcium supplements are taken in conjunction with vitamin D. These advantages include increased peak bone mass in early adulthood, maintenance of bone mineral density throughout adulthood, decreased risk of developing osteoporosis, and decreased incidence of fractures in individuals who already had osteoporosis. It is not necessary to take calcium and vitamin D supplements at the same time for them to work. But keep in mind that in order to encourage the bloodstream to contain and activate vitamin D, calcium absorption must occur. As a result, it's critical to continue consuming enough vitamin D.

6.3.4.3.3. The Calcium Debate

According to a recent British Medical Journal study, those who take calcium supplements without taking a vitamin D supplement and at doses of 500 mg or more daily are 30% more likely to experience a heart attack.

If you look more closely at the study, you will find that 5 points 8% of the 143 people who took calcium supplements experienced a heart attack, but so did 5 points 5% of the 111 people who took a placebo. Does this mean that taking calcium supplements is bad for you? Although this is a single study, a number of larger studies have not demonstrated that taking supplements containing calcium raises the risk of cardiovascular disease.

While the debate over this continues in the realm of science, we should focus on the things we do know:

1. There is overwhelming evidence that diets sufficient in calcium prevent osteoporosis and cardiovascular disease.
2. If a person has risk factors for osteoporosis and cannot get enough calcium from their diet, it is advised that they take supplements. Adults 50 years of age and older are advised by the National Osteoporosis Foundation to take 1,200 mg of calcium daily. This covers calcium from supplements as well as food sources.

3. Overindulging in calcium can have negative effects on your health and is not recommended. Overdosing on calcium, whether through food or supplements, can hinder the body's ability to absorb other vital minerals like iron and zinc in addition to calcium. To achieve the RDA of calcium, it is advised to take calcium supplements in divided doses rather than all at once, as the GI tract can only process approximately 500 mg of calcium at a time.

6.3.4.4. Dietary Reference Intake for Calcium

The dietary reference intakes (RDAs) for calcium are provided in Table 6.10, "Dietary Reference Intakes for Calcium." Since adolescence is the stage of life with accelerated bone growth, the RDA is increased to 1,300 mg per day during this time.

According to studies, a person's total amount of accumulated bone tissue increases during puberty when they consume more calcium.

For women over 50 and men over 71, the RDAs are also somewhat higher for a number of reasons.

These include a decrease in the gut's ability to absorb calcium with age, a decrease in vitamin D3 activation, and the necessity of maintaining adequate blood levels of calcium to prevent an acceleration of bone tissue loss, particularly during menopause.

For females over nine, the average dietary intake of calcium is currently lower than the RDA. According to the Institute of Medicine (IOM), consuming more calcium than 2,500 mg daily is not advised as it may have negative effects on certain individuals.

Table 6.10. *Dietary Reference Intakes for Calcium*

Age Group	Recommended Dietary Allowance (mg/day)	UL (mg/day)
Infants (0–6 months)	200*	–
Infants (6–12 months)	260*	–
Children (1–3 years)	700	2,500
Children (4–8 years)	1,000	2,500
Children (9–13 years)	1,300	2,500
Adolescents (14–18 years)	1,300	2,500
Adults (19–50 years)	1,000	2,500
Adult females (50–71 years)	1,200	2,500
Adults, male & female (> 71 years)	1,200	2,500

Source: https://courses.lumenlearning.com/sunyltnutrition/chapter/major-minerals-2/.

6.3.4.5. Dietary Sources of Calcium

The majority of the calcium in the average American diet comes from dairy products, particularly cheese. Just over 200 mg of calcium can be found in a slice of Swiss or cheddar cheese. A cup of nonfat milk has about 300 mg of calcium, which is roughly one-third of the average adult's RDA. Orange juice, soy milk, and cereals that have been fortified with calcium also supply at least one-third of the RDA for calcium. There are other excellent non-dairy sources of calcium, even though the average American diet mostly consists of dairy products (Table 6.11).

Table 6.11. *Calcium Content of Various Foods*

Food	Serving	Calcium (mg)	Percent Daily Value
Yogurt, low fat	8 oz.	415	42
Mozzarella	1.5 oz.	333	33
Sardines, canned with bones	3 oz.	325	33
Cheddar Cheese	1.5 oz.	307	31
Milk, nonfat	8 oz.	299	30
Soymilk, calcium fortified	8 oz.	299	30
Orange juice, calcium fortified	6 oz.	261	26
Tofu, firm, made with calcium sulfate	½ c.	253	25
Salmon, canned with bones	3 oz.	181	18
Turnip, boiled	½ c.	99	10
Kale, cooked	1 c.	94	9
Vanilla Ice Cream	½ c.	84	8
White bread	1 slice	73	7
Kale, raw	1 c.	24	2
Broccoli, raw	½ c.	21	2

Source: https://courses.lumenlearning.com/sunyltnutrition/chapter/major-minerals-2/.

6.3.4.6. Calcium Bioavailability

Most calcium absorption occurs in the duodenum of the small intestine when intake is low, but passive absorption also occurs in the jejunum and ileum, particularly when intake is higher. The body does not absorb all of the calcium from food, and surprisingly, calcium from certain vegetables like kale, brussel sprouts, and bok choy is more readily absorbed than calcium from dairy products. Approximately 30% of calcium is absorbed from milk and other dairy products.

Getting enough vitamin D has the biggest beneficial impact on calcium absorption. Individuals lacking in vitamin D absorb less than 15% of calcium from their diet. An additional factor that improves calcium bioavailability is the hormone estrogen. Therefore, a woman's absorption of calcium reduces and her risk of bone disease rises as she ages and experiences menopause, a time when estrogen levels drop. Certain fibers, like inulin, which is present in jicama, garlic, and onions, also encourage the intestinal uptake of calcium.

The bioavailability of calcium is reduced by substances that bind to it. The oxalates in some plants, the tannins in tea, the phytates in nuts, seeds, and grains, and some fibers are some of these substances that inhibit the absorption of calcium. Cocoa, beets, parsley, and spinach all contain high levels of oxalates. Food oxalate content is generally inversely correlated with calcium bioavailability. Diets high in fiber and low in fat also reduce the absorption of calcium, an effect that is probably caused by the way that fat and fiber affect how long food remains in the stomach. Anything that causes diarrhea, such as illness, drugs, and some age-related symptoms, shortens the time that calcium takes to pass through the gut, which reduces the amount of calcium absorbed. Age-related changes in the body include decreased stomach acidity, increased frequency of diarrhea, impaired kidney function, and compromised vitamin D activation and absorption. All of these factors can lower the body's ability to absorb calcium.

6.3.5. Magnesium

Measuring about 1% of mineralized bone tissue, the skeleton contains 60% of the magnesium present in the human body. Although it exists on the crystal's surface and aids in optimizing bone structure, magnesium is not a part of the hard mineral crystals themselves. A magnesium deficiency has been associated with a higher risk of osteoporosis, according to observational research. Insufficient intake of magnesium has been linked to lowered parathyroid hormone levels and increased vitamin D synthesis, potentially impairing bone remodeling. The results of a study involving 900 senior men and women did indicate a correlation between increased BMD in the hip and higher dietary intakes of magnesium. There have only been a small number of clinical trials examining the impact of magnesium supplements on bone health, and the findings point to some slight improvements in BMD.

Magnesium serves the body in a number of other ways besides helping to maintain bones. Magnesium is needed in all reactions involving the molecule that gives cells their energy, ATP. Magnesium is needed for over 300 enzymatic reactions. Magnesium is necessary for nerve transmission and muscle contraction. It also contributes to the synthesis of lipids, carbohydrates, and DNA and RNA. Magnesium may also lower blood pressure, which is a health benefit. The diets of many Americans do not provide them with the recommended amount of magnesium. A mild magnesium deficiency may be associated with an increased risk of cardiovascular disease, according to certain observational studies. A severe magnesium deficiency can cause tremors, muscle spasms, nausea, and loss of appetite.

6.3.5.1. Dietary Reference Intake and Food Sources for Magnesium

The RDA for magnesium in adults aged 19 to 30 is 400 mg for men and 310 mg for women. The RDA for adults over 30 rises marginally to 320 mg for females and 420 mg for males per day (Table 6.12).

Table 6.12. *Dietary Reference Intakes for Magnesium*

Age Group	Recommended Dietary Allowance (mg/day)	UL from Non-Food Sources (mg/day)
Infants (0–6 months)	30*	–
Infants (6–12 months)	75*	–
Children (1–3 years)	80	65
Children (4–8 years)	130	110
Children (9–13 years)	240	350
Adolescents (14–18 years)	410	350
Adults (19–30 years)	400	350
Adults (> 30 years)	420	350

Source: https://courses.lumenlearning.com/sunyltnutrition/chapter/magnesium-2/.

* denotes adequate intake

6.3.5.2. Dietary Sources of Magnesium

Since magnesium is a component of chlorophyll, a green pigment that is essential to photosynthesis in plants, green leafy vegetables are a good source of magnesium in the diet. Additionally, whole grains, nuts, dairy products, meats, and fish all contain high concentrations of magnesium. Hard water, coffee, and chocolate also have significant magnesium content. The majority of Americans do not consume enough magnesium in their diets to meet the RDA. Western diets tend to be low in fish and to consume refined grains and whole grains in an unbalanced manner (Table 6.13).

Table 6.13. *Magnesium Content of Various Foods*

Food	Serving	Magnesium (mg)	Percent Daily Value
Almonds	1 oz.	80	20
Cashews	1 oz.	74	19
Soymilk	1 c.	61	15
Black beans	½ c.	60	15
Edamame	½ c.	50	13
Bread	2 slices	46	12
Avocado	1 c.	44	11
Brown rice	½ c.	42	11
Yogurt	8 oz.	42	11
Oatmeal, instant	1 packet	36	9
Salmon	3 oz.	26	7
Chicken breasts	3 oz.	22	6
Apple	1 medium	9	2

Source: https://courses.lumenlearning.com/sunyltnutrition/chapter/magnesium-2/.

6.3.6. Phosphate

A molecule based on phosphorus, phosphate is essential for the movement of chemicals and molecules inside and outside of your cells. It is an essential component of the molecules known as nucleotides, which are the building blocks of your DNA, and it aids in the nutrient metabolism of your cells.

- When you have hyperphosphatemia (too much phosphate), your body tries to use calcium instead of phosphorus, which usually results in hypocalcemia. It typically does not show symptoms until it gets severe, and when that happens, hypocalcemia symptoms frequently follow. It may also be connected to persistent itching.
- Muscle weakness is typically the first symptom of hypophosphatemia, or not enough phosphate. The symptoms worsen with time and become more severe. These include breathing difficulties (due to muscle weakness), seizures, rhabdomyolysis (breakdown of muscle tissue, which can cause severe kidney damage), and reduced heart function.

6.3.7. Bicarbonate

Your body produces carbon dioxide, but not all of it is sent to your lungs where it is exhaled. Rather, a portion of it is recycled into bicarbonate, which is used by your body to maintain normal blood pH levels.

- **Acidosis:** Too little bicarbonate causes acidosis, where your blood is too acidic. This causes fatigue, nausea, and vomiting, and you will breathe faster and deeper. It can also cause confusion.
- **Alkalosis:** Too much bicarbonate causes alkalosis, where your blood becomes too alkaline. Symptoms include confusion, apathy, arrhythmias, and muscle twitching.

A Closer Look

Electrolyte Balance

Electrolyte balance reveals the intricate mechanisms by which the body regulates the levels of these essential minerals to maintain optimal physiological function. Electrolytes, including sodium, potassium, chloride, calcium, magnesium, and phosphate, play crucial roles in fluid balance, nerve function, muscle contraction, and pH regulation within the body. Sodium and potassium are two key electrolytes involved in regulating fluid balance and nerve transmission. Sodium, primarily found in ECF, helps maintain blood pressure, fluid balance, and nerve impulse transmission. Potassium, mainly located in intracellular fluid, regulates fluid balance, muscle contraction, and nerve signals. The body tightly regulates sodium and potassium levels through various mechanisms, including hormonal control by hormones such as aldosterone, which acts on the kidneys to regulate sodium and potassium excretion. Chloride, often found alongside sodium, plays a critical role in maintaining fluid balance and acid-base balance within the body. It helps regulate osmotic pressure, aids in digestion as part of hydrochloric acid in the stomach, and participates in the transport of carbon dioxide and oxygen in red blood cells. Calcium and magnesium are essential electrolytes for muscle contraction, nerve transmission, bone health, and enzymatic reactions. Calcium is crucial for muscle contraction, blood clotting, and bone formation, while magnesium is involved in muscle relaxation, energy metabolism, and DNA synthesis. Both electrolytes are regulated by hormones such as parathyroid hormone (PTH) and calcitonin, which help maintain calcium and magnesium balance in the body. Phosphate is another essential electrolyte involved in energy metabolism, bone mineralization, and acid-base balance. It is a component of ATP, the primary energy currency of cells, and plays a role in cell signaling, DNA synthesis, and maintaining pH balance in the body. Maintaining electrolyte balance is crucial for overall health and well-being, and imbalances can occur due to factors such as dehydration, excessive sweating, vomiting, diarrhea, kidney disorders, or certain medications. Electrolyte imbalances can lead to symptoms such as muscle cramps, weakness, fatigue, irregular heartbeat, confusion, and seizures. In severe cases, electrolyte imbalances can be life-threatening and require prompt medical attention. Replenishing electrolytes through a balanced diet rich in fruits, vegetables, whole grains, lean proteins, and adequate hydration is essential for supporting optimal physiological function and preventing electrolyte disturbances. Additionally, in cases of significant fluid loss or electrolyte imbalance, oral rehydration solutions or intravenous fluids may be necessary to restore proper balance and hydration status.

In conclusion, maintaining electrolyte balance is essential for overall health and well-being, as electrolytes play crucial roles in fluid balance, nerve function, muscle contraction, and pH regulation within the body. Understanding the importance of electrolytes and their regulation mechanisms can help individuals make informed decisions about their diet and hydration habits to support optimal health.

Summary

- Water, a primary component of body fluids, is the most abundant substance in the body. Water plays a vital role in several physiologic processes such as digestion, absorption and use of nutrients, distribution, waste excretion, and perfusion and maintenance of hemodynamics.
- The intracellular fluid (ICF) compartment is the system that includes all fluid enclosed in cells by their plasma membranes. Extracellular fluid (ECF) surrounds all cells in the body.
- Water is called the "universal solvent" because more substances dissolve in it than any other fluid. Molecules dissolve in water because of the hydrogen and oxygen molecules ability to loosely bond with other molecules.
- Water metabolism is a balance between intake and output. Intake consists of unregulated factors (ingested water in foods and liquids), water generated from the oxidation of ingested macronutrients, and regulated factors (consumption in response to thirst).
- Fluid homeostasis in the neonatal patient must account for the demands of transitioning from intrauterine to extrauterine existence as well as rapid growth and development.
- Electrolytes are minerals that have many functions in the body including maintaining water balance, helping your muscles (including your heart) contract and relax and helping transmit nerve impulses. The most common electrolytes are sodium, potassium, and chloride, which are lost in sweat along with water.
- Sodium, is vital not only for maintaining fluid balance but also for many other essential functions. In contrast to many minerals, sodium absorption in the small intestine is extremely efficient and in a healthy individual all excess sodium is excreted by the kidneys.

References

1. European Food Safety Authority (EFSA). (2010). Scientific opinion on principles for deriving and applying dietary reference values. *EFSA Journal, 8*, 1458.
2. European Commission. (2012). Commission regulation (EU) No 432/2012 of 16 May 2012 establishing a list of permitted health claims made on foods, other than those referring to the reduction of disease risk and to children's development and health. *Official Journal of the European Union, 136*, 1–40.
3. Griffiths, J. K. (2013). Vitamin deficiencies. In A. J. Magil, D. R. Hill, T. Solomon, E. T. Ryan (Eds.), *Hunter's Tropical Medicine and Emerging Infectious Disease* (9th ed., pp. 997–1002). Elsevier.
4. Rippin, H. L., Hutchinson, J., Jewell, J., Breda, J. J., & Cade, J. E. (2017). Adult Nutrient Intakes from Current National Dietary Surveys of European Populations. *Nutrients, 9*, 1288. https://doi.org/10.3390/nu9121288 (accessed on 18 May 2024).

5. Pedroza-Tobias, A., Hernandez-Barrera, L., Lopez-Olmedo, N., Garcia-Guerra, A., Rodriguez-Ramirez, S., Ramirez-Silva, I., Villalpando, S., Carriquiry, A., & Rivera, J. A. (2016). Usual Vitamin Intakes by Mexican Populations. *Journal of Nutrition, 146*, 1866S–1873S. https://doi.org/10.3945/jn.115.219162 (accessed on 18 May 2024).

6. Dietary Guidelines Advisory Committee. (2015). *Scientific Report of the 2015 Dietary Guidelines Advisory Committee: Advisory Report to the Secretary of Health and Human Services and the Secretary of Agriculture*. U.S. Department of Agriculture, Agricultural Research Service.

7. Sekhri, K., & Kaur, K. (2014). Public knowledge, use and attitude toward multivitamin supplementation: A cross-sectional study among general public. *International Journal of Applied and Basic Medical Research, 4*, 77–80. https://doi.org/10.4103/2229-516X.136780 (accessed on 18 May 2024).

8. Ryan, R. M., & Frederick, C. (1997). On energy, personality, and health: Subjective vitality as a dynamic reflection of well-being. *Journal of Personality, 65*, 529–565. https://doi.org/10.1111/j.1467-6494.1997.tb00326.x (accessed on 18 May 2024).

9. Aouizerat, B. E., Gay, C. L., Lerdal, A., Portillo, C. J., & Lee, K. A. (2013). Lack of energy: An important and distinct component of HIV-related fatigue and daytime function. *Journal of Pain and Symptom Management, 45*, 191–201. https://doi.org/10.1016/j.jpainsymman.2012.01.011 (accessed on 18 May 2024).

10. van Steenbergen, E., van Dongen, J. M., Wendel-Vos, G. C., Hildebrandt, V. H., & Strijk, J. E. (2016). Insights into the concept of vitality: Associations with participation and societal costs. *European Journal of Public Health, 26*, 354–359. https://doi.org/10.1093/eurpub/ckv194 (accessed on 18 May 2024).

11. Gledhill, J. (2005). A qualitative study of the characteristics and representation of fatigue in a French speaking population of cancer patients and healthy subjects. *European Journal of Oncology Nursing, 9*, 294–312. https://doi.org/10.1016/j.ejon.2004.11.002 (accessed on 18 May 2024).

12. Engberg, I., Segerstedt, J., Waller, G., Wennberg, P., & Eliasson, M. (2017). Fatigue in the general population - associations to age, sex, socioeconomic status, physical activity, sitting time and self-rated health: The northern Sweden MONICA study 2014. *BMC Public Health, 17*, 654. https://doi.org/10.1186/s12889-017-4623-y (accessed on 18 May 2024).

13. Enoka, R. M., & Duchateau, J. (2016). Translating fatigue to human performance. *Medicine & Science in Sports & Exercise, 48*, 2228–2238. https://doi.org/10.1249/MSS.0000000000000929 (accessed on 18 May 2024).

14. Bucher, E., Sandbakk, O., Donath, L., Roth, R., Zahner, L., & Faude, O. (2018). Exercise-induced trunk fatigue decreases double poling performance in well-trained cross-country skiers. *European Journal of Applied Physiology, 118*, 2077–2087. https://doi.org/10.1007/s00421-018-3938-4 (accessed on 18 May 2024).

15. Lin, C. F., Lee, W. C., Chen, Y. A., & Hsue, B. J. (2016). Fatigue-induced changes in movement pattern and muscle activity during ballet releve on demi-pointe. *Journal of Applied Biomechanics, 32*, 350–358. https://doi.org/10.1123/jab.2014-0263 (accessed on 18 May 2024).

16. Le Mansec, Y., Pageaux, B., Nordez, A., Dorel, S., & Jubeau, M. (2018). Mental fatigue alters the speed and the accuracy of the ball in table tennis. *Journal of Sports Sciences, 36*, 2751–2759. https://doi.org/10.1080/02640414.2017.1418647 (accessed on 18 May 2024).

17. Hanna, T. N., Zygmont, M. E., Peterson, R., Theriot, D., Shekhani, H., Johnson, J. O., & Krupinski, E. A. (2018). The effects of fatigue from overnight shifts on radiology search patterns and diagnostic performance. *Journal of the American College of Radiology, 15*, 1709–1716. https://doi.org/10.1016/j.jacr.2017.12.019 (accessed on 18 May 2024).

18. Mollicone, D., Kan, K., Mott, C., Bartels, R., Bruneau, S., van Wollen, M., Sparrow, A. R., & Van Dongen, H. P. A. (2019). Predicting performance and safety based on driver fatigue. *Accident Analysis & Prevention, 126*, 142–145. https://doi.org/10.1016/j.aap.2018.03.004 (accessed on 18 May 2024).

19. Rudin-Brown, C. M., Harris, S., & Rosberg, A. (2019). How shift scheduling practices contribute to fatigue amongst freight rail operating employees: Findings from Canadian accident investigations. *Accident Analysis & Prevention, 126*, 64–69. https://doi.org/10.1016/j.aap.2018.01.027 (accessed on 18 May 2024).

20. Sievertsen, H. H., Gino, F., & Piovesan, M. (2016). Cognitive fatigue influences students' performance on standardized tests. *Proceedings of the National Academy of Sciences of the United States of America, 113*, 2621–2624. https://doi.org/10.1073/pnas.1516947113 (accessed on 18 May 2024).

21. Mizuno, K., Tanaka, M., Fukuda, S., Imai-Matsumura, K., & Watanabe, Y. (2011). Relationship between cognitive functions and prevalence of fatigue in elementary and junior high school students. *Brain & Development, 33*, 470–479. https://doi.org/10.1016/j.braindev.2010.08.012 (accessed on 18 May 2024).

22. Liu, J., Zhou, G., Wang, Y., Ai, Y., & Pinto-Martin, J. (2012). Sleep problems, fatigue, and cognitive performance in Chinese kindergarten children. *The Journal of Pediatrics, 161*, 520–525. https://doi.org/10.1016/j.jpeds.2012.03.018 (accessed on 18 May 2024).

23. Wang, Z., Ying, Z., Bosy-Westphal, A., Zhang, J., Schautz, B., Later, W., Heymsfield, S. B., & Muller, M. J. (2010). Specific metabolic rates of major organs and tissues across adulthood: Evaluation by mechanistic model of resting energy expenditure. *The American Journal of Clinical Nutrition, 92*, 1369–1377. https://doi.org/10.3945/ajcn.2010.29885 (accessed on 18 May 2024).

24. Sahlin, K., Tonkonogi, M., & Soderlund, K. (1998). Energy supply and muscle fatigue in humans. *Acta Physiologica Scandinavica, 162*, 261–266. https://doi.org/10.1046/j.1365-201X.1998.0298f.x (accessed on 18 May 2024).

25. Sargeant, A. J. (2007). Structural and functional determinants of human muscle power. *Experimental Physiology, 92*, 323–331. https://doi.org/10.1113/expphysiol.2006.034322 (accessed on 18 May 2024).

26. Herculano-Houzel, S. (2011). Scaling of brain metabolism with a fixed energy budget per neuron: Implications for neuronal activity, plasticity and evolution. *PLoS ONE, 6*(3), e17514. https://doi.org/10.1371/journal.pone.0017514 (accessed on 18 May 2024).

27. Harris, J. J., Jolivet, R., & Attwell, D. (2012). Synaptic energy use and supply. *Neuron, 75*(5), 762–777. https://doi.org/10.1016/j.neuron.2012.08.019 (accessed on 18 May 2024).

28. Bordone, M. P., Salman, M. M., Titus, H. E., Amini, E., Andersen, J. V., Chakraborti, B., Diuba, A. V., Dubouskaya, T. G., Ehrke, E., Freitas, A. E., et al. (2019). The energetic brain—A review from students to students. *Journal of Neurochemistry, 151*, 139–165. https://doi.org/10.1111/jnc.14829 (accessed on 18 May 2024).

29. Raichle, M. E. (2015). The restless brain: How intrinsic activity organizes brain function. *Philosophical Transactions of the Royal Society B: Biological Sciences, 370*(1668), 20140172. https://doi.org/10.1098/rstb.2014.0172 (accessed on 18 May 2024).

30. Petit, J. M., & Magistretti, P. J. (2016). Regulation of neuron-astrocyte metabolic coupling across the sleep-wake cycle. *Neuroscience, 323*, 135–156. https://doi.org/10.1016/j.neuroscience.2015.12.007 (accessed on 18 May 2024).

31. Hogan, A. M., Pit-ten Cate, I. M., Vargha-Khadem, F., Prengler, M., & Kirkham, F. J. (2006). Physiological correlates of intellectual function in children with sickle cell disease: Hypoxaemia, hyperaemia and brain infarction. *Developmental Science, 9*, 379–387. https://doi.org/10.1111/j.1467-7687.2006.00503.x (accessed on 18 May 2024).

32. Rink, C., & Khanna, S. (2011). Significance of brain tissue oxygenation and the arachidonic acid cascade in stroke. *Antioxidants & Redox Signaling, 14*, 1889–1903. https://doi.org/10.1089/ars.2010.3474 (accessed on 18 May 2024).

33. Mairbaurl, H. (2013). Red blood cells in sports: Effects of exercise and training on oxygen supply by red blood cells. *Frontiers in Physiology, 4*, 332. https://doi.org/10.3389/fphys.2013.00332 (accessed on 18 May 2024).

34. Schneider, A. L., Jonassaint, C., Sharrett, A. R., Mosley, T. H., Astor, B. C., Selvin, E., Coresh, J., & Gottesman, R. F. (2016). Hemoglobin, anemia, and cognitive function: The Atherosclerosis Risk in Communities Study. *The Journals of Gerontology Series A: Biological Sciences and Medical Sciences, 71*, 772–779. https://doi.org/10.1093/gerona/glv158 (accessed on 18 May 2024).

35. Acaster, S., Dickerhoof, R., DeBusk, K., Bernard, K., Strauss, W., & Allen, L. F. (2015). Qualitative and quantitative validation of the FACIT-fatigue scale in iron deficiency anemia. *Health and Quality of Life Outcomes, 13*, 60. https://doi.org/10.1186/s12955-015-0257-x (accessed on 18 May 2024).

36. Scholey, A. B., Harper, S., & Kennedy, D. O. (2001). Cognitive demand and blood glucose. *Physiology & Behavior, 73*, 585–592. https://doi.org/10.1016/S0031-9384(01)00476-0 (accessed on 18 May 2024).

37. Scholey, A. B., Laing, S., & Kennedy, D. O. (2006). Blood glucose changes and memory: Effects of manipulating emotionality and mental effort. *Biological Psychology, 71*, 12–19. https://doi.org/10.1016/j.biopsycho.2005.02.003 (accessed on 18 May 2024).

38. Fairclough, S. H., & Houston, K. (2004). A metabolic measure of mental effort. *Biological Psychology, 66*, 177–190. https://doi.org/10.1016/j.biopsycho.2003.10.001 (accessed on 18 May 2024).

39. Scholey, A. B., Benson, S., Sela-Venter, S., Mackus, M., & Moss, M. C. (2019). Oxygen administration and acute human cognitive enhancement: Higher cognitive demand leads to a more rapid decay of transient hyperoxia. *Journal of Cognitive Enhancement, 3*(1), 1–6. https://doi.org/10.1007/s41465-019-00145-4 (accessed on 18 May 2024).

40. Sobrero, A., Puglisi, F., Guglielmi, A., Belvedere, O., Aprile, G., Ramello, M., & Grossi, F. (2001). Fatigue: A main component of anemia symptomatology. *Seminars in Oncology, 28*, 15–18. https://doi.org/10.1016/S0093-7754(01)90207-6 (accessed on 18 May 2024).

41. Butte, N. F., & Caballero, B. (2014). Energy needs: Assessment and requirements. In A. C. Ross, B. Caballero, R. J. Cousins, K. L. Tucker, & T. R. Ziegler (Eds.), *Modern Nutrition in Health and Disease* (11th ed., pp. 88–101). Wolters Kluwer-Lippincott, Williams & Wilkins.

42. Alberts, B., Johnson, A., Lewis, J., Morgan, D., Raff, M., Roberts, K., & Walter, P. (2017). Molecular Biology of the Cell: Cell Chemistry and Bioenergetics (Chapter 2, pp. 43–108). Garland Science/CRC Press.

Chapter

7

NUTRIENTS IMPORTANT FOR METABOLISM AND BLOOD FUNCTION

Contents

Unit Introduction

Nutrients play a vital role in supporting metabolism and blood function, ensuring the efficient functioning of the body and overall health. Among the essential nutrients crucial for these processes are vitamins, minerals, and macronutrients. Firstly, B vitamins, including B_1 (thiamine), B_2 (riboflavin), B_3 (niacin), B_6 (pyridoxine), B_{12} (cobalamin), and folate, are integral for metabolism. They act as coenzymes, aiding in energy production from carbohydrates, fats, and proteins. Additionally, they are involved in red blood cell formation and DNA synthesis, contributing to blood function. Secondly, minerals such as iron, zinc, and copper are indispensable for blood health. Iron is crucial for hemoglobin synthesis, and the protein in red blood cells responsible for oxygen transport. Zinc and copper are cofactors in various enzymes involved in red blood cell formation and antioxidant defense. Furthermore, macronutrients like protein and carbohydrates are essential for energy metabolism and blood glucose regulation. Protein provides amino acids necessary for tissue repair and enzyme synthesis, while carbohydrates serve as the primary energy source for cells, including red blood cells. Adequate hydration is also critical for blood volume maintenance and nutrient transport. A balanced diet rich in B vitamins, minerals, and macronutrients is essential for supporting metabolism and ensuring optimal blood function, thereby promoting overall health and well-being.

Orientation and Directional Terms

Term	Definition	Illustration
Red blood cells	A type of blood cell that is made in the bone marrow and found in the blood. Red blood cells contain a protein called hemoglobin, which carries oxygen from the lungs to all parts of the body. Checking the number of red blood cells in the blood is usually part of a complete blood cell (CBC) test.	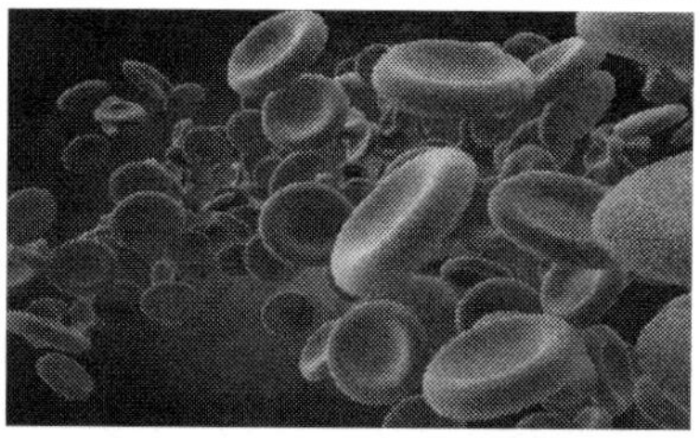
Food molecules	Carbohydrates, proteins, and lipids are the three most frequent types of molecules found in food. These molecules are also known as 'macronutrients,' and they are nutritionally important to us. The three groupings of molecules have quite different properties that will affect how your meal turns out.	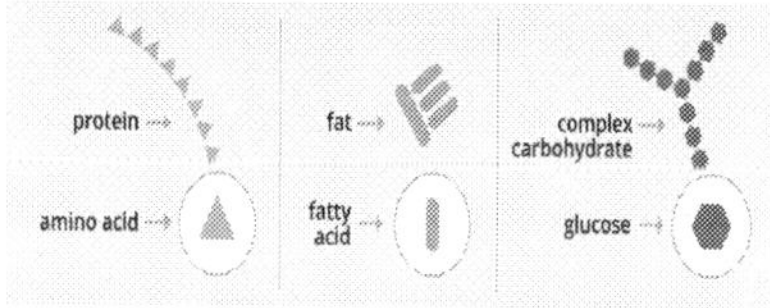
Flavin adenine dinucleotide	Flavin adenine dinucleotide is a redox-active coenzyme associated with various proteins, which is involved with several enzymatic reactions in metabolism. A flavoprotein is a protein that contains a flavin group, which may be in the form of FAD or flavin mononucleotide.	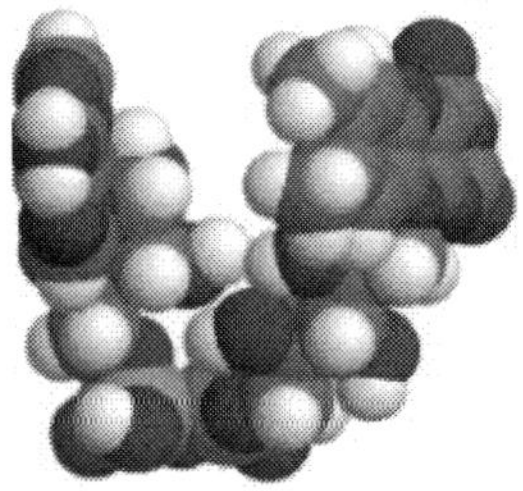
Nicotinamide adenine dinucleotide	Nicotinamide adenine dinucleotide is a coenzyme central to metabolism. Found in all living cells, NAD is called a dinucleotide because it consists of two nucleotides joined through their phosphate groups. One nucleotide contains an adenine nucleobase and the other, nicotinamide.	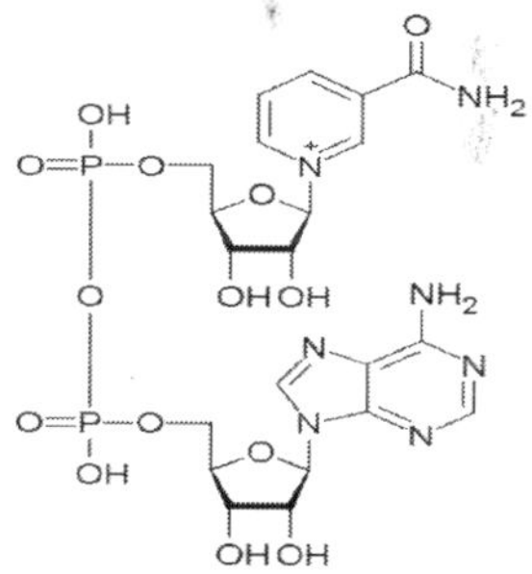
Glycogenesis	Glycogenesis is the process of glycogen synthesis, in which glucose molecules are added to chains of glycogen for storage. This process is activated during rest periods following the Cori cycle, in the liver, and also activated by insulin in response to high glucose levels.	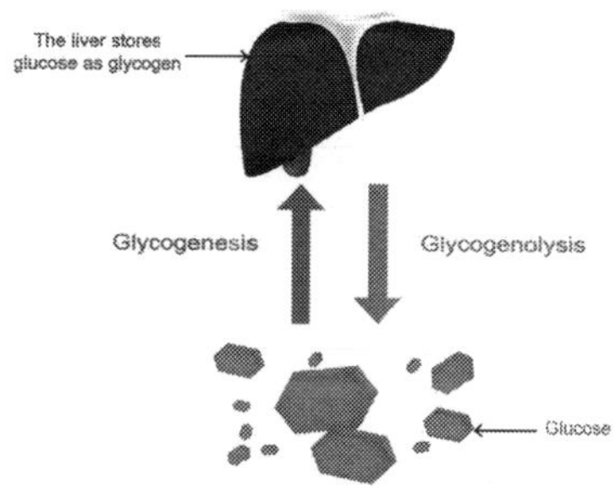

7.1. The Function of Blood in the Body and in Metabolism

The connective tissue and blood in circulatory system carry waste products out of cells and absorbed nutrients to cells. It moves waste materials and synthesized macromolecules to support cellular metabolism. It also moves chemicals, like hormones, which facilitates organ-to-organ communication. The blood that flows through an adult human body contains roughly 5 liters (1.3 gallons) and makes up about 8% of the body weight.

7.1.1. Prelude to Metabolism and Blood Function

Iron is essential to the body for a number of reasons. Its main function is to transport oxygen on behalf of the hemoglobin protein, which is present in red blood cells. Oxygen is necessary for the metabolism of cells. Reduced red blood cell ability to carry oxygen inhibits energy synthesis and, in turn, impairs cell function. Furthermore, iron is needed for the enzymatic synthesis of DNA and RNA as well as the production of energy. As a result, rapidly dividing cells are extremely vulnerable to iron deficiency. Low iron levels prevent red blood cells from being synthesized because the body is always renewing itself, which leads to anemia. Anemia can cause muscle weakness, pale skin, breathlessness, lightheadedness, and exhaustion. Iron-deficiency anemia in newborns and kids can affect their growth, motor skills, mental health, behavior, and academic achievement. The most common nutritional deficiency worldwide, iron deficiency affects many infants, children, and adolescents as well as 10% of women in the United States who are of childbearing age.

Iron-rich foods include chicken, red meats, leafy greens, egg yolks, lentils, clams, oysters, artichokes, prunes, raisins, and enriched cereal grains. Even though there are many iron-rich foods available, very little of the iron in food is actually absorbed. Using an iron skillet to cook food is one way to increase the amount of iron in your diet. Tomatoes and other acidic foods with a high moisture content absorb more iron when cooked than do non-acidic foods. Spaghetti sauce, for instance, can have a ten-fold increase in iron content when cooked in iron cookware. Cooking times also affect how much iron leaches into food; the longer food is cooked, the more iron is absorbed. Increased contact time from frequent stirring allows for greater absorption of iron from the cookware. Some international public health organizations have decided to reduce the global prevalence of iron-deficiency anemia by distributing iron cookware to high-risk populations in developing countries, based on the usefulness of iron cookware in increasing dietary intake of iron.

7.1.2. What Makes Up Blood and How Do These Substances Support Blood Function?

By volume, blood comprises roughly 78% water and 22% solids. The liquid component of blood, known as plasma, is composed primarily of water (95%), but it also includes waste products, gases, proteins, ions, glucose, lipids, vitamins, and minerals, as well as enzymes and hormones. The blood contains large amounts of the protein albumin. Both the pH of the blood and the fluid balance between the blood and tissues are maintained by albumin. The ability of blood to function as a transport medium depends on its water content, and the electrolytes it contains help to keep the pH level steady and fluid balance stable. Additionally, the high water content in the blood aids in regulating body temperature, and continuous blood flow distributes heat throughout the body. Because blood regulates temperature so well, cold air can be brought to body temperature before it reaches the lungs, thanks to the numerous tiny blood vessels in your nose.

Red blood cells, white blood cells, and platelets are the cellular components of blood. The most abundant of the constituents are red blood cells. Millions of them are present in each drop of blood. About 270 million hemoglobin proteins, which contain the mineral iron, which turns red when bound to oxygen, and impart red blood cells their distinctive red color. The primary function of red blood cells is to carry oxygen from the lungs to every cell in the body so that aerobic metabolism can produce energy. As a component of the immune system, white blood cells travel throughout the body searching for foreign invaders to eliminate. They comprise roughly 1% of the total volume of blood. In an emergency, platelets—fragments of cells—are constantly circulating in the blood. Platelets rush to the site of injury when blood vessels are damaged to seal the wound. Blood is made from stem cells found in the bone marrow and is constantly renewing itself. White blood cells can survive anywhere from 18 hours to a year or longer, while platelets have a lifespan of approximately 10 days. Red blood cells have an approximate lifespan of 120 days.

7.1.3. Nutrients In

All nutrients must be transported to the cells that require them after being absorbed from the small intestine. Furthermore, molecules produced in different cells occasionally need to be transported to different organ systems. All cells rely on blood as the conduit and blood vessels as the highway for the transportation of nutrients and molecules. Water-soluble substances, including many proteins, sugars, minerals, and vitamins, flow through the bloodstream on their own. Triglycerides, cholesterol, fat-soluble vitamins, and other lipids are all contained in lipoproteins, which enable their transportation through the aqueous environment of blood. Albumin is the main transport carrier that is required by a large number of proteins, medications, and hormones. Blood is responsible for carrying all of these chemicals as well as delivering oxygen from the lungs to every cell in the body. This is achieved by the hemoglobin molecule in red blood cells, which contains iron, as was previously mentioned.

7.1.4. Wastes Out

Water and carbon dioxide are waste products produced by cells during the metabolism of macronutrients to energy. The rate of blood flow is drastically decreased as blood passes through progressively smaller vessels, enabling an effective exchange of nutrients and oxygen for waste products from cells. The blood carries the carbon dioxide to the lungs, where it is exhaled, and the kidneys eliminate any extra water in the blood. Additionally, the liver detoxifies a variety of toxic substances that must be transported via the blood to the kidneys for excretion, as well as producing the waste product urea from the breakdown of amino acids (Figure 7.1).

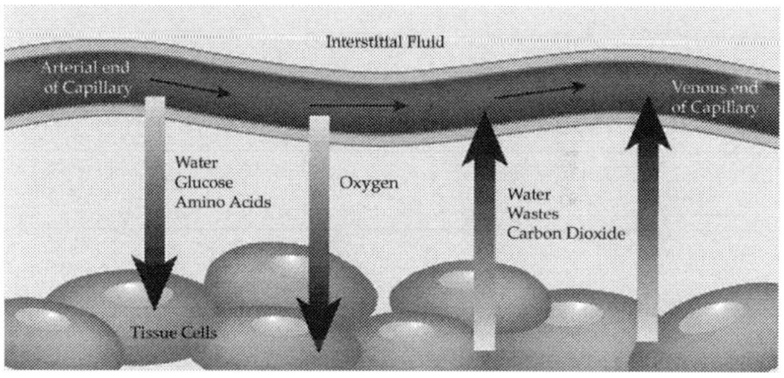

Figure 7.1. *The capillary exchange: Nutrients in and wastes out.*

Source: https://2012books.lardbucket.org/books/an-introduction-to-nutrition/s14-nutrients-important-for-metabo.html.

7.1.5. All for One, One for All

We'll talk about how our bodies function and collaborate to support life, rather than discussing the three Musketeers. The 11 organ systems in the body are entirely dependent upon one another to continue existing as a complex organism. Blood serves as a medium for communication between organ systems as well as the transportation of heat, nutrients, waste products, and water. The function of blood in delivering glucose, particularly to the brain, aptly illustrates the importance of blood to the rest of the body. An hourly average of 6 g of glucose is metabolized by the brain. The brain has to have constant access to glucose in order to prevent confusion, coma, and death. The pancreatic cells use their sense of blood glucose levels to carry out this function. The hormone glucagon, which signals the liver to accelerate glucose synthesis and glycogen breakdown, is released into the blood when blood glucose levels are low. Considering the liver, it releases glucose into the blood, which then carries it to the brain. In parallel, blood carries oxygen to help the brain's conversion of glucose into energy. Healthy blood works quickly to prevent hypoglycemia coma and death.

7.1.6. What Makes Blood Healthy?

Sustaining the wide range of vital functions of the blood requires maintaining blood health, including its ongoing renewal. When blood has the right concentrations of dissolved materials, such as albumin and electrolytes, and the right amounts of water and cellular components, it is considered healthy. Blood requires both macro- and micronutrients for optimum function, just like all other tissues. Amino acids are needed to assemble all of the enzymes and cellular organelles found in each red blood cell, as well as the enormous amount of hemoglobin packed within each red blood cell, in the bone marrow, the site of blood cell production. Like the brain, red blood cells only use glucose as fuel, and to support red blood cell metabolism, glucose must always be available. Like all other cells, blood cells are encased in a plasma membrane, primarily made of lipids. Acute sensitivity to certain vitamin and mineral deficiencies is also present in blood health.

7.1.7. Blood Tests Your Health

Because blood serves as a conduit for metabolic products and wastes, measuring the constituents and specific substances in the blood can provide information about the health of other organ systems in addition to the blood itself. Standard blood tests carried out as part of an annual physical can provide your doctor with information about the health of a specific organ or the likelihood of a disease (Figure 7.2).

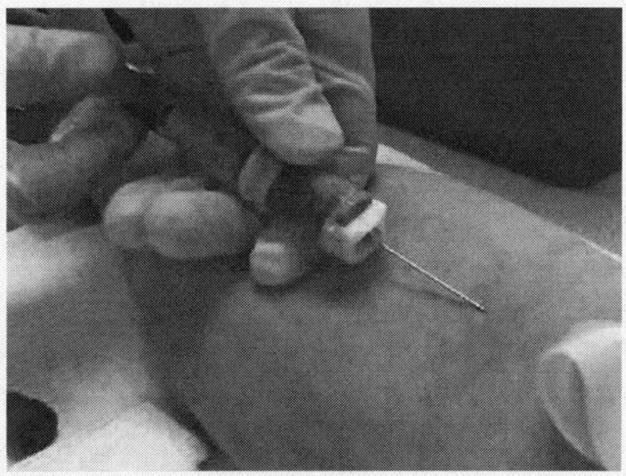

Figure 7.2. *Blood tests are helpful tools in diagnosing disease and provide much information on overall health.*

Source: https://med.libretexts.org/Courses/Chabot_College/Nutrition_1/11%3A_Nutrients_Important_for_Metabolism_and_Blood_Function/11.02%3A_Bloods_Function_in_the_Body_and_in_Metabolism_Support.

A measurable molecule or characteristic associated with a particular disease or health condition is called a biomarker. Blood biomarker concentrations indicate the likelihood of a disease. Prostate-specific antigen, glucose, triglycerides, and cholesterol are a few examples of biomarkers. The results of a blood test show the amounts of various substances in the blood as well as the typical ranges for that population. Results of blood tests outside of the "normal" range are not always a sign of health issues because a person's blood test levels can be influenced by a variety of factors, including diet, amount of physical activity, alcohol consumption, and medication use. Numerous blood parameters are evaluated because they provide information about overall health status and help diagnose disease risk. A partial list of substances measured in a standard blood test can be found in Table 7.1. Only a few of the health-related information that their levels provide is listed in this table.

Table 7.1. *Blood Tests*

Substance Measured	Indicates
Red-blood-cell count	Oxygen-carrying capacity
Hematocrit (red-blood-cell volume)	Anemia risk
White-blood-cell count	Presence of infection
Platelet count	Bleeding disorders, atherosclerosis risk
pH	Metabolic, kidney, and respiratory abnormalities
Albumin	Liver, kidney, and Crohn's disease, dehydration
Bilirubin	Liver-function abnormality
Oxygen/carbon dioxide	Respiratory or metabolic abnormality
Hemoglobin	Oxygen-carrying capacity
Iron	Anemia risk
Magnesium	Magnesium deficiency
Electrolytes (calcium, chloride, magnesium, potassium)	Many illnesses (kidney, metabolic, etc.)
Cholesterol	Cardiovascular disease risk
Triglycerides	Cardiovascular disease risk
Glucose	Diabetes risk
Hormones	Many illnesses (diabetes, reproductive abnormalities)

Source: https://2012books.lardbucket.org/pdfs/an-introduction-to-nutrition/s14-nutrients-important-for-metabo.pdf.

7.2. Metabolism

The totality of chemical reactions necessary to maintain cellular function and, by extension, an organism's life, is known as metabolism. Either all metabolic processes involved in breaking down molecules are referred to as catabolism, or all metabolic processes involved in building larger molecules are referred to as anabolism. Energy is typically released during catabolic processes and consumed during anabolic ones. Transporting matter and transferring energy are the two main objectives of metabolism. Food macronutrients provide energy that is converted into cellular energy, which powers cellular functions. Macroscopic nutrients are converted by metabolism into waste products and materials that cells can use for growth and reproduction.

Proteins called enzymes catalyze chemical reactions. (Remember that the definition of the word "catalyze" is to increase the rate of a chemical reaction while lowering the amount of energy needed to finish it, all without using up the catalyst itself. Enzymes are necessary for chemical reactions to occur quickly enough and consume enough energy for life to exist. A metabolic pathway is made up of a sequence of enzymatic reactions that convert a starting material, or substrate, into intermediates. These intermediates then serve as substrates for the subsequent enzymatic reactions in the pathway, and so on, until the last enzymatic reaction in the pathway synthesizes an end product. While some metabolic pathways are simple and only involve a few chemical reactions, others are complex and involve numerous enzymatic reactions. The metabolic pathways involved in catabolism and anabolism are coordinated by energy status, hormones, substrate, and end-product levels to maintain cellular efficiency. When a molecule is already available, cells cannot build it inefficiently because metabolic pathways are coordinatedly regulated. It is not metabolically efficient for a cell to synthesize fatty acids and break them down at the same time, just as it would be inefficient to build a wall and break it down simultaneously.

Food molecules start to break down as soon as it reaches the mouth because salivary amylase, an enzyme, starts to break down carbohydrates. The big polymers in food are broken down into absorbable monomers during the entire digestive process. The breakdown of proteins yields amino acids, lipids yield fatty acids, and carbohydrates yield monosaccharides. Like with monosaccharides and amino acids, these monomers are either directly absorbed into the bloodstream or, in the case of fatty acids and other fat-soluble molecules, are repackaged in intestinal cells for indirect transport through lymphatic vessels. Blood carries the nutrients to the cells after they are absorbed. The nutrients are taken up from the circulation and processed through either catabolic or anabolic pathways by the cells that need the energy or building blocks. The organ systems need fuel and building blocks, to carry out the various bodily processes—such as digestion, absorption, breathing, pumping blood, moving nutrients in and waste out of the body, regulation of body temperature, and producing new cells (Figure 7.3).

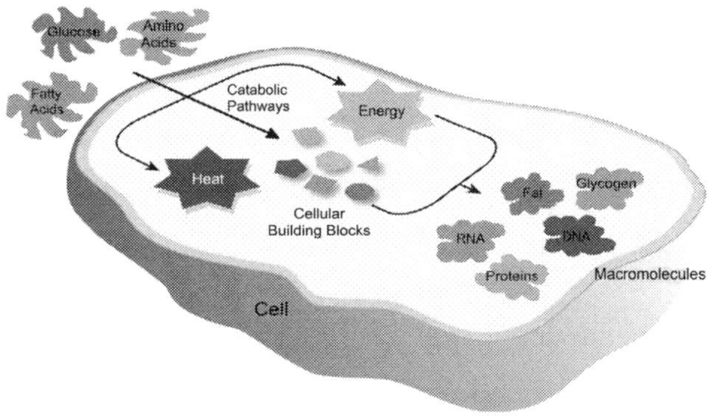

Figure 7.3. *Metabolism is categorized into metabolic pathways that break down the molecules that release energy (catabolism) and the molecules that consume energy by building bigger molecules (anabolism).*

Source: https://med.libretexts.org/Courses/Chabot_College/Nutrition_1/11%3A_Nutrients_Important_for_Metabolism_and_Blood_Function/11.03%3A_Metabolism_Overview.

Table 7.2. *Metabolic Pathways*

Catabolic Pathways	Function	Anabolic Pathways	Function
Glycolysis	Glucose breakdown	Gluconeogenesis	Synthesize glucose
Glycogenolysis	Glycogen breakdown	Glycogenesis	Synthesize glycogen
β-oxidation	Fatty-acid breakdown	Lipogenesis	Synthesize triglycerides
Proteolysis	Protein breakdown to amino acids	Amino-acid synthesis	Synthesize amino acids

Source: https://med.libretexts.org/Courses/Chabot_College/Nutrition_1/11%3A_Nutrients_Important_for_Metabolism_and_Blood_Function/11.03%3A_Metabolism_Overview.

More precisely, the metabolic processes that release or store energy are referred to as energy metabolism. Several of these involve catabolic pathways, such as amino acid catabolism, fatty acid breakdown, and glucose splitting (β-oxidation). The processes involved in producing triglycerides (lipogenesis) and storing excess energy (glycogenesis) are examples of anabolic pathways. A summary of some of the anabolic and catabolic pathways and how they work in energy metabolism can be found in Table 7.2.

7.2.1. Catabolism: The Breakdown

Every cell is aware of its energy balance. Cells produce molecules when their energy levels are high, and they start catabolic pathways to produce energy when their energy levels are low. Most tissues prefer to get their energy from glucose, but they can also catabolize fatty acids and amino acids to produce ATP, the molecule that powers cells. There are three distinct phases in the breakdown of nutrients into energy, and each one has its own unique metabolic pathway. The three phases of nutritional breakdown enable cells to reevaluate their energy needs since byproducts from each pathway can be directed into anabolic pathways or processed further to produce energy. Furthermore, after the needs of the cell for energy are satisfied, metabolic pathway intermediates can occasionally be switched to anabolic pathways. The three stages of nutrient breakdown are the following:

- **Stage 1:** Glycolysis for glucose, β-oxidation for fatty acids, or amino-acid catabolism.
- **Stage 2:** Citric acid cycle (or Kreb cycle).
- **Stage 3:** Electron transport chain and ATP synthesis.

Glycolysis is the first stage of the breakdown of glucose. It is a ten-step metabolic pathway that produces two ATP for every glucose molecule and occurs in the cytosol without the need for oxygen. Two three-carbon molecules known as pyruvate are among the byproducts of glycolysis in addition to ATP. In order to produce more ATP, pyruvate can either go through an anabolic pathway or be transferred to the citric acid cycle. When pyruvate is carried to the mitochondria in a negative-energy balance cell, one of its carbons is removed, producing acetyl-CoA. The citric acid cycle, the second stage of energy metabolism, receives acetyl-CoA, a two-carbon molecule involved in the metabolism of proteins, lipids, and glucose. The catabolic pathway, β-oxidation, starts the breakdown of fatty acids and occurs in the mitochondria. In this catabolic pathway, long chains of fatty acids undergo four consecutive enzymatic steps that remove two carbons from the chains to produce acetyl-CoA molecules. When nitrogen is taken out of an amino acid, the remaining carbon skeleton can be converted by an enzyme into acetyl-CoA or another intermediate of the citric acid cycle.

Acetyl-CoA is bonded to a four-carbon molecule in the citric acid cycle. Two carbons are lost as two molecules of carbon dioxide in this multistep process. The energy released during the citric acid cycle's breakage of chemical bonds is converted into two additional ATP molecules (or their equivalents) and high-energy electrons that are carried by the molecules flavin adenine dinucleotide (FADH2) and nicotinamide adenine dinucleotide (NADH). In what is known as the electron transport chain, NADH and FADH2 transport the electrons to the inner membrane of the mitochondria, where the third stage of energy synthesis occurs. This metabolic pathway results in the sequential transfer of electrons between several proteins and the synthesis of ATP. Chemically speaking, burning and the process of breaking down nutrients are identical because burning carbon molecules produces heat, carbon dioxide, and water. The breakdown of carbon molecules is slowed down by the numerous chemical reactions involved in nutrient catabolism, allowing for the capture of a large amount of energy rather than its conversion to heat and light. Given that complete nutrient catabolism is only 30–40% efficient, some energy is subsequently released as heat. Heat is an essential byproduct of the breakdown of nutrients and is responsible for regulating body temperature. Humans would not survive until their next meal if cells were too effective at converting nutrient energy into ATP, as they would succumb to hypothermia.

7.2.2. Anabolism: The Building

Catabolic pathways release energy that drives anabolic pathways, which in turn create proteins like DNA and RNA and even whole new cells and tissues. Anabolic pathways are necessary for the construction of new tissue, such as muscle, following extended physical activity or for the catabolic and anabolic pathways involved in bone remodeling. Triglycerides and glycogen are examples of molecules that store energy that are produced via anabolic pathways. Sometimes, intermediates in the catabolic pathways of energy metabolism are used as building blocks rather than as ATP. When a cell is in positive energy balance, this occurs. For instance, if needed, the amino acids glutamate or glutamine can be produced anabolically from the citric-acid-cycle intermediate α-ketoglutarate. Remember that 11 of the 20 amino acids that make up proteins can be synthesized by the human body. The particular amino acid that results from a particular pathway inhibits all of the metabolic pathways involved in amino acid synthesis. As a result, a cell will stop synthesizing glutamine if it has enough of it.

Although the end products of anabolic pathways influence them, the energy state of the cell has a greater influence. Larger molecules, like protein, RNA, and DNA, will be created as needed when there is an abundance of energy. On the other hand, proteins and other molecules will be broken down and catabolized to release energy when there is not enough of it. Children with Marasmus provide a striking illustration of this. The severely impaired bodies of these kids frequently result in infection-related death. Youngsters suffering from Marasmus are malnourished because these nutrients are necessary for the synthesis of macromolecules and energy. Children with Marasmus experience a breakdown of muscle and other organ tissues as a result of their negative energy balance, which is the survival attempt of the body. Children diagnosed with Marasmus appear malnourished or "muscle-wasted" due to a significant reduction in muscle mass" (Figure 7.4).

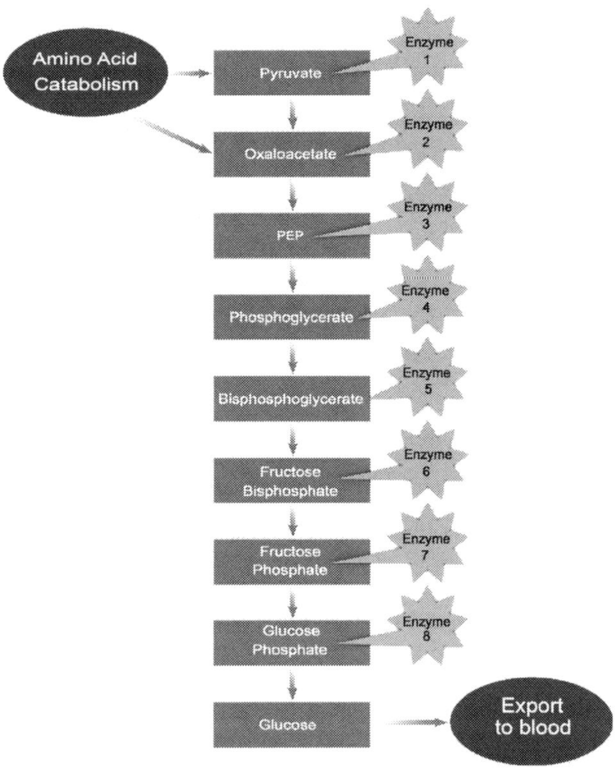

Figure 7.4. *Metabolic pathway of gluconeogenesis.*

Source: https://2012books.lardbucket.org/books/an-introduction-to-nutrition/s14-nutrients-important-for-metabo.html.

A person is also in negative energy balance in between meals, albeit in a much less severe example. Blood glucose levels start to decrease during this period. The anabolic pathway known as gluconeogenesis is triggered in order to return blood glucose levels to the normal range. The process of constructing glucose molecules from specific amino acids is known as gluconeogenesis, and it mostly takes place in the liver (Figure 7.4). The blood contains the glucose that the liver has produced and exported for use by other tissues.

7.2.3. Energy Storage

In contrast, more energy from nutrients will be stored when the body is "fed," or when energy levels are high. Only the tissues of the muscles and liver can store glucose. It is stored in these tissues as glycogen, a highly branching macromolecule made up of thousands of chemically bound glucose monomers. Glycogenesis is an anabolic process that connects the glucose monomers. One molecule of ATP is needed for every glucose molecule that is stored. As a result, energy storage is expensive. It does not take long for glycogen levels to reach their physiological limit, at which point extra glucose is turned into fat. Acetyl-CoA generated by catabolic pathways and a high concentration of ATP are detected by a cell in positive-energy balance. In response, the anabolic pathway known as lipogenesis is activated, resulting in the synthesis of triglycerides and the cessation of catabolism. The newly created triglycerides are delivered to adipocytes, which are cells that store fat. Since fat is more compact (per unit of energy) and the body does not store water with fat like it does with glycogen, fat is a preferable option for storing energy. Since water makes up a large portion of the weight of glycogen stores, an increase in water would result in a significant increase in body weight. Excess protein, fat, and lipids are all converted to fat by the body in a positive energy balance.

7.3. Vitamins Important for Metabolism and for Blood Function and Renewal

While vitamins and minerals are necessary as functional components of enzymes involved in energy release and storage, they play a different kind of role in energy metabolism than alcohol and macronutrients (carbohydrates, lipids, and proteins), which can be catabolized to release energy. Coenzymes and cofactors are the terms for the vitamins and minerals that are components of enzymes. Enzymes need coenzymes and cofactors to catalyze a particular reaction. They help transform a raw material into a final product (Figure 7.5). In addition to being important in many anabolic pathways, coenzymes and cofactors are also involved in catabolic pathways.

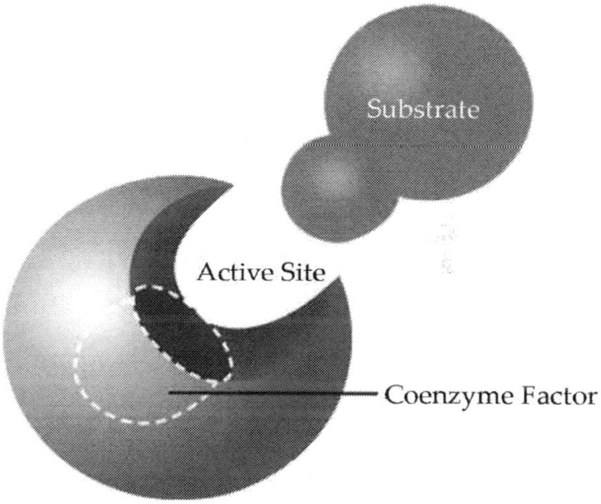

Figure 7.5. *Coenzymes and cofactors are the particular vitamin or mineral required for enzymes to catalyze a specific reaction.*

Source: https://med.libretexts.org/Courses/Chabot_College/Nutrition_1/11%3A_Nutrients_Important_for_Metabolism_and_Blood_Function/11.04%3A_Vitamins_Important_for_Metabolism_and_for_Blood_Function_and_Renewal.

Not only are vitamins and minerals crucial for metabolism, they are also necessary for the renewal and proper functioning of blood. When these essential nutrients are lacking in the diet, they can negatively impact blood health and hinder the delivery of nutrients, and allow wastes to accumulate, along with other important functions.

7.3.1. Vitamins: Functions in Catabolic Pathways, Anabolic Pathways, and Blood

7.3.1.1. Thiamine (B_1)

Thiamine is particularly crucial to the metabolism of glucose. It functions as a cofactor for the enzymes that metabolize glucose to produce energy. Furthermore, thiamine is necessary for the synthesis of RNA, DNA, and ATP because it contributes to the process of ribose from glucose. Thiamine deficiency primarily affects the heart and brain. Beriberi, another name for thiamine deficiency, is a condition that can result in symptoms such as heart failure, fatigue, disorientation, difficulty moving, lower extremity pain, and swelling. It is common in cultures where white rice is the primary food source. Along with what were referred to as "accessory factors" in the early 19th century but were essential for metabolism, the bran is removed from white rice during processing.

7.3.1.2. Riboflavin (B_2)

Flavoproteins are coenzymes involved in numerous metabolic pathways of protein, lipid, and carbohydrate metabolism. One of their main components is riboflavin. In the electron transport chain, flavoproteins help move electrons around. Moreover, the actions of flavoproteins are necessary for the proper functioning of other B-vitamin coenzymes, including vitamin B_6 and folate. The bright yellow color of riboflavin, attributed to the "flavin" portion of the molecule, played a significant role in its identification as a vitamin. Ariboflavin deficiency, also known as ariboflavinosis, is a common condition in individuals who suffer from alcoholism and is frequently accompanied by other dietary deficiencies, most notably protein deficiency. Dry, scaly skin, mouth sores and inflammation, sore throat, itchy eyes, and light sensitivity are some of its symptoms.

7.3.1.3. Niacin (B_3)

The coenzymes NADH and NADPH, which are involved in the catabolism and/or anabolism of proteins, lipids, and carbohydrates, include niacin. The main electron carrier, NADH, moves electrons to the electron-transport chain so that ATP can be produced. Additionally, the anabolic pathways of cholesterol and fatty acid synthesis depend on NADPH. Unlike other vitamins, niacin can be produced by humans from the amino acid tryptophan through an anabolic process that needs iron, vitamin B_6, riboflavin, and other dependent enzymes. Tryptophan is converted to niacin only when it has fulfilled all of the other requirements in the body. A few scientific studies have shown that diets high in tryptophan have very little effect on niacin deficiency. The contribution of tryptophan-derived niacin to niacin needs in the body varies widely. Common symptoms of pellagra, or niacin deficiency, include diarrhea, dermatitis, dementia, and occasionally even death.

7.3.1.4. Pantothenic Acid (B_5)

The primary transporter of carbon molecules in a cell, coenzyme A, is made from pantothenic acid. Acetyl-CoA enters the citric acid cycle as a carbon carrier for amino acids, fatty acids, and glucose (Figure 7.6). The synthesis of lipids, cholesterol, and the neurotransmitter acetylcholine is also aided by coenzyme A. Deficiency in vitamin B_5 is very uncommon. The following are some of the warning signs and symptoms: cramps, numbness, tiredness, and irritability. Pantothenic acid may be found in many ingredient lists for skin and hair care products, but there is no solid scientific proof that it makes skin or hair healthier in humans.

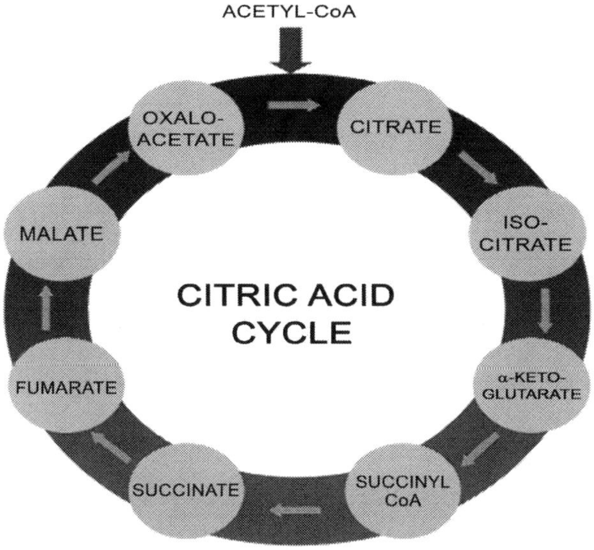

Figure 7.6. *Vitamin B_5 makes up coenzyme A, which carries the carbons of glucose, fatty acids, and amino acids into the citric acid cycle as Acetyl-CoA.*

Source: https://med.libretexts.org/Courses/Chabot_College/Nutrition_1/11%3A_Nutrients_Important_for_Metabolism_and_Blood_Function/11.04%3A_Vitamins_Important_for_Metabolism_and_for_Blood_Function_and_Renewal.

7.3.1.5. Pyroxidine (B_6)

Pyroxidine plays a part in the synthesis and catabolism of amino acids because it is the coenzyme that transfers nitrogen between amino acids. It also helps in the catabolic pathway of glycogenolysis by releasing glucose from glycogen, and enzymes need it to synthesize various neurotransmitters, including hemoglobin. Vitamin B_6 deficiency can manifest as fatigue, disorientation, mouth sores, dermatitis, and muscle weakness. Hemoglobin synthesis requires the coenzyme vitamin B_6. Although the symptoms are similar, anemia resulting from a vitamin B_6 deficiency is not the same as anemia caused by a deficiency in iron, cobalamin, or folate. Red blood cells have a normal or slightly smaller size, but their hemoglobin content is lower. This implies that each red blood cell can carry less oxygen, which leads to exhaustion, weakness in the muscles, and shortness of breath.

7.3.1.6. Biotin

As a coenzyme, biotin is necessary for both lipid metabolism and the citric acid cycle. Additionally, it is needed as an enzyme in the production of some unnecessary amino acids and glucose. For biotin to be absorbed in the gut, it must be released from protein using an enzyme called biotinidase. Although some biotin is produced by bacteria in the colon, this is not a major source of the vitamin. Although it is uncommon, eating a lot of egg whites over an extended period can result in biotin deficiency. This is due to a protein found in egg whites that firmly binds to biotin, preventing absorption. Biotin deficiency is also brought on by a rare genetic disease that causes the biotinidase enzyme to malfunction. When biotin deficiency is severe, hair loss may also occur in addition to symptoms similar to those of deficiency of other B vitamins.

7.3.1.7. Folate

Folate is a necessary coenzyme for the synthesis of DNA and RNA, as well as the amino acid methionine. Folate deficiency thus primarily affects rapidly dividing cells. In the bone marrow, dividing stem cells are constantly producing red blood cells, white blood cells, and platelets. A folate deficiency can result in macrocytic anemia, also referred to as megaloblastic anemia. Anemia is defined as having fewer red blood cells or red blood cells with less hemoglobin. Macrocytic and megaloblastic are terms for "big cell." Red blood cells with macrocytic anemia are larger and less numerous. It is brought on by red blood cells' inability to make DNA and RNA quickly enough; as a result, the cells enlarge but do not divide.

Folate is particularly important for the development and specialization of central nervous system cells. Neural tube birth defects are more common in offspring whose mothers were deficient in folate during their pregnancies. Spina bifida is a neural-tube defect that arises when the spinal cord is not entirely enclosed by the spine. It is causally linked to folate deficiency. Numerous mental and physical impairments can result from spina bifida (Figure 7.7). Compared to before enriched cereal grain products were fortified with folate in 1996 in the United States (and 1998 in Canada), observational studies demonstrate a decrease in the prevalence of neural-tube defects (Figure 7.7). Furthermore, clinical trial results show a significant reduction in neural-tube defects in the offspring of mothers who started taking folate supplements one month before getting pregnant and continued to do so throughout the pregnancy. The Food and Nutrition Board of the Institute of Medicine increased the RDA for folate for pregnant women to 600 µg in response to the scientific data. A few people were worried that consuming more folate could lead to colon cancer, but research has disproved this theory.

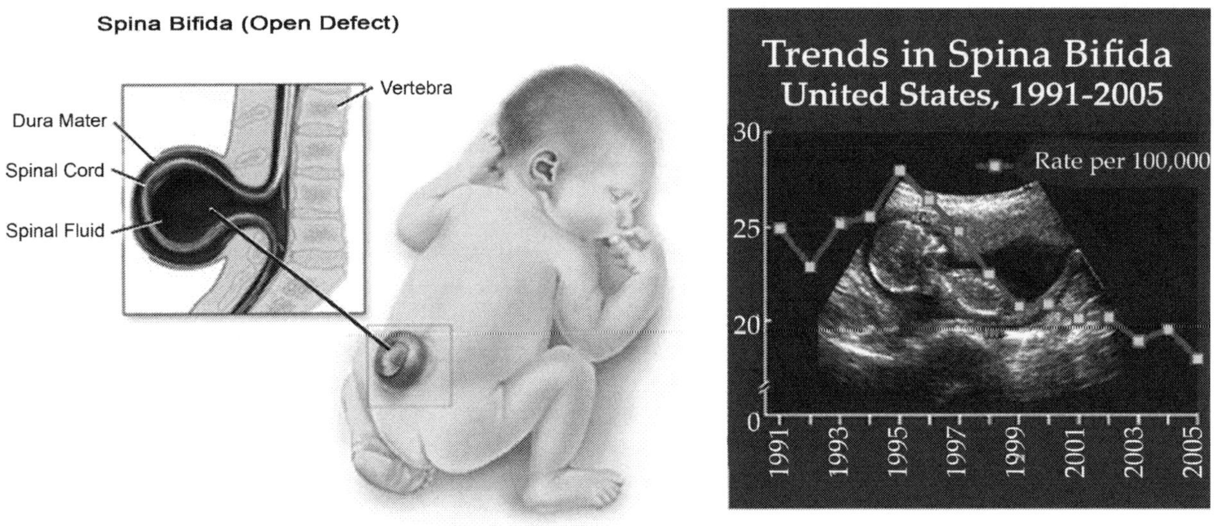

Figure 7.7. *Spina bifida is a neural-tube defect that can have severe health consequences.*

Source: https://med.libretexts.org/Courses/Chabot_College/Nutrition_1/11%3A_Nutrients_Important_for_Metabolism_and_Blood_Function/11.04%3A_Vitamins_Important_for_Metabolism_and_for_Blood_Function_and_Renewal.

7.3.1.8. Cobalamin (B_{12})

The only vitamin that has a metal ion in it is cobalamin, which comes from cobalt. An essential component of coenzymes is cobalamin. It is essential for the catabolism of fat and protein, the activity of the folate coenzyme, and the synthesis of hemoglobin. An enzyme that is dependent on folate needs cobalamin in order to synthesize DNA. Therefore, the health effects of a cobalamin deficiency are comparable to those of a folate deficiency. Macrocytic anemia is the result of cobalamin deficiency in both adults and children, and neural tube defects are more common in offspring of cobalamin-deficient mothers. Proper functioning of the stomach, pancreas, and small intestine is necessary for the human body to absorb cobalamin. The stomach cells secrete a protein known as intrinsic factor, which is required for the small intestine to absorb cobalamin. Pernicious anemia, a form of macrocytic anemia, can be brought on by a chronic stomach inflammation (like the one that some people experience due to *Helicobacter pylori* infection) or an autoimmune disease that impairs the secretion of this protein. The elderly are most likely to experience vitamin B_{12} malabsorption due to their potentially compromised digestive systems, which is a natural aspect of aging. Large oral doses of vitamin B_{12} or applying the vitamin under the tongue, where it is absorbed into the bloodstream without going through the intestines, are the two methods used to treat pernicious anemia. Vitamin B_{12} is injected into patients who do not respond to oral or sublingual therapy.

Table 7.3 provides an overview of the key roles that the B vitamins play in blood and metabolism, as well as the deficiencies associated with each vitamin.

Table 7.3. *B-Vitamin Functions in Metabolism and Blood, and Deficiency Syndromes*

B Vitamin	Function	Deficiency: Signs and Symptoms
B_1 (thiamine)	Coenzyme: assists in glucose metabolism, RNA, DNA, and ATP synthesis.	Beriberi: fatigue, confusion, movement impairment, swelling, heart failure.
B_2 (riboflavin)	Coenzyme: assists in glucose, fat and carbohydrate metabolism, electron carrier, other B vitamins are dependent on.	Ariboflavinosis: dry scaly skin, mouth inflammation and sores, sore throat, itchy eyes, light sensitivity.
B_3 (niacin)	Coenzyme: assists in glucose, fat, and protein metabolism, electron carrier.	Pellagra: diarrhea, dermatitis, dementia, death.
B_5 (pantothenic acid)	Coenzyme: assists in glucose, fat, and protein metabolism, cholesterol, and neurotransmitter synthesis.	Muscle numbness and pain, fatigue, irritability.
B_6 (pyroxidine)	Coenzyme; assists in amino-acid synthesis, glycogneolysis, neurotransmitter and hemoglobin synthesis.	Muscle weakness, dermatitis, mouth sores, fatigue, confusion.
Biotin	Coenzyme; assists in glucose, fat, and protein metabolism, amino-acid synthesis.	Muscle weakness, dermatitis, fatigue, hair loss.
Folate	Coenzyme; amino acid synthesis, RNA, DNA, and red blood cell synthesis.	Diarrhea, mouth sores, confusion, anemia, neural-tube defects.
B_{12} (cobalamin)	Coenzyme; fat and protein catabolism, folate function, red-blood-cell synthesis.	Muscle weakness, sore tongue, anemia, nerve damage, neural-tube defects.

Source: https://med.libretexts.org/Courses/Chabot_College/Nutrition_1/11%3A_Nutrients_Important_for_Metabolism_and_Blood_Function/11.04%3A_Vitamins_Important_for_Metabolism_and_for_Blood_Function_and_Renewal.

7.3.2. Do B-Vitamin Supplements Provide an Energy Boost?

This is a myth that is not supported by science, despite the claims of some marketers that taking a vitamin co-ntaining 1,000 times the daily value of certain B vitamins increases energy and performance. The high levels of added sugars, caffeine, and other herbal stimulants that come with high doses of B vitamins are what cause the "feeling" of having more energy that comes from energy-boosting supplements. As was previously mentioned, B vitamins are necessary for growth and energy metabolism; however, consuming more than is necessary will not increase your energy levels. The gas in your car is a great way to understand this phenomenon. The car will still drive at the same speed whether it has a half-full or full tank of gas; it does not matter. Likewise, energy metabolism issues arise from B vitamin deficiency; however, consuming more B vitamins than necessary does not accelerate metabolism. Customers who purchase B-vitamin supplements should exercise caution, as the body does not retain excess B vitamins, and any extra money spent will be thrown down the drain. Many foods naturally contain B vitamins, and many more are enhanced with them. B-vitamin deficiencies are uncommon in the United States, but many North Americans suffered from certain B-vitamin deficiencies in the 19th century. Pelagra, or niacin deficiency, was common among lower-class Americans whose primary food source was refined cornmeal. Severe symptoms included dementia, dermatitis, diarrhea, and even death. Because there is not enough niacin in the body to support metabolism, pellagra can have some negative health effects.

7.3.3. Dietary Reference Intakes and Sources of B Vitamins

Since they dissolve in water, B vitamins are not significantly stored in the body. As a result, the diet must provide them consistently. Thankfully, the gut normally absorbs B vitamins quite well. Table 7.4, which also provides some dietary sources for these micronutrients, lists the RDA or Adequate Intakes (AI) for the B vitamins as determined by the Institute of Medicine.

Table 7.4. *Dietary Reference Intakes and Food Sources for B Vitamins (RDA: Recommended Dietary Allowance)*

B Vitamin	**RDA (mg/day)**	**Food Sources**
B_1 (thiamine)	1.2 (males)	Whole grains, enriched grains, orange juice, milk, peanuts, dried beans and seeds.
	1.1 (females)	
B_2 (riboflavin)	1.3 (males)	Milk, yogurt, fortified breakfast cereals, organ meats, mushrooms, eggs, clams, spinach.
	1.1 (females)	
B_3 (niacin)	16 (males)	Meat, poultry, fish, whole grains, fortified breakfast cereals, enriched grains, mushrooms, peanuts.
	14 (females)	
B_5 (pantothenic acid)	5 (males)	Eggs, sunflower seeds, peanuts, meat, milk, vegetables.
	5 (females)*	
B_6 (pyroxidine)	1.3 (males)	Meats, whole grains, potatoes, fortified breakfast cereals, bananas, avocados.
	1.3 (females)	
Biotin	0.03 (males)	Egg yolks, peanuts, cheese.
	0.03 (females)*	
Folate	0.4 (males)	Green leafy vegetables, legumes, fortified breakfast cereals, orange juice, sunflower seeds, liver.
	0.4 (females)	
B_{12} (cobalamin)	0.0024 (males)	Animal derived foods, soy milk, and fortified breakfast cereals.
	0.0024 (females)	

Source: https://med.libretexts.org/Courses/Chabot_College/Nutrition_1/11%3A_Nutrients_Important_for_Metabolism_and_Blood_Function/11.04%3A_Vitamins_Important_for_Metabolism_and_for_Blood_Function_and_Renewal.

It should be remembered that food loses B vitamins when it is processed, cooked, and stored. Fruits and vegetables should be consumed more whole foods, steamed rather than boiled, and not kept in storage for extended periods in order to optimize B vitamin absorption. Alcohol also interferes with B vitamin absorption through the intestines.

7.3.4. Dietary Sources Rich in Folate and Vitamin B_{12}

Look over Table 7.5 for excellent dietary sources of these micronutrients to help ensure you are getting all the vitamin B_{12} and folate you require to support metabolism and blood-cell synthesis (Table 7.6).

Table 7.5. *Dietary Sources of Folate*

Food	Micrograms per Serving	Percent Daily Value
Liver	185 (3 oz.)	45
Calf liver	650 (3 oz.)	160
Fortified breakfast cereals	400 (¾ c.)	100
Spinach	100 (½ c., boiled)	25
Northern beans	100 (½ c., boiled)	25
Asparagus	85 (4 spears, boiled)	20
Vegetarian baked beans	60 (1 c.)	15
Broccoli	45 (2 spears)	10
Avocado	45 (½ c.)	10
Bread (enriched)	25 (1 slice)	6

Source: https://med.libretexts.org/Courses/Chabot_College/Nutrition_1/11%3A_Nutrients_Important_for_Metabolism_and_Blood_Function/11.04%3A_Vitamins_Important_for_Metabolism_and_for_Blood_Function_and_Renewal.

Table 7.6. *Dietary Sources of Vitamin B_{12}*

Food	Micrograms per Serving	Percent Daily Value
Liver	48 (1 slice)	800
Clams	34.2 (3 oz.)	570
Organic calf liver	31 (3 oz.)	520
Fortified breakfast cereals	6.0 (1 serving)	100
Trout (wild)	5.4 (3 oz.)	90
Trout (farmed)	3.5 (3 oz.)	58
Salmon (sockeye)	4.8 (3 oz.)	80
Cheeseburger	2.1	35
Yogurt (plain)	1.4 (1 c.)	23
Beef (top sirloin)	1.4 (3 oz.)	23
Milk	0.9 (1 c.)	15
Egg	0.6 (1 large)	10

Source: https://med.libretexts.org/Courses/Chabot_College/Nutrition_1/11%3A_Nutrients_Important_for_Metabolism_and_Blood_Function/11.04%3A_Vitamins_Important_for_Metabolism_and_for_Blood_Function_and_Renewal.

7.3.5. Vitamin K: Functions in Metabolism and Blood

Although there is growing evidence that vitamin K may be involved in energy metabolism, it is still unclear exactly what roles vitamin K-dependent enzymes play in this process. For the best possible metabolism of bone, vitamin K is needed. Additionally essential to blood function is vitamin K. It functions as a coenzyme with blood clotting-related enzymes. Blood-clotting proteins are always moving through the bloodstream. When a blood vessel is injured, platelets adhere to the wound and create a plug.

The fibrous protein fibrin is formed when the clotting factors in the surrounding blood flow react through a sequence of protein-protein interactions, strengthening the platelet plug and causing the blood-clotting cascade of events to be animated. Bleeding disorders are caused by a vitamin K deficiency. Vitamin K deficiency is comparatively uncommon, but it is more common in those with celiac disease, pancreatic or liver disease, and malabsorption disorders. Nosebleeds, easily bruised areas, broken blood vessels, bleeding gums, and heavy menstrual bleeding in women are among the signs and symptoms. Consumption of excess vitamin K from supplements compromises the effectiveness of the anticoagulant medication warfarin.

7.3.6. Dietary Reference Intakes and Sources of Vitamin K

Adult males' RDA for vitamin K is 120 mcg, while adult females' RDA is 90 mcg. While vitamin K can be found in a variety of foods, it is highest in green leafy vegetables. For a list of food sources of vitamin K, see Table 7.7.

Table 7.7. *Dietary Sources of Vitamin K*

Food	Micrograms per Serving	Percent Daily Value
Broccoli (½ c.)	160.0	133
Asparagus (4 spears)	34.0	28
Cabbage (½ c.)	56.0	47
Spinach (½ c.)	27.0	23
Green peas (½ c.)	16.0	13
Cheese (1 oz.)	10.0	8
Ham (3 oz.)	13.0	11
Ground beef (3 oz.)	6.0	5
Bread	1.1	<1
Orange	1.3	1

Source: https://med.libretexts.org/Courses/Chabot_College/Nutrition_1/11%3A_Nutrients_Important_for_Metabolism_and_Blood_Function/11.04%3A_Vitamins_Important_for_Metabolism_and_for_Blood_Function_and_Renewal.

7.4. Minerals Important for Metabolism and for Blood Function and Renewal

Minerals abound in a diet that is well-balanced, and minerals are abundant in herbs. To get the best possible mineral nutrition, add more flavor to your food, drink herbal teas, and eat more plants.

1. **Magnesium:** As the body's 11th most abundant element, magnesium is known to take part in hundreds of metabolic reactions as a cofactor. Since ATP and magnesium form a complex, magnesium is necessary for all reactions involving the synthesis of ATP, such as those involving the synthesis of carbohydrates, lipids, proteins, RNA, and DNA. Many Americans' diets do not provide them with the recommended amount of magnesium. A mild

magnesium deficiency may be associated with an increased risk of cardiovascular disease, according to certain observational studies. A severe magnesium deficiency can cause tremor, muscle spasms, nausea, and loss of appetite.

2. **Iron:** Hemoglobin, a protein that carries oxygen, is found in red blood cells. It is made up of four globular peptides, one heme complex per peptide. Iron is located in the middle of each heme (Figure 7.8). Hundreds of metabolic enzymes depend on iron as a critical component. Iron-sulfur clusters are present in a large number of the electron-transport chain proteins and are essential for the transfer of high-energy electrons and, eventually, the synthesis of ATP. Additionally, iron is involved in a variety of metabolic processes that primarily occur in the liver and detoxify toxic substances. Iron is also necessary for the synthesis of DNA. The vast majority of iron that the body uses comes from red blood cell recycling, which occurs continuously.

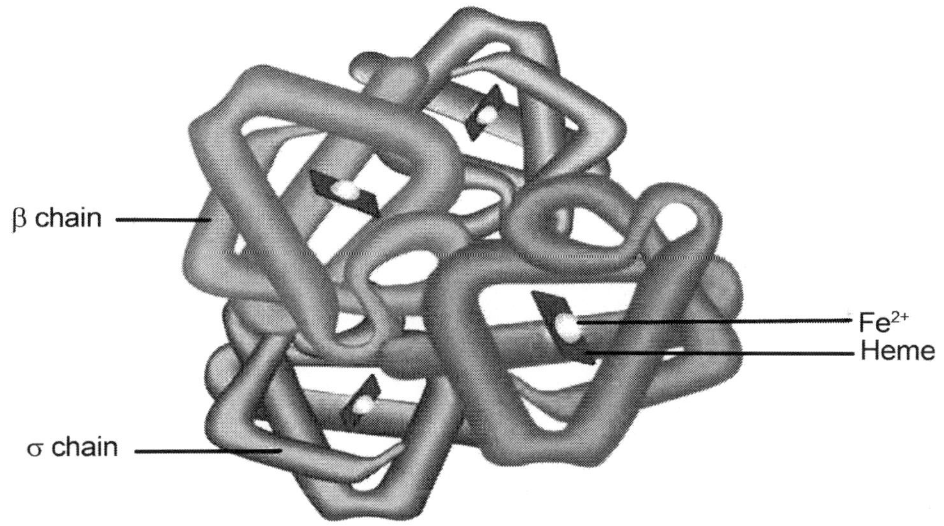

Figure 7.8. *Hemoglobin is composed of four peptides. Each contains a heme group with iron in the center.*

Source: https://med.libretexts.org/Courses/Chabot_College/Nutrition_1/11%3A_Nutrients_Important_for_Metabolism_and_Blood_Function/11.05%3A_Minerals_Important_for_Metabolism_and_for_Blood_Function_and_Renewal.

The iron in hemoglobin binds to oxygen in the capillaries of lungs and carries it to the cells, where it is released. Anemia is caused by insufficient hemoglobin synthesis and decreased red blood cell oxygen carrying capacity when iron levels are low. In an attempt to make up for low dietary intake, the small intestine absorbs iron more effectively when iron levels are low. However, this process is unable to offset the excessive iron loss that results from low intake or chronic blood loss. The body recycles iron back into the bone marrow, which produces red blood cells, when blood cells are no longer needed. The skeletal muscle, liver, spleen, and bone marrow all contain some iron that is stored by the body. Iron is expelled in relatively small amounts when skin and small intestine lining cells perish and blood is lost, as occurs during menstruation. Dietary sources must supply the lost iron.

The sources of iron in the diet have a significant impact on its bioavailability. Heme iron is more bioavailable than nonheme iron, and approximately 60% of iron in diets derived from animals is bound to hemoglobin. Nonheme, the only iron source in plant-based diets, accounts for the remaining 40% of iron found in animal-based foods. Certain plant substances, like phytate, oxalates, tannins, and polyphenols, prevent the absorption of iron. However, consuming vitamin C-rich fruits and vegetables along with foods high in iron significantly improves iron absorption. The bioavailability of vegetarian diets is between 5 and 12%, while that of mixed diets is between 14 and 18%.

3. **Zinc:** It is directly involved in the synthesis of RNA, DNA, and proteins and is a cofactor for more than 200 enzymes in the human body. Moreover, zinc cofactors with enzymes that are part of the metabolism of energy. Zinc plays important roles in energy metabolism and anabolism, so deficiencies in this mineral stunt growth in infants and young children. Early in the 1960s, research in the Middle East connected diets high in phytate to adolescent nutritional dwarfism, demonstrating how growth depends on sufficient dietary zinc. Certain chemicals, such as phytate, found in cereal grains and some vegetables prevent the gut from absorbing zinc and other minerals. This is primarily a result of the diet's deficiency in red meat and seafood and its reliance on cereal grains as the primary food source. Serious zinc deficiency in adults can result in weight loss, diarrhea, skin sores, loss of appetite, and hair loss. Zinc is a necessary cofactor for an enzyme that produces the heme component of hemoglobin; anemia can arise from diets that are severely zinc deficient.

4. **Iodine:** Goiter is a severe enlargement of the thyroid gland in the neck; iodine can help prevent this condition. Thyroid hormone, which controls growth, development, and basal metabolism, is synthesized with the help of iodine. Fatigue, cold sensitivity, constipation, weight gain, depression, dry, itchy skin, and paleness are just a few of the numerous signs and symptoms of low iodine levels and, by extension, hypothyroidism. Although goiter is frequently the most obvious symptom of a chronic iodine deficiency, low thyroid hormone can have serious effects on all phases of growth and development during infancy, childhood, and adolescence. A severe iodine deficiency causes cretinism in fetuses and infants, a condition that can cause severe physical and neurological impairment. Thyroid hormone is important for brain development and growth. Iodine deficiency is the leading preventable cause of brain damage globally, according to estimates from the World Health Organization (WHO), affecting over two billion people.

5. **Selenium:** Because selenium is a cofactor of the enzymes that allow cells to release active thyroid hormone, low levels of the mineral can have symptoms that are similar to those of iodine deficiency. Antioxidant activity is one of 'the other vital roles of selenium.
6. **Copper:** Similar to iron, copper aids in the electron-transport chain's electron transfer. Moreover, copper cofactors with enzymes necessary for the uptake and transportation of iron. Antioxidant properties are one of copper's other vital roles. Rarely do mild to moderate copper deficiency symptoms appear. Anemia can result from a more severe copper deficiency because the body is unable to mobilize iron for the synthesis of red blood cells. Further indications and symptoms include neurological issues and stunted growth in children, as copper is a cofactor for an enzyme that produces myelin, which coats many nerves.
7. **Manganese:** It is a cofactor for the enzymes in the liver that catabolize amino acids and produce glucose (gluconeogenesis). It is rare to be deficient in manganese.

Table 7.8. *Mineral Functions in Metabolism and Blood and Deficiency Syndrome*

Mineral	**Function**	**Deficiency: Signs and Symptoms**
Macro		
Magnesium	ATP synthesis and utilization, carbohydrate, lipid, protein, RNA, and DNA synthesis.	Tremor, muscle spasms, loss of appetite, nausea.
Trace		
Iron	Assists in energy production, DNA synthesis required for red blood cell function.	Anemia: fatigue, paleness, faster heart rate.
Zinc	Assists in energy production, protein, RNA and DNA synthesis; required for hemoglobin synthesis.	Growth retardation in children, hair loss, diarrhea, skin sores, loss of appetite, weight loss.
Iodine	Making thyroid hormone, metabolism, growth, and development.	Goiter, cretinism, other signs, and symptoms include fatigue, depression, weight gain, itchy skin, low heart-rate.
Selenium	Essential for thyroid hormone activity.	Fatigue
Copper	Assists in energy production, iron metabolism.	Anemia: fatigue, paleness, faster heart rate.
Manganese	Glucose synthesis, amino-acid catabolism.	Impaired growth, skeletal abnormalities, abnormal glucose metabolism.
Chromium	Assists insulin in carbohydrate, lipid, and protein metabolism.	Abnormal glucose metabolism.

Source: https://med.libretexts.org/Courses/Chabot_College/Nutrition_1/11%3A_Nutrients_Important_for_Metabolism_and_Blood_Function/11.05%3A_Minerals_Important_for_Metabolism_and_for_Blood_Function_and_Renewal.

8. **Chromium:** Compared to most other minerals, the utilization of chromium by the body is less well understood. It contributes to the metabolism of proteins, fats, and carbohydrates by improving the effects of insulin. As of right now, most scientific research assessing the effectiveness of chromium supplementation in treating and preventing type 2 diabetes has produced conflicting results. To find out more about whether and at what doses chromium is beneficial in treating specific chronic diseases, more research is required. Table 7.8 provides an overview of the key roles that minerals play in metabolism and the corresponding deficiency syndromes.

7.4.1. Dietary Reference Intakes for Minerals and Dietary Sources

Table 7.9 lists the RDA for adults for the minerals that are involved in metabolism as determined by the IOM. The dietary sources of these micronutrients are also included in the table. Foods' mineral content is primarily determined by their geographic location because the soil in which they are grown has a significant impact on it. For example, since iodine is mostly found in seawater, the soil's iodine content decreases with increasing distance from the sea.

Table 7.9. *Dietary Reference Intakes and Food Sources for Minerals Important for Metabolism*

Mineral	Recommended Dietary Allowance (mg/day)	Food Sources
Macro		
Magnesium	420.000 (males)	Nuts, vegetables, coffee and tea, cocoa.
	320.000 (females)**	
Trace		
Iron	8.000 (males)	Animal products, fortified breakfast cereals, beans, spinach, peas.
	18.000 (females)	
Zinc	11.000 (males)	Red meat, poultry, seafood, fortified breakfast cereals, beans, nuts, whole grains.
	8.000 (females)	
Iodine	0.150 (males)	Seafood, dairy products.
	0.150 (females)	
Selenium	0.055 (males)	Tuna, beef, chicken, nuts, dairy products.
	0.055 (females)	
Copper	0.900 (males)	Whole grains, liver, legumes, seeds, cocoa.
	0.900 (females)	
Manganese	2.300 (males)	Whole grains, brown rice, spinach, nuts, tea.
	1.800 (females)*	
Chromium	0.035 (males)	Egg yolks, whole grains, meats, organ meats, mushrooms, nuts, broccoli.
	0.025 (females)*	

Source: https://med.libretexts.org/Courses/Chabot_College/Nutrition_1/11%3A_Nutrients_Important_for_Metabolism_and_Blood_Function/11.05%3A_Minerals_Important_for_Metabolism_and_for_Blood_Function_and_Renewal.

7.4.2. Bioavailability

Mineral bioavailability can be very low because they are not as efficiently absorbed as most vitamins. Foods derived from plants frequently contain substances like phytate and oxalate that bind to minerals and prevent them from being absorbed. Mineral absorption is generally improved by eating foods derived from animals. Generally speaking, absorption of a given mineral will decrease with increased dietary intake. Certain minerals affect how others are absorbed. For example, an excess of zinc in the diet can hinder the absorption of copper and iron. On the other hand, some vitamins improve the absorption of minerals. For instance, vitamin D increases the absorption of calcium and magnesium, while vitamin C increases the absorption of iron. As with vitamins, some gastrointestinal conditions and diseases, like Crohn's disease and kidney disease, as well as aging, affect how well minerals are absorbed, increasing the risk of mineral deficiencies in those with malabsorption conditions and the elderly.

A Closer Look

Riboflavin (B2)

Riboflavin, commonly known as vitamin B_2, plays a crucial role in maintaining overall health and well-being. As a water-soluble vitamin, riboflavin is not stored in the body in significant amounts, necessitating regular dietary intake to meet daily requirements. One of its primary functions is its involvement in energy metabolism. Riboflavin serves as a precursor for the synthesis of two coenzymes: flavin mononucleotide (FMN) and flavin adenine dinucleotide (FAD). These coenzymes are essential for the conversion of carbohydrates, fats, and proteins into adenosine triphosphate (ATP), the body's main source of cellular energy. Therefore, riboflavin plays a vital role in supporting energy production and metabolic function.

In addition to its role in energy metabolism, riboflavin acts as an antioxidant, helping to protect cells and tissues from oxidative damage. It participates in the regeneration of other antioxidants, such as glutathione, which neutralize harmful free radicals and reactive oxygen species. This antioxidant activity helps maintain cellular integrity and may contribute to reducing the risk of chronic diseases associated with oxidative stress, such as cardiovascular disease and certain cancers.

Riboflavin is also essential for the production of red blood cells and overall hematological function. It is involved in the synthesis of heme, the iron-containing component of hemoglobin, which transports oxygen in the blood. Adequate riboflavin intake is necessary for preventing anemia and supporting optimal blood health. Furthermore, riboflavin plays a role in maintaining healthy skin, hair, and mucous membranes. It contributes to the production of collagen, a structural protein that provides strength and elasticity to the skin and connective tissues. Riboflavin deficiency may lead to skin disorders such as dermatitis and contribute to symptoms such as cracked lips and inflammation of the tongue.

Dietary sources rich in riboflavin include dairy products, meat, poultry, fish, eggs, green leafy vegetables, nuts, and enriched grains and cereals. However, riboflavin can be sensitive to light and heat, so cooking and processing may lead to some loss of the vitamin in foods. While riboflavin deficiency is relatively rare in developed countries, certain populations, such as vegans, vegetarians, and individuals with malabsorption disorders, may be at higher risk. Overall, ensuring an adequate intake of riboflavin through a balanced diet is essential for supporting energy metabolism, antioxidant defense, blood health, and overall well-being.

Summary

- Blood is a connective tissue of the circulatory system, transporting absorbed nutrients to cells and waste products from cells. It supports cellular metabolism by transporting synthesized macromolecules and waste products.
- Dietary sources of iron include red meats, poultry, leafy green vegetables, prunes, raisins, egg yolks, lentils, oysters, clams, artichokes, and enriched cereal grains. While there are many food sources of iron, only a small fraction of dietary iron is absorbed.
- Blood is about 78 percent water and 22 percent solids by volume. The liquid part of blood is called plasma and it is mostly water (95 percent), but also contains proteins, ions, glucose, lipids, vitamins, minerals, waste products, gases, enzymes, and hormones.
- Since blood is the conduit of metabolic products and wastes, measuring the components of blood, and particular substances in blood, can reveal not only the health of blood, but also the health of other organ systems.
- Metabolism is defined as the sum of all chemical reactions required to support cellular function and hence the life of an organism. Metabolism is either categorized as catabolism, referring to all metabolic processes involved in molecule breakdown, or anabolism, which includes all metabolic processes involved in building bigger molecules.
- The energy released by catabolic pathways powers anabolic pathways in the building of macromolecules such as the proteins RNA and DNA, and even entire new cells and tissues.
- Thiamine is especially important in glucose metabolism. It acts as a cofactor for enzymes that break down glucose for energy production. Additionally, thiamine plays a role in the synthesis of ribose from glucose and is therefore required for RNA, DNA, and ATP synthesis.
- Niacin is a component of the coenzymes NADH and NADPH, which are involved in the catabolism and/or anabolism of carbohydrates, lipids, and proteins. NADH is the predominant electron carrier and transfers electrons to the electron-transport chain to make ATP.
- Biotin is required as a coenzyme in the citric acid cycle and in lipid metabolism. It is also required as an enzyme in the synthesis of glucose and some nonessential amino acids. A specific enzyme, biotinidase, is required to release biotin from protein so that it can be absorbed in the gut.
- Cobalamin contains cobalt, making it the only vitamin that contains a metal ion. Cobalamin is an essential part of coenzymes. It is necessary for fat and protein catabolism, for folate coenzyme function, and for hemoglobin synthesis.

References

1. Rippin H.L., Hutchinson J., Jewell J., Breda J.J., Cade J.E. Adult Nutrient Intakes from Current National Dietary Surveys of European Populations. Nutrients. 2017;9:1288. doi: 10.3390/nu9121288.

2. Pedroza-Tobias A., Hernandez-Barrera L., Lopez-Olmedo N., Garcia-Guerra A., Rodriguez-Ramirez S., Ramirez-Silva I., Villalpando S., Carriquiry A., Rivera J.A. Usual Vitamin Intakes by Mexican Populations. J. Nutr. 2016;146:1866S–1873S. doi: 10.3945/jn.115.219162.

3. Bailey R.L., Gahche J.J., Miller P.E., Thomas P.R., Dwyer J.T. Why US adults use dietary supplements. JAMA Int. Med. 2013;173:355–361. doi: 10.1001/jamainternmed.2013.2299.

4. Ryan R.M., Frederick C. On energy, personality, and health: Subjective vitality as a dynamic reflection of well-being. J. Pers. 1997;65:529–565. doi: 10.1111/j.1467-6494.1997.tb00326.x.

5. Aouizerat B.E., Gay C.L., Lerdal A., Portillo C.J., Lee K.A. Lack of energy: An important and distinct component of HIV-related fatigue and daytime function. J. Pain Symptom Manag. 2013;45:191–201. doi: 10.1016/j.jpainsymman.2012.01.011.

6. van Steenbergen E., van Dongen J.M., Wendel-Vos G.C., Hildebrandt V.H., Strijk J.E. Insights into the concept of vitality: Associations with participation and societal costs. Eur. J. Public Health. 2016;26:354–359. doi: 10.1093/eurpub/ckv194.

7. Gledhill J. A qualitative study of the characteristics and representation of fatigue in a French speaking population of cancer patients and healthy subjects. Eur. J. Oncol. Nurs. 2005;9:294–312, discussion 294–312. doi: 10.1016/j.ejon.2004.11.002.

8. Engberg I., Segerstedt J., Waller G., Wennberg P., Eliasson M. Fatigue in the general population-associations to age, sex, socioeconomic status, physical activity, sitting time and self-rated health: The northern Sweden MONICA study 2014. BMC Public Health. 2017;17:654. doi: 10.1186/s12889-017-4623-y.

9. Sahlin K., Tonkonogi M., Soderlund K. Energy supply and muscle fatigue in humans. Acta Physiol. Scand. 1998;162:261–266. doi: 10.1046/j.1365-201X.1998.0298f.x.

10. Sargeant A.J. Structural and functional determinants of human muscle power. Exp. Physiol. 2007;92:323–331. doi: 10.1113/expphysiol.2006.034322.

Chapter

MEDICAL NUTRITION THERAPY AND EVIDENCE-BASED NUTRITION CARE

8

Contents

Unit Introduction

Medical nutrition therapy (MNT) is the evaluation of a patient's nutritional status for the purpose of improving their own health and lowering medical expenses if they have a disease, injury, or condition related to diet. MNT entails establishing treatment objectives for the patient and creating a customized nutrition plan that incorporates self-management education and patient education. Therapeutic nutrition, or MNT, is a term that has gained importance in modern integrated health care systems. The goal of creating MNT was to raise awareness of the value of therapeutic nutrition. Thus, nutritional diagnostic, therapeutic, and counseling services for the management of disease are referred to as MNT, or nutrition therapy. Studies indicate that patients who received MNT intervention had better health and a higher quality of life. According to the Academy of Nutrition and Dietetics, MNT is an "integral component" of healthcare and the management of a variety of illnesses, including cancer, diabetes, heart disease, osteoporosis, and chronic kidney disease (Figure 8.1).

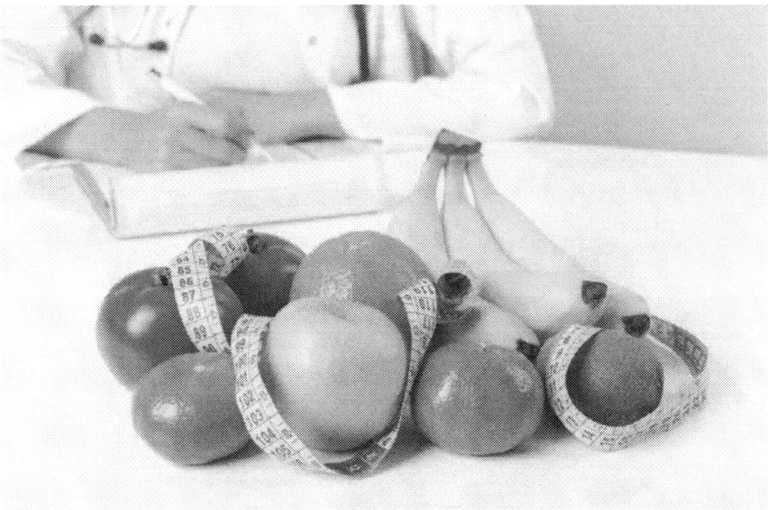

Figure 8.1. *Naturopathic nutrition therapy.*

Source: https://aanmc.org/tag/relationship-with-food/.

The goal of MNT is to identify patients who may have serious health issues related to nutrition and to suggest dietary changes that will improve their quality of life and health outcomes. Patterns of eating and drinking are linked to eight of the top 10 causes of death in the United States, including diabetes mellitus, coronary heart disease, stroke, and certain cancers. MNT is beneficial for other significant patient populations, such as low birth weight babies, the elderly, and obese patients. In addition to raising the risk of stroke, cardiovascular disease, gout, osteoarthritis, sleep apnea, and hypertension, obesity also increases the risk of malnutrition in the elderly. The biggest risk to a newborn's health is a low birth rate. In addition, MNT is also utilized to treat conditions like bulimia nervosa and anorexia, cystic fibrosis, irritable bowel syndrome, hyperlipidemia, gastric ulcers, sprue (a malabsorption syndrome), and (in pediatric patients) failure to thrive. To lower morbidity and mortality from these and other acute or chronic conditions, adequate nutrition is crucial. By providing alternatives to more costly medication treatments and reducing the need for surgery or extended hospital stays, the MNT helps to control healthcare costs while directly benefiting patients.

Medical nutritional therapy is utilized in acute or long-term care facilities, as well as in home care and outpatient settings. A thorough review of the patient's medical history and a dietary assessment with laboratory results and anthropometric measurements are standard components of MNT in the majority of these settings.

An evaluation of the patient's past and present dietary history is a crucial component of MNT. A dietary assessment is frequently carried out to ascertain the macronutrient (energy or calorie, protein, and fat) and micronutrient (vitamin and mineral) content of the patient's food intake. Food records, dietary recalls, food frequency questionnaires, diet histories, and various other data collection techniques, such as biochemical indices, are some of the most widely used dietary assessment instruments. Data gathered from clinical assessments, biochemical testing, and dietary information can be combined to create a scientific evaluation of nutritional status.

Measurements of the patient's height, weight, and body fat percentage (ascertained by skinfolds or hydrostatic weighing) are part of the clinical evaluation. A clinical evaluation may also involve looking for indications of nutritional deficiencies in the nails, skin, eyes, and mouth. Together with the findings of the biochemical tests and dietary assessment, the data gathered from a clinical evaluation paints a complete picture of the patient's current nutritional status and relative risk factors for diet-related illnesses. The patient's specific ailment or diet-related condition can then be treated with an MNT.

MNT is a key element of diabetes self-management education and management. That being said, there are a lot of myths about diabetes and nutrition. Moreover, people with diabetes have been and continue to be given dietary recommendations in clinical practice that are not well supported by research. In light of this, this position statement offers guidelines and suggestions for diabetes MNT that are supported by evidence.

In the past, dietary guidelines for diabetes and its complications were developed using clinical expertise, scientific understanding, and expert consensus. Nevertheless, it was frequently challenging to determine the quality of the evidence that went into creating these guidelines. In order to address this issue, the American Diabetes Association evidence grading system is used to classify the principles and recommendations in this position statement and the 2002 technical review according to the quality of the available evidence. The diabetic patient should be included in the decision-making process, and the best available evidence must still take into account their unique circumstances, preferences, and cultural and ethnic preferences. By raising clinicians' and patients' knowledge of beneficial nutrition therapies, evidence-based recommendations aim to improve diabetes care.

Orientation and Directional Terms

Term	Definition	Illustration
Medical nutrition therapy (MNT)	Medical nutrition therapy (MNT) is a nutrition-based treatment for many temporary and long-term health conditions. A registered dietitian builds a plan tailored to your individual needs. This may involve changes to the foods you eat or the delivery of nutrients through a tube or IV.	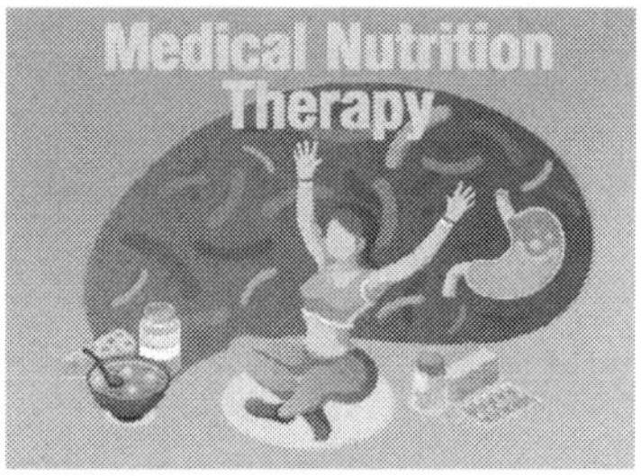
Registered dietitian nutritionist (RDN)	A registered dietitian nutritionist (RDN) is a credentialed healthcare professional who applies evidence-based information about nutrition and diet to contribute to the health and wellness of individuals, groups, and communities.	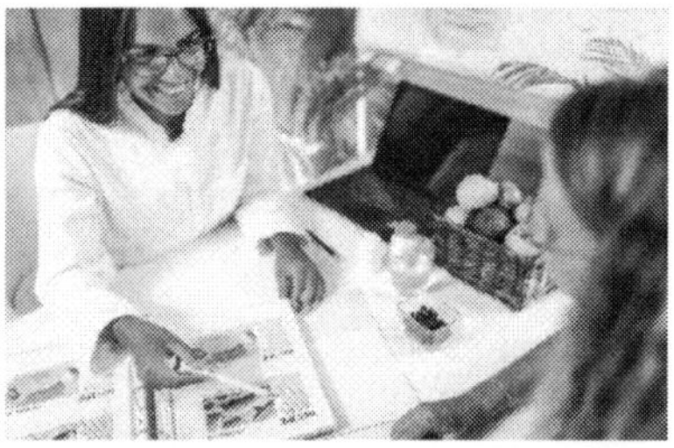
Hypoglycemia	Hypoglycemia (low blood sugar) is common in people who have diabetes. But it can also sometimes affect people without diabetes. You need to treat hypoglycemia as soon as possible by consuming carbohydrates. If it's left untreated, severe low blood sugar can be life-threatening.	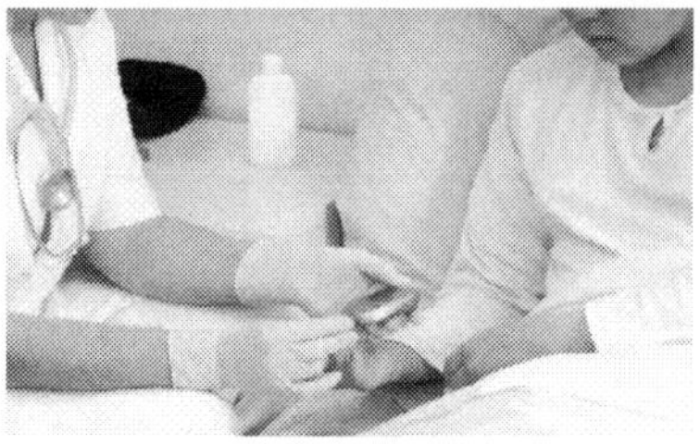
Resistant starch	Resistant starch (RS) is starch, including its degradation products, that escapes from digestion in the small intestine of healthy individuals. Resistant starch occurs naturally in foods, but it can also be added as part of dried raw foods, or used as an additive in manufactured foods.	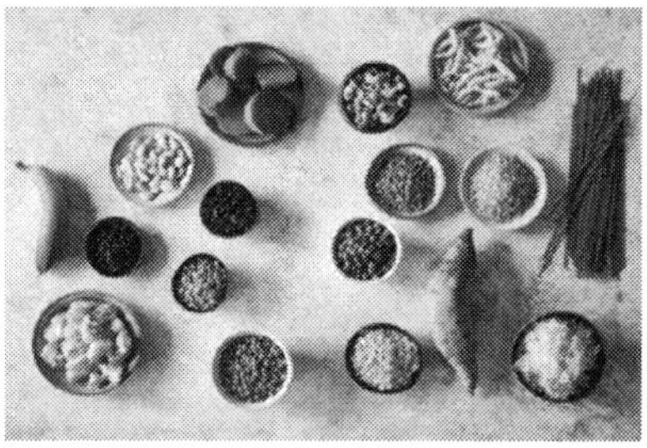
Protein metabolism	Protein metabolism occurs in liver, specifically, the deamination of amino acids, urea formation for removal of ammonia, plasma protein synthesis, and in the interconversions between amino acids.	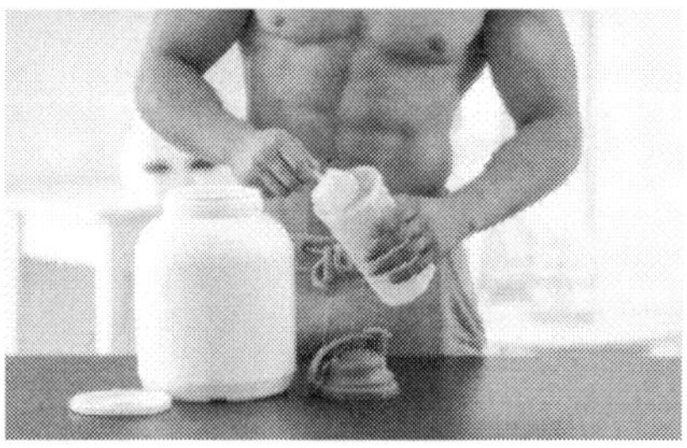

8.1. Concept of Medical Nutrition Therapy

MNT is a personalized approach to managing chronic health conditions, focusing on weight loss or weight maintenance. This therapeutic method can help alleviate symptoms of specific conditions and prevent further health issues by following a customized diet and meal plan. Through nutritional counseling, also known as MNT, your Registered Dietitian Nutritionist (RDN) will collaborate with you to design a nutrition plan that suits your dietary requirements, providing guidance along the way. Though embarking on a new diet or meal plan may feel daunting to some, your dietitian will equip you with the necessary tools to effectively manage your chronic condition through dietary modifications.

Your doctor may suggest nutritional therapy if you have one of these conditions:

- Diabetes;
- Heart disease;
- Renal disease;
- Obesity;
- Gastrointestinal disorders;
- Osteoporosis;
- Cancer;
- History of heart attack.

1. **Nutrition and Diabetes:** MNT is beneficial to those who have diabetes. Given that diabetes is largely influenced by diet, medical nutritional therapy frequently works in conjunction with standard diabetes care. A customized diabetes and nutrition plan can assist you in keeping your blood glucose levels within normal bounds. MNT can aid in lowering diabetes symptoms like weight gain and frequent urination.
2. **Weight Loss:** A helpful strategy for those who wish to reduce weight is nutrition therapy. Nutrition and weight management go hand in hand, so MNT can assist you in examining the foods and eating patterns you currently consume. If you are obese, your doctor might suggest MNT since reducing weight can help avoid additional health issues like:

- High blood pressure;
- Heart disease;
- Diabetes;
- Liver disease;
- Infertility;
- Stroke;
- Certain cancers;
- Mental health problems.

8.1.1. Medical Nutrition Therapy Work

MNT is a vital component of healthcare aimed at treating and managing various medical conditions through personalized nutrition interventions. MNT involves the assessment of an individual's nutritional status, dietary habits, medical history, and health goals to develop tailored nutrition plans. These plans are designed to address specific health needs, prevent or manage chronic diseases, and optimize overall well-being. These plans are designed to address specific health needs, prevent or manage chronic diseases, and optimize overall well-being.

The process of MNT typically involves several key steps:

- **Assessment:** This involves gathering information about the individual's health status, including medical history, current medications, dietary habits, physical activity level, anthropometric measurements (such as weight, height, and body composition), and biochemical data (such as blood tests). This comprehensive assessment helps to identify nutritional risk factors, nutrient deficiencies, and specific dietary needs.

- **Diagnosis:** Based on the assessment findings, healthcare professionals, such as registered dietitians or nutritionists, establish a diagnosis related to the individual's nutritional status and medical condition. This involves identifying nutrition-related problems or concerns that can be addressed through dietary intervention.
- **Goal Setting:** Collaboratively, healthcare providers and patients establish realistic and achievable nutrition goals. These goals may include weight management, blood sugar control, blood pressure regulation, cholesterol reduction, improved digestion, or overall dietary optimization.
- **Intervention:** Using evidence-based nutrition guidelines and principles, healthcare professionals develop individualized nutrition plans tailored to meet the specific needs and goals of the patient. These plans may include recommendations for dietary modifications, meal planning, portion control, nutrient supplementation, behavior change strategies, and lifestyle modifications.
- **Monitoring and Evaluation:** Regular monitoring and follow-up assessments are essential to track progress, evaluate the effectiveness of the nutrition intervention, and make any necessary adjustments to the nutrition plan. This ongoing support helps to ensure patient adherence, address barriers to success, and optimize outcomes.

MNT is used in the management of a wide range of medical conditions, including diabetes, cardiovascular disease, obesity, gastrointestinal disorders, renal disease, cancer, eating disorders, food allergies, and metabolic disorders. By addressing the nutritional aspects of these conditions, MNT aims to improve clinical outcomes, enhance quality of life, and promote long-term health and wellness. It is an integral part of interdisciplinary healthcare teams, collaborating with physicians, nurses, pharmacists, and other allied health professionals to provide comprehensive patient care.

8.1.2. Benefits of Medical Nutrition Therapy

The advantages of nutrition therapy are numerous. MNT can assist you in managing your chronic illness as well as averting further health problems. With the assistance of an RDN, you can develop a personalized diet plan that can help reduce your risk of developing conditions like obesity, diabetic neuropathy, and heart disease. Even though losing weight is frequently the aim, doing so can also lead to improved habits and higher energy levels. When working with an RDN, you'll probably observe that you begin to:

- Increase your physical activity;
- Make healthier choices;
- Read food labels;
- Reduce the amount of fried or processed foods you eat;
- Drink more water instead of sugary drinks.

8.1.3. Medical Nutrition Therapy for Diabetes Mellitus

The objectives of MNT for diabetes mellitus are to maximize health through optimal nutrition, maintain a desirable body weight, and improve overall metabolic outcomes (glucose and lipid levels). Consistent carbohydrate intake, adjustments to fat intake, and regular meal and snack scheduling are all included in the consistent-carbohydrate meal planning approach (if needed). The consistent-carb meal planning strategy is preferred by the American Diabetes Association over the standardized energy-level meal patterns determined by the exchange lists (Figure 8.2).

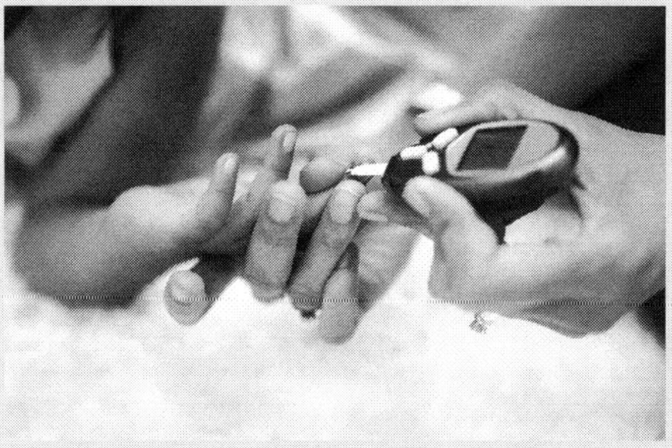

Figure 8.2. *Medical nutrition therapy for diabetes mellitus.*

Source: https://www.hopkinsmedicine.org/health/conditions-and-diseases/diabetes/type-1-diabetes-in-children.

Diabetes is identified and categorized in accordance with the findings of pertinent laboratory and medical examinations.

The A1C test is now approved for use in the diagnosis of diabetes mellitus by the expert committee on diabetes mellitus diagnosis and classification.

In order to diagnose diabetes mellitus, an A1C test result of greater than 6.5% is required.

The classification of diabetes mellitus includes four clinical classes:

- Type 1 diabetes (caused by beta-cell destruction that usually leads to absolute insulin deficiency).
- Type 2 diabetes (caused by progressive insulin secretory defect on the background of insulin resistance).
- Other specific types (due to other causes, e.g., genetic defects in beta-cell function, genetic defects in insulin action, diseases of the exocrine pancreas, or drug or chemical induced).
- Gestational diabetes mellitus (diabetes mellitus diagnosed during pregnancy.

The type of diabetes and the unique needs of each patient as indicated by the signs and symptoms related to nutrition will dictate the MNT, nutrition diagnosis, and self-management training strategy. The overall goal of nutrition intervention is to assist and facilitate individual lifestyle and behavior changes that will lead to improved metabolic control.

The following goals of MNT apply to all persons with diabetes:

- Attain and maintain optimal metabolic outcomes including:
  - a blood glucose level in the normal range, or as close to the normal range as safely possible, to reduce the risk of diabetic complications,
  - lipid and lipoprotein profile that reduces the risk of macrovascular disease, and
  - blood pressure levels that reduce the risk of vascular disease.

- Prevent, treat, or delay the development of obesity, dyslipidemia, cardiovascular disease, hypertension, nephropathy, retinopathy, and neurologic complications associated with diabetes mellitus.
- Improve health through healthy food choices and physical activity.
- Address individual nutrition needs, taking into consideration the patient's personal and cultural preferences and willingness to change.
- Maintain the pleasure of eating by only limiting food choices when indicated by scientific evidence.
- Contribute to normal outcomes of pregnancies for women with preexisting diabetes and gestational diabetes.
- Provide adequate energy and nutrients for increased needs during pregnancy and lactation.
- Provide adequate energy to maintain normal growth and development rates in children and adolescents with diabetes.

8.1.3.1. Nutritional Adequacy

The physician may specify one of the following:

1. **Consistent-Carbohydrate Meal Plan:** The meal plan includes changes to fat intake, regular meal and snack timing, and a consistent carbohydrate intake (±15 g/ meal or snack), but not specific energy levels. The plan calls for four choices of carbohydrates (60 g) at breakfast and five choices of carbohydrates (75 g) at lunch and dinner. The remaining choices come from vegetables, lean meats, and healthy fats. This diet, which excludes midday and evening snacks, is the typical hospital meal plan for patients with diabetes. The daily calorie intake from the meal plan ranges from 1,500 to 1,800 kcal, of which roughly half come from carbohydrates, 20% from protein, and 30% from fat.

If the patient asks for more food, offer options from the vegetable and lean meat categories. Snacks between meals will be given based on the patient's specific nutritional requirements and preferences, or to support medical treatment such as medications to regulate blood sugar. Snacks are not automatically provided to all patients. There is no significant difference in long-term glucose levels, lipid levels, or insulin responses in type 2 diabetes based on meal frequency (e.g. three meals vs smaller meals and snacks). Therefore, meal division should be based on individual preferences. Evening snacks may be appropriate for pregnant or lactating individuals, those with diabetes who have higher energy and protein needs, or those taking medications that increase the risk of low blood sugar.

2. **Nutrition Prescription per the Recommendations of a Registered Dietitian:** The patient's energy and protein requirements, fat tolerance, dietary preferences, and eating patterns are all taken into consideration when the dietitian creates a customized diet plan. Patients on insulin are catered for with snacks, or they are served in accordance with facility policies. With this order, meal plans based on carb counting or exchange lists may be used. The focus is on

meal pattern customization rather than adhering to a set standard macronutrient distribution. Dietary fat is adjusted based on blood glucose, lipid, and body weight objectives. Dietary protein, carbohydrate, and mineral content can be adjusted to meet specific metabolic and therapeutic objectives.

3. **Regular Diet:** Patients who require more protein and energy due to other medical conditions like burns, sepsis, cancer, pressure ulcers, or surgery may want to think about this (Figure 8.3).

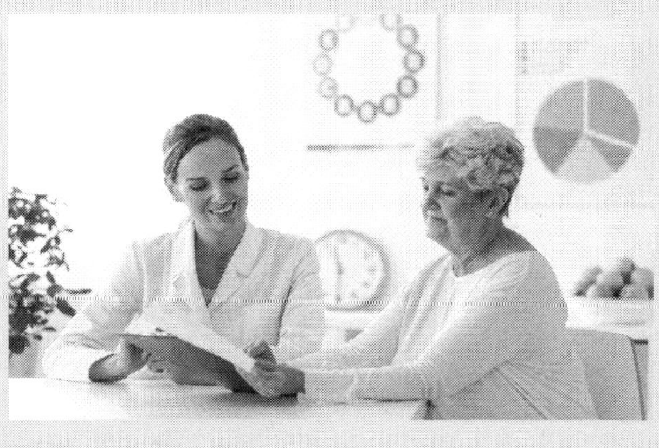

Figure 8.3. *Preventing and managing malnutrition in older adults.*

Source: https://www.nephrocare.com/careers/working-in-the-nephrocare-team.

8.1.4. Nutrition Intervention and Planning for Medical Nutrition Therapy: Carbohydrates and Diabetes

It is preferable to refer to carbohydrates as sugars, starches (e.g., amylase, amylopectin, modified starches), and fiber (eg. hydrocolloids, pectin, cellulose, and hemicellulose). The main objective of diabetes management is blood glucose regulation to reach near-normal levels. Reducing hyperglycemia after meals through diet is crucial to reducing the complications associated with diabetes.

Blood glucose levels are influenced by a food's carbohydrate content as well as its quantity (in g). Compared to other macronutrients, the total amount of carbohydrates consumed at meals and snacks has a bigger impact on the postmeal glucose response. The quantity of carbohydrates consumed at meals, the blood glucose response afterward, and the amount of rapid-acting or short-acting insulin needed before meals to maintain target blood glucose levels are all directly correlated. Thus, tracking the total grams of carbohydrates consumed—whether through the use of exchanges or carbohydrate counting—remains a crucial tactic in attaining glycemic control, as it is a strong predictor of glycemic response. Research has shown that, when the total amount of carbohydrates consumed stays constant, people with type 1 or type 2 diabetes mellitus do not significantly differ in their glycemic response when they consume a range of sugars or starches. When sucrose is used in place of isoenergetic amounts of starch, it does not adversely affect glycemic or lipid responses in individuals with type 1 or type 2 diabetes at doses between 10 and 35% of total energy intake. Based on these findings, sugar (e.g., sucrose) intake does not have to be avoided. Instead, sugar intake should be based on the total amount of carbohydrate needed to achieve optimal metabolic control and the nutritional contribution to the diet. Recently, the use of low–glycemic index foods or low-glycemic diets has received renewed interest. Factors that influence the glycemic response to food include: the type and amount of carbohydrate, type of sugar, nature of starch, cooking, and food processing, as well as other food components (e.g., fat and natural substances that slow digestion—lectins, phytates, tannins, and starch-protein and starch-lipid combinations).

The degree of glucose intolerance, the lente effect, fasting and preprandial glucose concentrations, and the second meal are additional variables that impact the glycemic response to food. The use of low-glycemic diets or not in improving metabolic outcomes is still not well supported by science due to the multitude of factors that can affect a food's glycemic response and the paucity of long-term studies. A meta-analysis of studies involving low-glycemic index diets in individuals with diabetes revealed that these diets resulted in a 0.4% decrease in hemoglobin A1C (HbA1C) in contrast to high-glycemic index diets. High-fiber, low-glycemic index foods can improve glycemic control temporarily, according to some studies, when added to meals or snacks. When combined with an analysis of total carbohydrate intake, the glycemic index and/or glycemic load may offer more advantages than when the total carbohydrate intake is the only factor taken into account. Thus, taking the glycemic index into account could be beneficial as a supplement for certain people. Measuring blood glucose levels before and after meals is the only way for people to determine whether the glycemic index is helpful in helping them maintain their glycemic goals.

An individual's energy goals to reach or maintain a desired body weight, eating habits, and glucose and lipid goals should all be taken into consideration when determining the appropriate total amount of carbohydrates to consume. The metabolic profile of the patient and the need for weight loss should be taken into account when calculating the carbohydrate and monounsaturated fat content of the diet in people with type 2 diabetes mellitus. A low-fat, energy-restricted diet or a low-carb diet may be beneficial for weight loss in the short term (up to one year). It is crucial to monitor lipid profiles, renal function, and protein intake (in patients with nephropathy) for patients following low-carb diets. Hypoglycemia therapy should be adjusted as necessary (Figure 8.4).

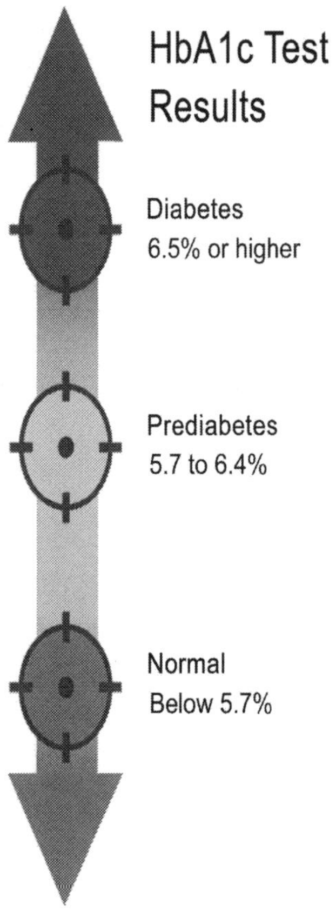

Figure 8.4. *The HbA1c test.*

Source: https://vitrosens.com/what-is-the-hba1c-test/.

8.1.4.1. Fiber

The American Diabetes Association and the evidence-based nutrition practice guidelines recommend that individuals with diabetes consume the same amount of fiber as the general population. Dietary fiber intake should be 14 g per 1,000 kcal, or 25 g for adult women and 38 g for adult men, according to the Dietary Reference Intake (DRI). On the other hand, new research indicates that people with diabetes might gain from eating more fiber in their diet. A recent review of the literature found that, in comparison to low-fiber diets, diets containing 30 to 50 g of fiber per day from whole food sources consistently resulted in lower serum glucose levels. In order to help people with type 2 diabetes mellitus with both immediate postprandial glucose metabolism and long-term glucose control, viscous dietary fibers are added. These fibers slow down the rate at which the stomach empties, digests, and absorbs glucose. Supplemental fiber with doses ranging from 10 to 29 g daily might also help with glycemic management. Consuming dietary fiber in the form of whole foods or supplements has been shown to have a positive impact on serum lipid levels, blood pressure, and inflammation markers. A daily intake of 12 to 33 g of fiber from whole foods or up to 42 g from supplements may have benefits. Consuming a high-fiber diet can help patients with diabetes who have lipid metabolism disorders, especially hypercholesterolemia, by lowering their cholesterol levels. When incorporating fiber into meal planning, one should take into account the possible gastrointestinal side effects of excessive dietary fiber intake. To avoid unfavorable side effects, a gradual increase in fiber from whole foods and supplements within recommended ranges, is advised. Unlike sugars and starches, fiber is not absorbed and digested. When calculating the amount of carbohydrates available in a serving, half the grams of fiber should be deducted from the total carbohydrates (in g) when there are more than 5 g of fiber per serving.

8.1.4.2. Resistant Starch

In the small intestine, resistant starch (nondigestible oligosaccharides and the starch amylase) is not absorbed as glucose because it is not digested. Legumes are the main dietary source of resistant starch; 2 to 3 g of resistant starch can be found in 100 g of cooked legumes, and approximately 6 g can be found in 100 g (dry weight) of cornstarch. Resistant starch has been proposed to correlate with lower insulin levels and to cause a smaller increase in postprandial glucose than digestible starch. Research involving individuals with diabetes has concentrated on raw cornstarch and its ability to avert hypoglycemia during the night. There is limited evidence, though, that eating cornstarch snacks reduces the risk of hypoglycemia. As of right now, resistant starch has no known health benefits for diabetics.

8.1.4.3. Timing of Carbohydrate and Food Intake: Type 1–Diabetes

In individuals who are insulin-dependent, the total amount of carbohydrates in meals and snacks takes precedence as it dictates the amount of insulin administered prior to meals and the amount of insulin released after meals. To keep their blood glucose targets within reach, people on intensive insulin therapy can modify their premeal insulin dosage according to the quantity of carbohydrates they eat at meals. Time of meal and snack consumption, interval between insulin injection and food intake, and quantity of meals and snacks should all be determined by individual needs. The achievement of ideal blood glucose control and the prevention or postponement of the onset of diabetic complications require self-monitoring of blood glucose levels. Either way, regardless of diabetes type or treatment, better glycemic control has been linked to testing blood glucose three to eight times a day. To achieve blood glucose goals, the American Diabetes Association advises pregnant women taking insulin or those with type 1 diabetes to check their blood glucose levels three times a day or more. For those who inject a fixed daily dosage of insulin, maintaining daily consistency in food consumption is essential. Consuming carbohydrates consistently should be the top priority for those on fixed insulin regimens who do not modify their premeal insulin dosages. Insulin dosages should be changed to reflect the quantity of food needed or typically consumed by individuals on insulin therapy. Patients should also eat at regular intervals that coincide with the action time of their insulin preparation and blood glucose readings. Following a review of blood glucose records, consultation with the patient's doctor, and collaboration with the coordinating healthcare team, the decision to modify insulin dosages should be made.

8.1.4.4. Intensified Insulin Therapy (Multiple Daily Injections or Insulin Pump Therapy)

Intensified insulin therapy aims to achieve the closest possible blood glucose readings to the normal range for each patient. Insulin infusion pumps enable meal timing and size flexibility by imitating the body's natural insulin delivery system. Insulin pump or rapid-acting insulin users should modify their insulin dosages for meals and snacks according to the amount of carbohydrates they contain. When done correctly, advanced carb counting can significantly improve meal planning flexibility. According to the Diabetes Control and Complications Trial, people with lower A1C levels (0.5% statistically significant) than those who did not modify their preprandial insulin dosages had a premeal insulin regimen based on the amount of carbohydrates in their meals. Increased insulin therapy may cause hypoglycemia and weight gain, among other possible issues. Preventing weight gain is desirable because it can have a negative impact on blood pressure, glycemia, dyslipidemia, and general health. Decreases in A1C and blood glucose levels can lead to hypoglycemia, which is more common in people with type 1 diabetes. Individuals receiving insulin pump therapy or multiple-dose insulin (MDI) should self-monitor their blood glucose (SMBG) before meals and snacks, and sometimes postprandially at bedtime and before exercising. Furthermore, SMBG should be carried out when a patient has low blood sugar suspicions, following treatment of low blood sugar until normoglycemic, and before performing crucial tasks like operating a vehicle. Based on the results of the SMBG, changes in food intake or medication should be made. Treatment for hypoglycemia needs to be appropriate.

8.1.5. Diabetes Nutrition Management: Meal Planning Approaches

Dietitians can teach patients how to achieve their nutrition goals more effectively if they are familiar with the range of meal planning techniques available. The goals for metabolic outcomes as well as the patient's dietary requirements, literacy level, motivation, and lifestyle, should all be taken into consideration when choosing an approach. Current diabetes treatment guidelines form the basis of the patient education publications produced by the American Diabetes Association. Approaches that can be used for teaching meal planning include:

- **Basic Nutrition Guidelines:** These guidelines provide the patient with an understanding of the basic principles of nutrition and guidance in selecting an adequately balanced diet for optimal health, e.g., dietary guidelines for Americans, food guide pyramid, and guide to good eating.
- **Basic Diabetes Guidelines:** The patient gains an understanding of the relationship between food intake and metabolic outcomes from these guidelines. They instruct the patient on how to choose foods that are appropriate for controlling their diabetes, e.g., the diabetes food guide pyramid, healthy food options, and the initial step in meal planning for those who have just been diagnosed with the disease, according to the American Diabetes Association and American Dietetic Association.

- **Menu Approaches to Meal Planning:** These approaches provide simple examples to assist patients with meal planning, e.g., the new family cookbook for people with diabetes and the American diabetes association's month of meals cookbook series and individualized menus.
  - **Exchange Lists for Meal Planning:** The goal of this method is to give patients direction and structure when it comes to meal planning. Exchanges are arranged according to calorie levels, which is useful when creating meal plans with calorie restrictions. Foods with comparable amounts of fat, protein, and carbohydrates are grouped together to form food groups. This aids the patient in organizing their meals and achieving their desired intake levels of carbohydrates and nutrients. The American Diabetes Association/Academy of Nutrition and Dieetics' "Eating Healthy with Diabetes" exchange list is the most widely used.
- **Counting Approaches:** These approaches provide structure with specific rules that are clearly identified. They allow optimal flexibility with food choices and meal planning.

Weight loss is advised for people with diabetes who are overweight or obese as well as those who are at risk of developing diabetes because energy balance, overweight, and obesity in diabetes all have an impact on insulin resistance and metabolic outcomes. Short-term research has shown that lowering blood pressure, improving glycemia and dyslipidemia measurements, and decreasing insulin resistance are all linked to weight loss in individuals with type diabetes.

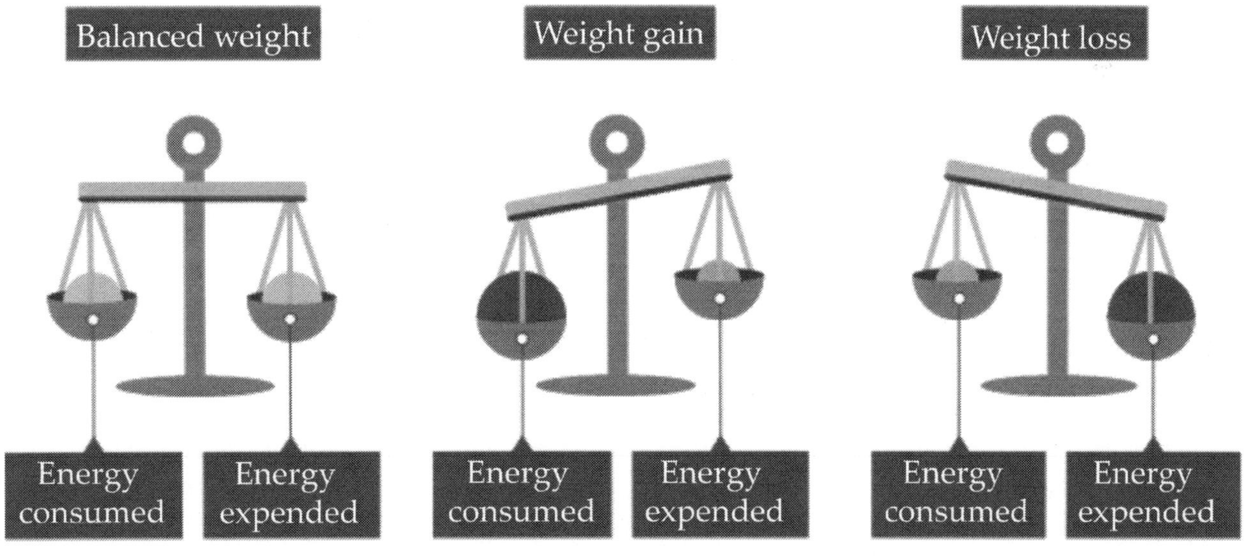

Figure 8.5. *Energy in = energy out → healthy weight.*

Source: https://hipatiabioygeologia.wordpress.com/2019/10/08/diet-and-nutrition-2/.

According to the evidence-based nutrition guidelines, a reasonable body weight is one that the patient and the medical team agree is both attainable and sustainable. A five to 10% reduction in body weight from baseline improves metabolic outcomes. To determine healthy weight ranges and determine the ideal body weight, one can utilize the body mass index. Individuals with diabetes who are overweight or obese and for whom losing weight is a primary health goal may follow national guidelines for weight management. Bariatric surgery should be taken into consideration for patients with type 2 diabetes whose BMI is greater than 35 kg/m^2, particularly if their diabetes is hard to control with lifestyle changes and medication (Figure 8.5).

A typical weight-loss diet will initially result in 1 to 2 pounds of weight loss per week if it modifies total energy intake to create an energy deficit of 500 to 1,000 kcal/day. Even though many people can lose weight with these standard diets—up to 10% of their starting weight in just 6 months—without ongoing support and follow-up, the majority of those who lose weight end up gaining it back. The conventional wisdom on weight loss advocates low-fat, low-energy diets, but three randomized controlled trials revealed that at 6 months, low-carb diet participants lost more weight than low-fat diet participants. In contrast to low-fat diets, low-carb diets were linked to larger improvements in triglyceride levels and HDL cholesterol concentrations at 6 months, according to a meta-analysis. However, the LDL cholesterol level was significantly higher on the low-carb diets. Similar results, except for elevated LDL levels, were found in a more recent meta-analysis of patients with type 2 diabetes following restricted-carb diets. According to the analysis, the level of triglycerides is predicted to drop by about 23% when the amount of carbohydrates consumed is reduced from 65% to 35% of total energy. A comparison of the studies showed that the amounts of carbohydrates consumed varied, ranging from 4% to 45% of total energy, and that the majority of the studies' carbohydrate intake was below the RDA of 130 g/day. It was concluded that a lower-carb diet can help treat type 2 diabetes because it can have positive effects on triglyceride, glucose, and A1C levels. It is yet unknown how these diets will affect cardiovascular outcomes.

Most studies start a low-carb diet with an induction phase wherein 55% of the diet's energy comes from carbohydrates. Low-carb diets come in a wide range of variations, so it's critical that the dietitian collaborate with the doctor and patient to create a meal plan that best supports the desired metabolic outcomes. When recommending a low-carb diet to patients with diabetes, it is wise to provide an amount of carbohydrates that satisfies the RDA of 130 g/day because lower intakes exclude a number of foods that are significant sources of energy, fiber, fat-soluble vitamins A and E, water-soluble vitamins folate, thiamin, and pyridoxine, and minerals like calcium, potassium, and magnesium. Reduced uric acid levels in gout patients as well as other associated side effects like constipation, diarrhea, headaches, halitosis, and insomnia raise safety concerns about low-carb diets. Diets low in carbohydrates might not be appropriate for women in their reproductive years, children, or people with high blood pressure. Furthermore, because high-protein diets increase the risk of glomerular hyperfiltration and hasten renal complications linked to diabetes, the American Diabetes Association does not support their use. The macronutrient distribution for a low-carb meal plan should therefore generally take into account the ratio of protein, which should not be greater than 20% of total energy. When given a low-carb meal plan, patients should be closely watched and have regular evaluations of their renal function, lipid profile, protein intake, glucose, and ketone levels in their urine, and, in cases where gout is present, their uric acid levels. To avoid hypoglycemia episodes, the hypoglycemic risk also needs to be evaluated.

In selected patients, drug therapy as an adjunct to lifestyle change may be appropriate to achieve weight loss. However, it is common for patients to regain weight after the discontinuation of medications. In patients with severe obesity, surgical options, such as gastric bypass and gastroplasty, may be appropriate and allow significant improvement in glycemic control with reduction or discontinuation of medications.

8.1.6. Protein and Diabetes

Protein intake makes up 15–20% of the average amount of calories consumed, is generally constant from early childhood to old age, and seems to be similar in people with diabetes. It has long been believed that insulin resistance and insufficiency have a greater impact on glucose metabolism in diabetics than they do on abnormalities of protein metabolism. Nonetheless, it has been shown that mild hyperglycemia in individuals with type 2 diabetes can lead to an elevated turnover of protein, indicating a higher requirement for protein. Short-term kinetic studies have shown increased protein catabolism in type 1 diabetic subjects treated with conventional insulin therapy, indicating the need for near-normal glycemia and sufficient protein intake. People with diabetes appear to be protected against protein malnutrition when consuming a typical diet because the majority of adults consume at least 50% more protein than is necessary.

Patients with and without nephropathy are said to consume similar amounts of protein through diet; however, in every study, the amount of protein consumed fell within the usual range and infrequently topped 20% of total energy consumed. The onset of diabetic nephropathy does not seem to be linked to protein intake within the normal range. It may be wise to avoid protein intakes exceeding 20% of total daily energy as there is no information on the long-term effects of this consumption on the development of nephropathy.

Protein does not raise plasma glucose concentrations because glucose from ingested protein does not appear in the general circulation, as shown by a number of studies conducted in both healthy individuals and people with controlled type 2 diabetes. Furthermore, it appears that protein does not impede the absorption of carbohydrates because the peak glucose response to carbohydrates alone is comparable to that of carbohydrates and protein. After receiving treatment with either carbohydrate alone or carbohydrate and protein, the subjects with type 1 diabetes showed similar rates of restoration of euglycemia following hypoglycemia, time to peak glucose levels, and subsequent rate of glucose fall. There hasn't been enough research done on how protein affects satiety, long-term weight loss, and the control of energy intake. It is unknown how safe and effective high-protein, low-carb diets will be in the long run.

8.1.7. Dietary Fat and Diabetes

8.1.7.1. Fatty Acids and Dietary Cholesterol

Reducing consumption of saturated fat and cholesterol is the main objective when it comes to diet in people with diabetes. The main dietary factor that affects plasma LDL cholesterol is saturated fat. Additionally, compared to the general population, people with diabetes seem to be more sensitive to dietary cholesterol. Low-saturated-fat and low-cholesterol diets reduce plasma total cholesterol, LDL cholesterol, and triglycerides in non-diabetic individuals, but they have conflicting effects on HDL cholesterol.

Positive correlations have been noted between changes in plasma total cholesterol, LDL and HDL cholesterol, and dietary total and saturated fat. Increased exercise prevents the drop in HDL cholesterol linked to low-fat diets and produces greater reductions in plasma total, LDL cholesterol, and triglycerides. Studies on diabetes patients, however, are lacking in terms of demonstrating the effects of particular dietary cholesterol and saturated fatty acid percentages. As a result, the objective for people with diabetes is still the same as it is for everyone else.

Diets high in carbohydrates and low in saturated fat, or enriched with cis-monounsaturated fatty acids (monounsaturated fat) reduce plasma LDL cholesterol in an equivalent manner in metabolic research diets when energy intake and weight are held constant. Low-fat content, when compared in metabolic studies to isocaloric high monounsaturated fat diets, high carbohydrate diets (>10% of energy) raise postprandial levels of plasma glucose, insulin, triglycerides, and, in some studies, decrease plasma HDL cholesterol. Diets heavy in monounsaturated fats, however, have not been demonstrated to lower HbA1c or fasting plasma glucose levels. When diets high in monounsaturated fat are consumed freely outside of regulated environments, there is worry that this could lead to an increase in energy intake and weight gain. Therefore, recommendations for nutrition therapy will depend on both the metabolic profile and the need to lose weight. Moreover, whether to replace saturated fat with monounsaturated fat or carbohydrates may depend on ethnic or cultural preferences.

Diabetes patients' consumption of polyunsaturated fats has not been thoroughly researched. Polyunsaturated fats seem to lower plasma total and LDL cholesterol when compared to saturated fat, but not as effectively as monounsaturated fats. Supplements containing N-3 polyunsaturated fatty acids have been demonstrated to reduce type 2 diabetics' plasma triglyceride levels. While the corresponding increase in plasma LDL cholesterol is concerning, their use is unlikely to have a negative impact on glucose metabolism. It's possible that N-3 supplements work best when treating severe hypertriglyceridemia. Although the majority of n-3 fatty acid studies conducted on diabetics have used supplements, there is evidence from the general public that n-3 fatty acid-containing foods have cardioprotective benefits.

It is recommended to consume two to three servings of fish per week as a source of dietary n-3 polyunsaturated fat. Trans-unsaturated fatty acids, which result from processing vegetable oils to increase their solidity (a process known as hydrogenation), have an effect on plasma LDL cholesterol that is comparable to that of saturated fats.

Trans-fatty acids also reduce HDL cholesterol in plasma. As a result, consumption of trans-fatty acids ought to be restricted. Dietary and biliary cholesterol cannot be absorbed through the intestinal wall by means of plant sterol and stanol esters. It has been demonstrated that plant sterols/stanols can reduce LDL and total cholesterol in doses of about 2 g/day.

8.1.7.2. Low-Fat Diets

A transient reduction in energy intake and a modest loss of weight to a new equilibrium body weight are linked to low-fat, high-carb diets in studies assessing the effect of ad libitum energy intake as a function of dietary fat content.

There is a rise in HDL cholesterol and a fall in plasma total cholesterol and triglycerides with this slight weight loss. This is supported by the long-term, low-fat, high-carb diets that have been linked to modest weight loss and no rise in plasma triglycerides.

8.1.7.3. Fat Replacements

Reducing the amount of high-fat foods in the diet, offering lower-fat or fat-free options, and using fat replacers—ingredients that mimic the qualities of fat but contain much fewer calories—in food formulations are some ways to reduce the amount of fat consumed daily. The Food and Drug Administration certifies that the fat substitutes and replacers available today are safe to use in food products. Frequent consumption of foods containing fat substitutes may aid in lowering cholesterol and other dietary fat intake, but it may not have any effect on overall energy intake or weight. To evaluate the impact of foods containing fat substitutes on energy intake and the macronutrient composition of diabetics' diets, long-term research is required.

8.1.8. Energy Balance and Obesity

For people with type 2 diabetes, losing weight is a key therapeutic goal because obesity has an impact on insulin resistance. Short-term research has shown that lowering blood pressure, improving glycemia and dyslipidemia measurements, and decreasing insulin resistance are all linked to weight loss in individuals with type 2 diabetes. Nevertheless, there are no long-term data available to determine how much these improvements can be sustained. The central nervous system regulates energy intake, energy expenditure, and body weight, which is why most people find it difficult to lose weight over the long term. Genetic factors appear to have an impact on this regulation. Furthermore, for people who are genetically predisposed to obesity, environmental factors frequently make weight loss difficult.

Research indicates that in order to achieve long-term weight loss of up to 5–7% of initial weight, participants must participate in structured, intensive lifestyle programs that include education, individual counseling, a reduction in dietary fat and energy intake, regular physical activity, and frequent participant contact. Fat is probably the most important nutrient to restrict when dieting to lose weight. A high-fat diet causes an increase in spontaneous food consumption, while a low-fat diet causes a decrease in total energy intake. Exercise has very little effect on weight loss on its own. Exercise, however, should be promoted since it enhances insulin sensitivity, sharply lowers blood sugar, and is critical to the long-term maintenance of weight loss. Behavioral therapy alone hasn't produced much weight loss either, and it's possible that behavioral methods work best when combined with other weight loss techniques. Nevertheless, the best methods for treating and preventing obesity in the long run are still unknown.

Conventional diets for weight loss offer 500–1,000 fewer calories than what is thought to be required for weight maintenance. While many people using these diets can lose some weight (up to 10% of starting weight), the medical literature shows that long-term results are poor when the other elements of an intensive lifestyle program are not included. Most people who lose weight eventually gain it back. Meal replacements, which are frequently formula products, offer a predetermined quantity of energy. Significant weight loss can be achieved by using meal replacements once or twice a day in place of a regular meal, but maintenance of weight loss requires sticking to the meal replacement therapy plan. For people with type 2 diabetes, very low calorie diets (VLCDs), which limit daily caloric intake to 800 calories or less, result in significant weight loss and quick improvements in glycemia and lipemia. Weight gain is typical when self-selected meals are resumed after stopping VLCDs. Consequently, it seems that VLCDs are not very effective in treating type 2 diabetes, and they should only be used in conjunction with a regimented weight-maintenance program.

The information that is currently available indicates that treating overweight people with type 2 diabetes may benefit from the use of weight loss pills. They do have some effect, though. Furthermore, the information at hand indicates that these drugs are only effective when taken, and they should be combined with lifestyle modifications. Only those with a BMI of greater than 27.0 kg/m^2 should use these medications. Patients with a BMI of at least 35 kg/m^2 should only be considered for gastric reduction surgery, despite the fact that it can be an effective weight loss treatment for severe obesity (including severe obesity in people with type 2 diabetes). The relative advantages and risks of surgical approaches to weight loss are unknown because there is a lack of data comparing them with medical approaches. Thus, it is best to view gastric reduction surgery as an unproven diabetes treatment.

8.1.9. Micronutrients and Diabetes

It is important to inform people with diabetes about the potential toxicity of taking excessive amounts of vitamin and mineral supplements, as well as the importance of getting enough of these nutrients from natural food sources. Even though it can be challenging to determine, supplementation may be helpful if vitamin and mineral deficiencies are found. A multivitamin preparation may be beneficial as a supplement for certain populations, including the elderly, women who are pregnant or nursing, strict vegetarians, and people following low-calorie diets.

There has been interest in prescribing antioxidant vitamins to individuals with diabetes because the condition may be characterized by elevated oxidative stress. Megadoses of dietary antioxidants, such as beta carotene, vitamin C, vitamin E, selenium, and other carotenoids, have not, in general, been shown to protect against cancer, diabetes, or cardiovascular disease. Large placebo-controlled trials have failed to demonstrate a benefit and, in some cases, have suggested negative effects of antioxidant vitamins, despite the fact that large observational studies have linked the consumption of antioxidants in food or supplements with benefits for the cardiovascular system.

Although it is generally acknowledged that folate can prevent birth defects, it is unclear how folate supplements can lower homocysteine and lower the risk of cardiovascular events. It is not possible to recommend vitamins B_1, B_6, and B_{12} as a regular therapeutic option because their role in the treatment of diabetic neuropathy has not been established. Nicotinamide is being studied to maintain β-cell mass in individuals with type 1 diabetes who have recently been diagnosed; however, its benefits have not been satisfactorily shown. Deficiencies in some minerals, like magnesium, potassium, and maybe zinc and chromium, can make carbohydrate intolerance worse. The need for zinc or chromium supplementation is more difficult to identify than the need for potassium or magnesium replacement, which can be determined based on low serum levels.

There have been reports of chromium supplementation having positive effects on glycemia. However, it's possible that the populations under investigation had slightly low baseline chromium levels, and in the largest study, chromium levels weren't assessed before or after supplementation. Other carefully planned research has not been able to demonstrate that supplementing with chromium improves glycemic control in individuals with diabetes in any appreciable way. The benefits of chromium supplementation for people with diabetes have not yet been proven beyond a reasonable doubt. It is advised to consume 1,000–1,500 mg of calcium daily, particularly for older individuals with diabetes. This suggestion seems safe and should help older people with osteoporosis. It's unclear if supplementing with calcium is beneficial for younger people. It has been investigated how vanadium salts relate to diabetes. There is a chance for toxicity and no conclusive proof of effectiveness. Numerous herbal remedies have been demonstrated to have somewhat positive effects on blood sugar levels. The active ingredient content of commercially available products, however, varies widely and is not well standardized. There is no proof that herbal preparations are beneficial over the long term for people with diabetes. They might also interfere with the way that medications work. It is crucial that medical professionals are informed when patients with diabetes use these products.

Supplementing with vitamins or minerals does not appear to be beneficial for diabetics without underlying deficiencies. There are two exceptions: calcium to prevent bone disease and folate to prevent birth defects.

8.1.10. Alcohol and Diabetes

The same alcohol consumption guidelines that apply to the general public also apply to people with diabetes. Women who are pregnant or who suffer from other medical conditions like pancreatitis, advanced neuropathy, severe hypertriglyceridemia, or alcohol addiction should refrain from drinking. If people decide to drink, it is advised that they limit how many drinks they have each day—two for adult males and one for adult women—if they choose to do so. A standard definition of a drink is an alcoholic beverage that contains approximately 15 g of alcohol, such as 12 ounces of beer, 5 ounces of wine, or 1.5 ounces of distilled spirits. It doesn't seem that the kind of alcohol a person drinks affects its cardioprotective properties.

For diabetics, alcohol consumption can have both hypoglycemic and hyperglycemic effects. The amount of alcohol consumed acutely, whether it is done so with or without food, and whether it is used excessively or chronically all influence these effects. Alcohol did not acutely affect blood glucose or insulin levels in people with type 1 or type 2 diabetes in studies where moderate amounts of alcohol were consumed with food. For this reason, all diabetics should include alcoholic beverages in their regular food and meal plans; no food should be excluded.

In the United States, heavy or excessive alcohol use is one of the main preventable causes of death. S. Nonetheless, light-to-moderate alcohol consumption in adults is linked to improved insulin sensitivity and a lower risk of type 2 diabetes, coronary heart disease, and stroke, according to epidemiological data in non-diabetic individuals. Chronic light-to-moderate intake (5–15 g/day) was linked to a lower risk of coronary heart disease in adults with diabetes, most likely because it concurrently raised plasma HDL cholesterol. The relationship between blood pressure and alcohol consumption appears to be U- or J-shaped. Although moderate to light alcohol consumption does not increase blood pressure, there is a strong correlation between blood pressure in men and women and long-term excessive alcohol consumption (>30–60 g/day).

8.2. Medical Nutrition Therapy for Special Populations

8.2.1. Children and Adolescents with Diabetes

In order to maintain normal growth and development in children and adolescents with type 1 diabetes, blood glucose goals should be met without causing excessive hypoglycemia. Individualized meal and food planning, adaptable insulin dosage schedules and algorithms, self-blood glucose monitoring, and outcome-driven, education-driven decision-making are ways to achieve this. It seems that children and adolescents with type 1 or type 2 diabetes have similar dietary needs to other children and adolescents of the same age. When calculating a child's energy needs, it is important to take their appetite into careful consideration. Assuming that growth and development are within normal bounds, the best way to estimate a child's or adolescent's energy needs is a food/nutrition history of a typical daily intake. Recording height and weight on pediatric growth charts is the first step in evaluating weight gain and growth at the time of diagnosis. By regularly monitoring weight gain and growth patterns, one can assess the adequacy of energy intake.

It is not advisable to suppress a child's appetite or have them eat constantly in an attempt to regulate their blood sugar levels. The prescription for nutrition should have a customized macronutrient composition based on the needs for growth and development as well as blood glucose and plasma lipid targets. The main objectives of treatment for young people with type 2 diabetes are to normalize glycemia and promote a healthy lifestyle.

The achievement of blood glucose targets and the cessation of excessive weight gain with normal linear growth are signs of a successful treatment involving nutrition therapy and physical activity. Recommendations for nutrition should also take related cardiovascular risk factors like dyslipidemia and hypertension into account. It is important to think about behavior modification techniques that reduce the consumption of high-energy, high-fat foods while promoting a healthy diet and regular exercise for the whole family. For children and adolescents with diabetes, individualized food/meal plans and strict insulin regimens can offer flexibility to accommodate changing activity levels, varying appetites, and irregular meal times and schedules.

8.2.2. Pregnancy and Lactation with Diabetes

An adequate diet for both the mother and the fetus, energy intake for a suitable weight gain, and the administration of any required vitamin and mineral supplements are the objectives of MNT during pregnancy. Achieving and maintaining ideal glycemic control during pregnancy is further aided by MNT if the pregnancy is complicated by diabetes. First trimester energy needs do not increase unless a woman has exhausted her body before becoming pregnant. For increases in maternal blood volume and in the size of the breast, uterus, and adipose tissue, as well as for placental growth, fetal growth, and amniotic fluids, an extra 300 kcal per day are advised during the second and third trimesters. Lower energy intakes have, however, been linked to successful pregnancy outcomes.

Pregnant women should consume a healthy diet that includes enough protein (0.75 g·kg−1 day−1 plus an extra 10 g/day) in addition to enough calories. The amount of nutrients required by women with and without diabetes during pregnancy and lactation is comparable. 400 µg/day of folic acid from fortified foods and/or supplements, along with food folate from a variety of foods, is recommended for all women who are capable of becoming pregnant in order to prevent neural tube defects and other congenital abnormalities. A balanced diet that produces a suitable amount of weight gain usually provides all the vitamins and minerals required during pregnancy. Prenatal vitamin and mineral supplements are frequently recommended despite the lack of evidence supporting their use due to uncertainty regarding a baby's nutritional status and intake. Analyzing the pregnant woman's eating habits may reveal unique requirements for her. Four non-nutritive sweeteners have been approved by the Food and Drug Administration as safe to use during pregnancy. During pregnancy, women with diabetes, like those without the disease, should abstain from alcohol consumption.

8.2.2.1. Pregnancy with Prior-Onset Type 1 or Type 2 Diabetes

A customized prenatal food and meal plan is part of prepregnancy nutrition therapy, which aims to improve blood glucose control. The allocation of energy intake and carbohydrates in the meal plan should be customized for each pregnant woman based on her food and eating habits, blood glucose levels, and the anticipated physiological changes that pregnancy will bring about in her body. Frequent meals and snacks help prevent hypoglycemia because the fetus continuously takes glucose from the mother. Generally speaking, an evening snack is required to reduce the risk of fasting ketosis and hypoglycemia during the night. Monitoring blood sugar levels and keeping daily food logs give important information for adjusting insulin dosage and meal plans.

8.2.2.2. Gestational Diabetes Mellitus

In order to achieve and maintain normoglycemia, avoid ketones, and provide enough energy for a healthy gestational weight gain, nutrition therapy for gestational diabetes encourages these behaviors. Throughout the day, carbohydrates are broken down into three small-to-moderate-sized meals and two to four snacks. To avoid accelerating ketosis over night, you might need to eat something in the evening. Generally speaking, breakfast is a worse time of day to consume carbohydrates than other meals. Based on information from self-blood glucose monitoring and individual assessments, specific dietary and nutrition recommendations are established and adjusted.

A desirable weight gain during pregnancy should be achieved by energy intake. Obese women with gestational diabetes who follow hypocaloric diets develop ketonemia and ketonuria. Lowering mean blood glucose levels without increasing plasma-free fatty acids or causing ketonuria seems to be possible with a more moderate energy restriction of 30% of estimated energy needs. Individual energy recommendations and whether a woman is undereating to avoid insulin therapy can be ascertained through daily food records, weekly weight checks, and ketone testing.

Frequent aerobic exercise can help improve maternal glycemia by lowering postprandial and fasting glucose concentrations. It can also be used as an adjuvant to nutrition therapy. Not enough research has been done to support any particular kind of exercise. Blood glucose data are required to assess the efficacy of nutritional therapy, exercise, and the necessity of pharmaceutical therapy. Maintaining carbohydrate consistency at meals and snacks to enable insulin adjustments becomes a primary goal if insulin therapy is added to nutrition therapy. Despite the fact that the majority of women with gestational diabetes return to normal glucose tolerance after giving birth, they are more likely to have type 2 diabetes later in life and to develop gestational diabetes in future pregnancies. It is advised to make lifestyle changes to decrease or avoid weight gain and to increase physical activity after pregnancy, as these actions can lower the risk of developing diabetes later in life.

8.2.2.3. Lactation

For women with gestational diabetes or pre-existing diabetes, breastfeeding is advised; however, care coordination and planning are necessary for a successful lactation. Breastfeeding lowers blood glucose levels, so it's common for insulin-treated women to need to have a carbohydrate snack before or during nursing. An extra approximately 200 calories should be consumed during the first 6 months of lactation in addition to the pregnancy meal plan. Nonetheless, approximately 1,800 kcal per day suffices to meet lactation's nutritional needs and may facilitate a gradual reduction in body weight.

8.2.3. Older Adults with Diabetes

There is very little research on how a person's nutritional needs change as they age and almost none on people who have diabetes. Therefore, it is necessary to extrapolate dietary guidelines for older adults with diabetes from general population knowledge. A change in body weight is probably the most reliable indicator of poor nutritional status in older adults. Generally, an involuntary gain or loss of more than 10 pounds or 10% of body weight in less than 6 months calls for an assessment to see whether nutrition may be the cause. When it comes to overweight older adults, it's important to assess whether they need to lose weight. Rather than being overweight, older adults with diabetes—especially those residing in long-term care facilities—tend to be underweight. In this age group, lower body weight has been linked to higher rates of morbidity and mortality. For older adults with diabetes, exercise training can improve risk factors for atherosclerosis, slow the decline in age-related lean body mass, decrease central adiposity, and improve insulin sensitivity. It can also significantly slow the decline in maximal aerobic capacity (V_{o2}) that comes with aging. For older adults, especially those with lower energy intake, a daily multivitamin supplement may be appropriate. It should be recommended that older adults consume at least 1,200 mg of calcium per day. It is not appropriate for long-term care facilities to impose dietary restrictions on their elderly diabetic residents. Not having enough food options, eating poorly, and unneeded restrictions can all lead to malnutrition and dehydration. It seems that in these situations, standard (regular) diets are not any more effective than specialized diabetic diets. Because of this, it is advised that residents be given the regular (unrestricted) menu, with the amount and timing of carbohydrates being consistent. Diets like "no concentrated sweets" or "no sugar added," which are frequently provided to senior citizens in long-term care facilities, have no supporting data. Additionally, changing prescription regimens rather than imposing dietary restrictions may frequently be the better course of action for controlling blood sugar.

8.3. Medical Nutrition Therapy for the Treatment/Prevention of Acute Complications of Diabetes and Co-Morbid Conditions

MNT plays a crucial role in both the treatment and prevention of acute complications of diabetes and co-morbid conditions. For individuals with diabetes, proper nutrition management can help regulate blood glucose levels, reducing the risk of hyperglycemia and hypoglycemia, which are common acute complications. A diet rich in fiber, whole grains, lean proteins, and healthy fats can help stabilize blood sugar levels and improve insulin sensitivity. Additionally, MNT can address co-morbid conditions such as cardiovascular disease and obesity, which often accompany diabetes. For instance, a heart-healthy diet low in saturated fats and sodium can help manage blood pressure and cholesterol levels, reducing the risk of cardiovascular complications. Furthermore, weight management through nutrition therapy can alleviate strain on the cardiovascular system and improve overall metabolic health. In sum, personalized MNT tailored to individual needs is essential in managing diabetes and preventing acute complications while addressing co-morbid conditions to optimize overall health outcomes.

8.3.1. Acute Complications

8.3.1.1. Hypoglycemia

Hypoglycemia may arise as a result of modifications to vitamin and/or medication intake, physical activity, and food consumption. Eating foods high in glucose or carbohydrates is necessary to treat hypoglycemia. The acute glycemic response is more closely correlated with the glucose content in the food than its carbohydrate content. 10 g of oral glucose can raise blood glucose levels by about 40 mg/dl (2.2 mmol/l) over 30 minutes in insulin-induced hypoglycemia, and 20 g of oral glucose can raise blood glucose levels by about 60 mg/dl (3.3 mmol/l) over 45 minutes. In all cases, the glucose levels start to drop about 60 minutes after the glucose is consumed.

Any type of carbohydrate that contains glucose will cause blood glucose to rise, even though pure glucose might be the best option. The glycemic response and subsequent hypoglycemia are unaffected by adding protein to the carbohydrate treatment of hypoglycemia. However, adding fat might cause the acute glycemic response to be delayed. Gastric emptying rates are comparable for liquids and solid foods and double during hypoglycemia compared to euglycemia.

8.3.1.2. Acute Illness

Individuals with type 1 diabetes may be more susceptible to diabetic ketoacidosis if they have an acute illness. The need for insulin does not go away during a severe illness. Additionally, the need for insulin may rise due to related elevated levels of counterregulatory hormones. Acute illness patients should test their blood glucose, check for ketones in their blood or urine, drink plenty of fluids, and consume carbohydrates, particularly if their blood glucose level is less than 100 mg/dl (5.5 mmol/l). To maintain glucose within the target range and avoid starvation ketosis in adults, ⍰150–200 g of carbohydrates per day (45–50 g, or three to four carbohydrate choices, every 3–4 h) should be consumed in addition to medication adjustments.

8.3.1.3. Hypertension

Reducing weight and sodium consumption have been the main goals of MNT for the treatment of hypertension. Alcohol, potassium, calcium, and the composition of the diet (total fat, saturated fat, and cholesterol) are other factors that have been taken into account. A low-fat diet high in fruits and vegetables (five to nine servings per day) and low-fat dairy products (two to four servings per day) will lower blood pressure slightly and be high in calcium, magnesium, and potassium. Few researches have been conducted solely on individuals with diabetes. Subjects who are "salt sensitive," a characteristic that may apply to many diabetics, may respond better to sodium reduction. As of right now, there is no standard clinical test to identify people who might be sensitive to salt. The association between blood pressure and sodium intake has been confirmed by numerous meta-analyses and reviews. According to reports, a moderate sodium restriction has a mean effect of reducing blood pressure in hypertensive subjects by approximately 5 mmHg for systolic and diastolic blood pressure and in normotensive subjects by approximately 3 mmHg for systolic and 1 mmHg for diastolic blood pressure. A diet low in total fat, saturated fat, and cholesterol that included fruits, vegetables, and low-fat dairy products was compared to three different levels of sodium intake. The more sodium one consumes, the more their blood pressure will drop. There is a general association in people with diabetes between weight reduction and a reduction in blood pressure, but there is great variability in the response. Reduction in blood pressure can occur with a modest amount of weight loss. An association between high alcohol intake ($\geq$3 drinks/day) and elevated blood pressure has been reported; however, there is no major difference in blood pressure between people who consume <3 drinks/day and nondrinkers. Clinical trials have reported a beneficial effect of potassium supplementation on lowering blood pressure, whereas evidence for a beneficial effect from calcium and magnesium supplementation are lacking.

8.3.1.4. Dyslipidemia

Individuals with type 1 and type 2 diabetes frequently have dyslipidemia, which is defined as abnormal lipid levels, lipoprotein composition, or both. Effective insulin therapy typically lowers plasma triglycerides and returns lipid levels to normal for the majority of people with type 1 diabetes. There may be a slight drop in plasma LDL cholesterol as well. Limit the amount of saturated and trans-unsaturated fats in adult individuals with elevated plasma LDL cholesterol to less than 10%, preferably less than 7%, of total energy intake. Monounsaturated fats or carbohydrates can be used in place of saturated fat if necessary. Increases in soluble (viscous) fiber and plant stanols/sterols can both improve the reduction of plasma LDL cholesterol.

Despite better glycemic control, dyslipidemia—characterized by elevated plasma triglycerides, decreased HDL cholesterol, and small, dense LDL particles—is a common symptom of obesity-related type 1 diabetes and many types of type 2 diabetes. Increased viscerally distributed body adiposity in the abdomen is closely linked to this dyslipidemia. For these individuals, suggested lifestyle modifications include: 1) cutting dietary cholesterol to less than 200 mg per day and saturated fat to less than 7% of energy; 2) increasing soluble fiber (10–25 g/day) and plant stanols/sterols (2 g/day) to improve the lowering of plasma LDL cholesterol; 3) losing a small amount of weight; and 4) increasing physical activity. Reduced plasma LDL cholesterol and lowered plasma triglycerides are the results of diet-induced weight loss and fat restriction. Most studies, though not all of them, have demonstrated that substituting carbohydrates for saturated fat improves plasma LDL cholesterol while having either positive or neutral effects on plasma triglycerides. Saturated fat can also be replaced with monounsaturated fat. On the other hand, eating more fat in the diet may result in consuming more calories and gaining weight. Besides lowering plasma triglycerides, regular exercise also increases insulin sensitivity.

Supplementing with fish oils that contain n-3 fatty acids may be advised for patients whose plasma triglycerides remain elevated even after taking medication. Fish oils, however, have the potential to raise plasma LDL cholesterol, so caution must be used. Individuals who have plasma triglycerides greater than 1,000 mg/dl should be prescribed lipid-lowering medication and have all forms of dietary fat restricted because they are more likely to develop pancreatitis and chylomicronemia syndrome.

8.3.1.5. Nephropathy

Numerous dietary components have been found to play a part in preventing nephropathy. Even modest reductions in protein intake have been demonstrated to improve glomerular filtration rate and lower urinary albumin excretion rates in individuals with microalbuminuria and type 1 or type 2 diabetes. Research on individuals with macroalbuminuria (overt nephropathy) and type 1 diabetes revealed that dietary protein reduction to 0.8 g kg^{-1} day^{-1} slowed the decline in glomerular filtration rate. Nonetheless, these decreases ought to consider the necessity of preserving a healthy nutritional state in individuals suffering from persistent kidney failure. Meal plans for renal disease and protein restriction should be created by a registered dietitian with experience in MNT for diabetes. The potential advantages of plant protein over animal protein in the case of renal insufficiency have been examined in a number of studies. It will take long-term clinical trials involving patients with nephropathy and diabetes to ascertain whether consuming more or less of a particular type of protein is beneficial.

8.3.1.6. Catabolic Illness

States of catabolic disease produce changes in bodily compartments, which can include an increase in the ECF compartment (often accompanied by a rise in body weight) and a corresponding decrease in body cell mass and body fat. The amount of weight loss that has occurred recently, the amount of extra fluid present, the existence or lack of clinical stress markers, and the duration of the patient's fasting period should all be considered when determining whether or not nutrition intervention is necessary. A recent weight loss of more than 10% warrants a detailed nutritional evaluation. Unintentional weight loss of 10–20% indicates a moderate malnutrition in terms of protein and calories, while weight loss of more than 20% typically denotes severe malnutrition. For patients with diabetes, a standard enteral formula (containing 50% carbohydrates) or a lower-carb formula (containing 33–40% carbohydrates) may be used. It is crucial to closely monitor weight, fluid balance, acid-based status, hemodynamic data, plasma glucose, and electrolytes. It might be necessary to modify medication—typically insulin—to preserve glycemic control. The majority of hospitalized patients can have their needs satisfied with 25–35 kcal/kg body weight. Avoid overfeeding as this can worsen hyperglycemia, lead to aberrant liver function, and raise the production of carbon dioxide and oxygen. Protein requirements are approximately 1.0 g kg^{-1} body $weight^{-1}$ for individuals under mild stress and 1.5 g kg^{-1} for individuals under moderate to severe stress who have normal renal and hepatic function. Fats should make up no less than 30% of the total energy provided.

8.3.1.7. Diabetes Prevention

The significant global rise in diabetes prevalence in recent years emphasizes the significance of diabetes prevention in high-risk individuals. In some populations, type 2 diabetes seems to be strongly influenced by genetic susceptibility. But since population gene pools change very slowly, the current epidemic most likely represents significant lifestyle changes. Changes in lifestyle, marked by less physical activity and more energy consumption, have contributed to the rise in obesity, a major risk factor for diabetes that is influenced by both behavior and genetics. Even though it can be challenging to keep a lower body weight over time, a number of studies have shown that moderate, sustained weight loss can significantly lower the risk of type 2 diabetes. Clinical trial information from the U.S. and Finland now firmly believes that losing a moderate amount of weight can lower one's risk of developing diabetes. Numerous prospective studies have also shown that leading an active lifestyle can either delay or prevent the onset of type 2 diabetes. Exercise reduces the risk of type 2 diabetes and impaired glucose tolerance, both at moderate and high intensities.

Lowering total fat consumption, especially that of saturated fat, may lower the risk of diabetes. Increasing dietary fat intake is linked to a higher incidence of diabetes, regardless of total calorie intake; however, not all studies show this relationship. All forms of dietary fat appear to have the potential to negatively impact insulin sensitivity, except for omega-3 fatty acids. The biggest impact might come from saturated fat. When combined with a suitable total energy intake for managing weight, a higher intake of polyunsaturated fat may lower the risk of type 2 diabetes.

There is evidence from recent studies that consuming more whole grains and dietary fiber lowers the risk of diabetes. While certain micronutrients may influence the metabolism of glucose and insulin, there is a lack of consistent or sufficient data to support their involvement in the onset of diabetes. Reduced risk of diabetes and enhanced insulin sensitivity have been linked to moderate alcohol consumption. Nevertheless, there is not enough information to make a specific recommendation for moderate alcohol consumption to prevent type 2 diabetes. It is not possible to make dietary recommendations to prevent type 1 diabetes. Breastfeeding could be advantageous. There is not enough information available at this time to support any specific recommendations for the prevention of type 2 diabetes in youth, even though rising childhood obesity may be linked to rising type 2 diabetes prevalence, especially in minority adolescents. Reducing energy and fat intake, increasing physical activity, and managing weight as a result could be advantageous.

8.4. International Dietetics and Nutrition Terminology (IDNT)

The IDNT is a standardized language that can be used in the NCP, providing standardized definitions and terminology related to nutrition care. This guarantees accurate definitions of terminology regardless of the location of a dietitian's practice. The IDNT is being adopted by numerous Canadian health provider organizations and is advised as a practice tool by the International Confederation of Dietetic Associations (ICDA). Dietitians in the 21st century are expected to have a solid understanding of the scientific principles that guide their work, as well as a solid foundation in the methods used to determine those principles through rigorous research methodology, analysis, ethical approaches, and the application of critical skills. Dietetics is a discipline that depends entirely on a robust evidence base to shape clinical practice. This requirement is fully recognized in the current dietetics training curriculum, and the dietetic profession is increasingly empowered globally to influence clinical decision-making through critical applications of research.

Increasingly, dietitians are expanding on their clinical practice through active involvement in research and increasingly through research leadership. This increases the standing of the profession, refines therapeutic approaches and develops the knowledge connections with medicine and other health professions allied to medicine.

"The application of the science of nutrition to the human being in health and disease" is the definition of dietetics. However, the term "dietitian," which refers to a dietetics practitioner, was in use long before nutrition science was recognized as a legitimate field of study. The term "dietitian" was first used in the USA in 1899, despite Florence Nightingale's claim to be the first dietitian due to her emphasis during the Crimean War that the sick men under her care would not recover if they were not well fed. The definition of a dietitian was then given as someone who worked in a hospital and fed patients healthy meals; the majority of the first dietitians were home economists. The 20th century saw a significant expansion in the role of the dietitian, who is now thought to play more than just supplying food. The breadth of knowledge and abilities needed to qualify and register as a dietitian reflects the belief that dietitians are the experts in the planning and assessment of nutritional care for both the general public and patients in need of therapeutic diet regimens.

The American Dietetic Association (ADA) was established in 1917, marking the formal establishment of the dietetics profession in the United States. The first dietetic department was established in the Edinburgh Royal Infirmary in 1924, and the first dietitians in the UK were nurses. After multiple failed attempts, the British

Dietetic Association (BDA) was finally founded in 1936. A number of the pioneers of British dietetics were able to travel to the USA in the 1920s to observe the work of established dietetic departments there. Following suit, other nations registered more than 30 dietetic associations with the International Committee of Dietetic Associations (ICDA) in 2000.

8.4.1. Dietetic and Nutritional Policy

In Nordic food cultures, health and dietetics are major concerns. Certain nations, such as Norway, may view health as the most essential aspect of food culture, which is to say, a view of food in which customs and normative discourses are continuously entwined. A strong nutrition policy is supported by public discourse on nutrition and health, as well as state regulations. Nutrition policies ought to tackle the twin burden of malnutrition by averting diet-related illnesses, ensuring a safe and sustainable food supply, and incorporating associated risk factors. The 1992 Plan of Action on Nutrition and the World Declaration on Nutrition served as the foundation for the global development of nutrition policies. Policies pertaining to nutrition can be enacted at the family, community, state, and federal levels, as well as in a variety of industries, including the food environment, mass media, healthcare, workplaces, and schools. It is crucial to use an evidence-based nutrition action approach, make decisions, develop, implement, and evaluate PHN policy, and implement interventions based on globally harmonized criteria for various population groups.

To compare the development of nations, to track dietary consumption and the population's nutritional status, to assess the effects of interventions, and to supply information for political decision-making, surveillance and monitoring data on nutrition and health indicators are crucial. More than 90% of nations in each region have policies and programs covering topics like undernutrition, obesity and diet-related non-communicable diseases (NCDs), nutrition for infants and young children, and vitamins and minerals, according to the World Health Organization's (WHO) global nutrition policy review. Significant gaps were found in the governance of nutrition, the design and content of some policies and programs, the implementation of policies, monitoring, and evaluation. Nutrition policies fall short of addressing the issues that nations and areas are currently dealing with, particularly the dual burden of malnutrition (i.e., undernutrition, obesity, and NCDs linked to diet). The lack of human resources for implementing nutrition programs, who are primarily in charge of delivering nutrition programs, limits the national capacity of PHN.

8.4.1.1. A Standardized Nutrition Care Process and Language Are Essential Components of a Conceptual Model

Because patient outcomes are receiving more attention and because accrediting agencies, third-party payers, researchers, and others are requiring more information in their evaluations of patient care, the documentation of clinical services within healthcare systems has grown in importance. It is essential that clinical nutrition practitioners implement a standardized nutrition care process and language to document thoroughly and communicate meaningful information regarding their role in improving patient outcomes, given the multitude of users who rely on healthcare information in the patient record. A standardized nutrition care process has been developed and adopted by the dietetics profession as a result of a body of work. In order to articulate a conceptual model for clinical nutrition practice and documentation and to distinguish the unique body of knowledge that is clinical dietetics, two essential components are needed: a standardized nutrition care process that adheres to the scientific method and a standardized language. In order to standardize and direct nutrition practitioners' clinical judgments or critical thinking processes and to record data relating nutrition care to patient outcomes, the conceptual model acts as an organizing framework.

Nutritionists who specialize in dietetics use food science and nutrition to help people become healthier. Dietitian nutritionists collaborate with nutrition and dietetic technicians to offer patients care and guidance. General nutrition education can also be given by nutrition and dietetic technicians as well as dietitian nutritionists. Both hold national credentials and play a crucial role in foodservice and healthcare management teams.

Professionals in the field of dietetics often focus their efforts on specific populations, facilities or initiatives, including:

- Designing individual nutritional therapies to address specific health issues, such as unhealthy weight, diabetes or hypertension
- Developing facility-wide nutrition programs for health care, educational, correctional and other institutions
- Increasing public awareness of proper nutritional standards and habits
- Improving the accuracy and comprehension of food labels
- Ensuring the safety of our food supply
- Researching how changes in diet (such as reducing salt intake) affect health (by reducing blood pressure)
- Working with food manufacturers to improve the nutritional quality of prepared foods

8.5. Principles of Evidence-Based Nutrition

The process of formulating dietary recommendations using the most up-to-date scientific data is known as evidence-based nutrition. This approach to nutrition aims to dispel myths and misinformation about nutrition that are not supported by current scientific evidence, emphasizing the value of rigorous scientific research in determining what constitutes a healthy diet and nutritional needs. This nutritional approach is predicated on the idea that looking at the evidence is the best way to Figure out what is generally beneficial for our health.

An essential component of evidence-based practice in nutrition is the systematic reviews of recent studies. This is a methodical approach to gather research on a particular subject or query and ascertain the conclusions drawn from all current and pertinent research. This means that to determine the most appropriate nutritional recommendations, we should look to the body of the most recent and reliable scientific evidence rather than depending solely on our own personal opinions or beliefs about nutrition.

8.5.1. Anecdotal Evidence vs. Scientific Evidence

Anecdotal evidence and scientific evidence represent two distinct forms of evidence that serve different purposes in assessing the validity and reliability of claims or hypotheses. Anecdotal evidence typically consists of personal stories, testimonials, or accounts of individual experiences. While anecdotal evidence can be compelling and emotionally resonant, it is inherently subjective and prone to biases, including selective memory, confirmation bias, and the placebo effect. Anecdotal evidence alone is generally not considered robust or reliable enough to draw broad conclusions or inform decision-making in scientific or clinical contexts. On the other hand, scientific evidence relies on systematic observation, experimentation, and rigorous analysis following the scientific method. Scientific evidence is typically gathered through controlled studies, clinical trials, meta-analyses, and peer-reviewed research publications. It aims to minimize bias, account for variability, and establish causal relationships between variables. Scientific evidence undergoes scrutiny and validation by the scientific community, which helps ensure its accuracy, reproducibility, and generalizability.

While anecdotal evidence can provide initial insights or generate hypotheses, scientific evidence is essential for confirming or refuting those hypotheses and informing evidence-based practice in fields such as medicine, psychology, and public policy. Ultimately, scientific evidence carries more weight in decision-making processes due to its objectivity, reliability, and ability to draw valid conclusions about cause-and-effect relationships.

8.5.2. Evidence-Based Nutrition and Levels of Evidence

Evidence-based nutrition relies on the systematic integration of the best available scientific evidence, clinical expertise, and patient values and preferences to inform nutrition-related decisions and interventions. Within the framework of evidence-based practice, different levels of evidence exist to categorize the strength and reliability of research findings. These levels help guide practitioners and researchers in assessing the quality and validity of evidence when making recommendations or formulating guidelines. The hierarchy of evidence typically includes the following levels:

- **Systematic Reviews and Meta-Analyses:** Considered the highest level of evidence, systematic reviews and meta-analyses compile and analyze data from multiple primary studies on a particular topic. They provide a comprehensive summary of the available evidence, often including statistical analyses to quantify the overall effect size.
- **Randomized Controlled Trials (RCTs):** These are experimental studies where participants are randomly assigned to different interventions or control groups. They are designed to minimize bias and establish cause-and-effect relationships between interventions and outcomes.
- **Cohort Studies:** These follow a group of individuals over time to assess the association between exposure to certain factors (e.g., dietary habits) and subsequent health outcomes. They can provide valuable insights into long-term effects but are susceptible to biases such as confounding variables.
- **Case-Control Studies:** These compare individuals with a particular condition (cases) to those without the condition (controls) to identify potential risk factors or associations. While useful for studying rare outcomes, they are prone to recall bias and do not establish causality.
- **Cross-Sectional Studies:** These assess exposure and outcome variables at a single point in time to examine associations or prevalence rates. While they provide valuable epidemiological data, they cannot establish temporal relationships or causality.

- **Expert Opinion and Consensus Statements:** Expert opinions and consensus statements reflect the collective judgment of professionals in the field based on their clinical experience and knowledge. While less rigorous than empirical research, they can provide valuable guidance when empirical evidence is lacking or inconclusive.

In evidence-based nutrition, recommendations and guidelines are typically based on findings from high-quality studies such as systematic reviews and RCTs whenever possible. However, in the absence of such evidence, lower levels of evidence may still contribute to the overall body of knowledge, albeit with greater caution and consideration of potential biases.

A Closer Look

Nutritional Diagnosis

Nutritional diagnosis is a critical component of MNT, providing a systematic framework for assessing an individual's nutritional status, identifying nutrition-related problems, and formulating targeted interventions to address them. This process involves a comprehensive evaluation of various factors, including dietary intake, anthropometric measurements, biochemical markers, and clinical indicators, to determine the individual's nutritional health and specific nutrition-related needs. The first step in nutritional diagnosis is to gather relevant information through a thorough assessment. This includes obtaining a detailed dietary history, which involves documenting the types and amounts of foods and beverages consumed, meal patterns, eating behaviors, and dietary preferences. Anthropometric measurements, such as height, weight, BMI, waist circumference, and body composition, provide valuable insights into the individual's body composition and nutritional status. Biochemical markers, such as blood glucose levels, lipid profiles, electrolyte levels, and markers of nutrient deficiencies, offer objective measures of nutrient status and metabolic health. Clinical indicators, such as medical history, medications, symptoms, and physical examination findings, provide additional context for understanding the individual's overall health and nutritional needs. Once the assessment data has been collected and analyzed, a nutritional diagnosis is made based on the identification of specific nutrition-related problems or needs that require intervention. This involves synthesizing the information obtained from the assessment to identify patterns, trends, and areas of concern related to the individual's dietary intake, nutritional status, and health outcomes. Common nutrition-related problems may include inadequate or excessive nutrient intake, malnutrition, overweight or obesity, micronutrient deficiencies, dyslipidemia, diabetes, gastrointestinal disorders, and food allergies or intolerances, among others. The next step in nutritional diagnosis is to formulate a problem list, which prioritizes the identified nutrition-related problems based on their significance, urgency, and potential impact on the individual's health outcomes. This helps guide the development of a personalized nutrition care plan that targets the most pressing issues and addresses the individual's specific needs and goals. The nutrition care plan may include specific dietary recommendations, meal plans, portion control strategies, nutrient supplementation, behavior change interventions, and education on healthy eating habits. Finally, ongoing monitoring and evaluation are essential components of nutritional diagnosis, allowing for the assessment of progress and adjustment of the nutrition care plan as needed. Regular follow-up visits enable healthcare professionals to track changes in dietary intake, anthropometric measurements, biochemical markers, and clinical outcomes, and to provide ongoing support, guidance, and encouragement to the individual. By systematically evaluating nutritional status, identifying nutrition-related problems, and implementing personalized interventions, nutritional diagnosis plays a crucial role in optimizing health outcomes and promoting overall well-being through targeted nutrition interventions tailored to individual needs.

Summary

- Medical nutrition therapy (MNT) refers to the assessment of the nutritional status of patients with an illness, diet-related condition, or injury, in order to benefit the patient's own health and reduce health-care costs.
- Medical nutrition therapy (MNT) is an effective intervention for the management of obesity, prediabetes, and diabetes, which have all increased dramatically in the United States and worldwide over the last 30 years.
- The purpose of MNT is to identify patients at risk for major nutrition-related health problems and recommend dietary adjustments leading to better health outcomes and improved quality of life.
- The goals of medical nutrition therapy for diabetes mellitus are to improve overall metabolic outcomes (glucose and lipid levels), provide appropriate energy to maintain desirable body weight, and improve overall health through optimal nutrition.
- Resistant starch (nondigestible oligosaccharides and the starch amylase) is not digested and therefore not absorbed as glucose in the small intestine.
- The IDNT is a standardized language, with standardized nutrition care terms and definitions that can be used in the NCP. This ensures a reliable definition of terms regardless of where a dietitian is practicing.
- Nutrition and dietetic technicians work with dietitian nutritionists to provide care and consultation to patients.
- Academy of nutrition and dietetics suggests that the MNT is an "integral component" of the health care and the management of the different diseases such as diabetes, heart diseases, osteoporosis, chronic kidney disease and cancer.

References

1. Brown, J. E., et al. (2007). *Nutrition Through The Life Cycle* (3rd ed.). Belmont, CA: Wadsworth Publishing, Co.
2. Byham-Gray, L. D., Gilbride, J. A., Dixon, L. B., & Stage, F. K. (2005). Evidence-based practice: What are dietitians' perceptions, attitudes, and knowledge? *Journal of the American Dietetic Association, 105*(10), 1574–1581.
3. Cataldo, C. B. (2003). *Nutrition and Diet Therapy* (6th ed.). Belmont, CA: Wadsworth Publishing Company.
4. Chiu, Y. W., Weng, Y. H., Wahlqvist, M. L., Yang, C. Y., & Kuo, K. N. (2012). Do registered dietitians search for evidence-based information? A nationwide survey of regional hospitals in Taiwan. *Asia Pacific Journal of Clinical Nutrition, 21*(4), 630–637.
5. Diekman, C. B. (2007). Evidence-based practice: Key to success. *Journal of the American Dietetic Association, 107*(7), 1088.
6. Dudek, S. G. (2006). *Nutrition essentials for nursing practice* (5th ed.). Philadelphia: Lippincott.

7. Elia, M., & Cummings, J. H. (2007). Physiological aspects of energy metabolism and gastrointestinal effects of carbohydrates. *European Journal of Clinical Nutrition, 61*(Suppl 1), S40–S74.

8. Escott-Stump, S. (2007). *Nutrition and Diagnosis-Related Care* (6th ed.). Philadelphia: Lippincott.

9. Furst, P., & Stehle, P. (2004). What are the essential elements needed for the determination of amino acid requirements in humans? *Journal of Nutrition, 134*, 1558S–1565S.

10. Hall-McMahon, E. J., & Campbell, K. L. (2012). Have renal dietitians successfully implemented evidence-based guidelines into practice? A survey of dietitians across Australia and New Zealand. *Journal of Renal Nutrition, 22*(6), 584–591.

11. Hand, R. K., & Abram, J. K. (2016). Sense of competence impedes uptake of new academy evidence-based practice guidelines: Results of a survey. *Journal of the Academy of Nutrition and Dietetics, 116*(4), 695–705.

12. Hu, F. B., Manson, J. E., Stampfer, M. J., Colditz, G., Liu, S., Solomon, C. G., & Willett, W. C. (2001). Diet, lifestyle, and the risk of type 2 diabetes mellitus in women. *The New England Journal of Medicine, 345*, 790–797.

13. Laramee, S. H. (2005). Evidence-based practice: A core competency for dietetics. *Journal of the Academy of Nutrition and Dietetics, 105*(3), 333.

14. Lutz, C. A., & Rutherford, K. P. (2006). *Nutrition and Diet Therapy* (4th ed.). Philadelphia: Davis.

15. Mahan, L. K., & Escott-Stump, S. (2007). *Krause's Food Nutrition and Diet Therapy* (11th ed.). Philadelphia: Saunders.

16. Hankinson, S. E., & Speizer, F. E. (1996). Prospective assessment of breastfeeding and breast cancer incidence among 89,887 women. *Lancet, 347*, 431–436.

17. Mitchell, M. K. (2002). *Nutrition Across the Life Span* (2nd ed.). Philadelphia: Saunders.

18. Myers, E. F. (2005). ADA evidence analysis library. *Journal of the Academy of Nutrition and Dietetics, 105*(supp), S79–S.

19. Olfert, M. D., & Arnold, S. J. (2012). Beyond Google: Helping nutrition students achieve information literacy. *Journal of the Academy of Nutrition and Dietetics, 112*(sup), A18–A.

20. Papoutsakis, C., Moloney, L., Sinley, R. C., Acosta, A., Handu, D., & Steiber, A. L. (2017). Academy of Nutrition and Dietetics Methodology for developing evidence-based nutrition practice guidelines. *Journal of the Academy of Nutrition and Dietetics, 117*(5), 794–804.

21. Rand, W. M., Pellett, P. L., & Young, V. R. (2003). Meta-analysis of nitrogen balance studies for estimating protein requirements in healthy adults. *The American Journal of Clinical Nutrition, 77*, 109–127.

22. Rodner, M., Long, S., & DeYoung, S. (2004). *Foundations and Clinical Applications of Nutrition: A Nursing Approach* (3rd ed.). St. Louis, MO: Mosby.

23. Sizer, S., & Whitney, E. (2007). *Nutrition: Concepts and Controversies* (11th ed.). Salt Lake City, UT: Brooks Cole Publishing Company.

24. Smith, S. C., & Penumetcha, M. (2010). Librarian involvement in a nutrition undergraduate research course: Preparing nutrition students for evidence-based practice. *Journal of Allied Health, 39*(2), e69–e76.

25. Steiber, A., & Barkoukis, H. (2006). Individualized research experiences in a dietetic internship program. *Topics in Clinical Nutrition, 21*(3), 176–181.
26. Trahms, C. M., & Pipes, P. (2001). *Nutrition in Infancy and Childhood* (7th ed.). New York: McGraw-Hill.
27. Vogt, E. A. M., Byham-Gray, L. D., & Touger-Decker, R. (2013). Perceptions, attitudes, knowledge, and clinical use of evidence-based practice among US registered dietitians. *Topics in Clinical Nutrition, 28*(3), 283–294.
28. Wardlaw, G. M., & Insel, P. M. (2002). *Perspectives in Nutrition* (6th ed.). New York: Mosby-Year Book.
29. Whelan, K., Thomas, J. E., & Madden, A. M. (2006). Undertaking a research project improves student dietitians' confidence in their research skills. *Journal of Human Nutrition and Dietetics, 19*(6), 474–475.
30. World Health Organization. (2007). *Protein and Amino Acid Requirements in Human Nutrition. Report of a Joint WHO/FAO/UNU Expert Consultation* (WHO Technical Report Series: No. 935). Geneva: WHO.
31. Browning, R., & Kram, R. (2005). Energetic cost and preferred speed of walking in obese vs. normal weight women. *Obesity Research, 13*, 891–899.
32. Franz, M. J., Bantle, J. P., Beebe, C. A., Brunzell, J. D., Chiasson, J.-L., Garg, A., Holzmeister, L. A., Hoogwerf, B., Mayer-Davis, E., Mooradian, A. D., Purnell, J. Q., & Wheeler, M. (2002). Evidence-based nutrition principles and recommendations for the treatment and prevention of diabetes and related complications (Technical Review). *Diabetes Care, 25*, 148–198.
33. The American Diabetes Association. (2002). Diabetes mellitus and exercise (Position Statement). *Diabetes Care, 25*(Suppl. 1), S64–S68.
34. American Diabetes Association. (2000). Type 2 diabetes in children and adolescents (Consensus Statement). *Diabetes Care, 23*, 381–389.
35. Cryer, P. E., Fisher, J. N., & Shamoon, H. (1994). Hypoglycemia (Technical Review). *Diabetes Care, 17*, 734–755.
36. Sacks, F. M., Svetkey, L. P., Vollmer, W. M., Appel, L. J., Bray, G. A., Harsha, D., Obarzanek, E., Conlin, P. R., Miller, E. R., Simons-Morton, D. G., Karanja, N., & Lin, P.-H., for the DASH-Sodium Collaborative Research Group. (2001). Effects on blood pressure of reduced dietary sodium and the dietary approaches to stop hypertension (DASH) diet. *New England Journal of Medicine, 344*, 3–10.
37. Hu, F. B., & Willett, W. C. (2018). Current and future landscape of nutritional epidemiologic research. *JAMA, 320*(20), 2073–2074.
38. Adams, K. M., Lindell, K. C., Kohlmeier, M., & Zeisel, S. H. (2006). Status of nutrition education in medical schools. *American Journal of Clinical Nutrition, 83*(4), 941S–944S.
39. Kris-Etherton, P. M., Akabas, S. R., & Bales, C. W. (2014). The need to advance nutrition education in the training of health care professionals and recommended research to evaluate implementation and effectiveness. *American Journal of Clinical Nutrition, 99*(5 suppl), 1153S–1166S.
40. Devries, S., Dalen, J. E., & Eisenberg, D. M. (2014). A deficiency of nutrition education in medical training. *American Journal of Medicine, 127*(9), 804–806.

41. McClinchy, J., Dickinson, A., & Barron, D. (2013). Practitioner and patient experiences of giving and receiving healthy eating advice. *British Journal of Community Nursing, 18*(10), 498–504.

42. Johnston, B. C., Kanters, S., & Bandayrel, K. (2014). Comparison of weight loss among named diet programs in overweight and obese adults: A meta-analysis. *JAMA, 312*(9), 923–933.

43. Poole, C. D., Halcox, J. P., & Jenkins-Jones, S. (2013). Omega-3 fatty acids and mortality outcome in patients with and without type 2 diabetes after myocardial infarction: A retrospective, matched-cohort study. *Clinical Therapeutics, 35*(1), 40–51.

44. Aung, T., Halsey, J., & Kromhout, D., for the Omega-3 Treatment Trialists' Collaboration. (2018). Associations of omega-3 fatty acid supplement use with cardiovascular disease risks: Meta-analysis of 10 trials involving 77,917 individuals. *JAMA Cardiology, 3*(3), 225–234.

45. Manson, J. E., Cook, N. R., Lee, I. M., & VITAL Research Group. (2019). Vitamin D supplements and prevention of cancer and cardiovascular disease. *New England Journal of Medicine, 380*(1), 33–44.

46. Johnston, B. C., Lytvyn, L., & Lo, C. K. (2018). Microbial preparations (probiotics) for the prevention of Clostridium difficile infection in adults and children: An individual patient data meta-analysis of 6,851 participants. *Infection Control & Hospital Epidemiology, 39*(7), 771–781.

Chapter

NUTRITION COUNSELING AND DOCUMENTATION

9

Contents

Unit Introduction

In nutrition counseling, a client and a qualified counselor work together to interpret the findings of a nutrition assessment, determine unique nutrition needs and goals of the client, talk about how to achieve those goals, and decide on the best course of action. Nutrition counseling concentrates on actionable steps to address clients' nutritional needs and the advantages of behavior modification, while also assisting clients in understanding critical health information. Nurses, other facility-based healthcare professionals, volunteers, or community health workers can all serve as nutrition counselors. Effective counseling plays a role in achieving favorable nutrition and health outcomes. Counseling should ideally take place in a private, comfortable setting for the client. In a busy medical facility as opposed to a community setting, this might be more difficult, but things can be improved. Counselors should receive training on how to properly interpret and utilize support tools including flipcharts, counseling cards, brochures for take-home work, data collection forms, and referral forms. Dietary counseling offers personalized nutritional support to promote eating habit changes. Additionally, it might help prevent or treat diseases like cancer, obesity, diabetes, hyperlipidemia, heart disease, and other nutrition-related conditions (Figure 9.1).

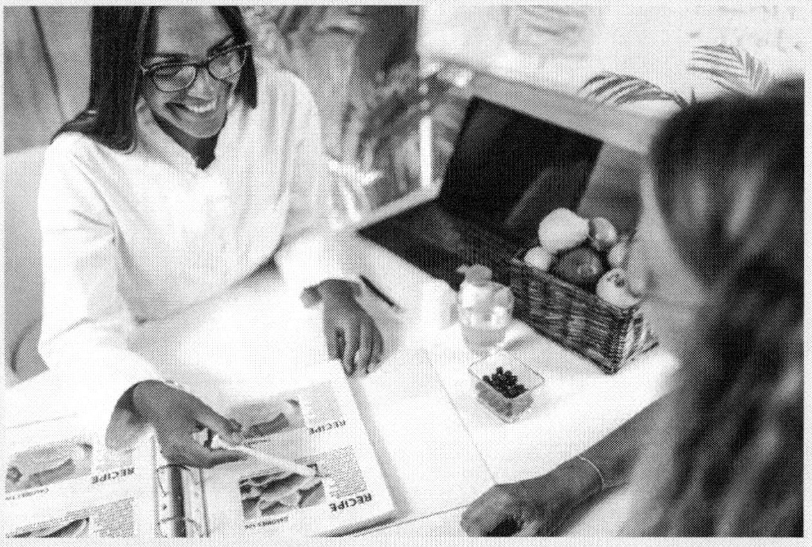

Figure 9.1. *Nutrition counseling programs.*

Source: https://www.nutritioned.org/wp-content/uploads/2022/11/online-nutrition-counseling.jpg.

The main health issues of today are more often caused by acute and chronic illnesses associated with inadequate diet and/or excessive consumption. Obesity and poor eating habits are major contributors to cancer and coronary heart disease. The prevalence of chronic illnesses is still rising in America as a result of issues like the rising obesity rate in the country. Tailored dietary advice can give the patient valuable understanding of food-associated ailments and information about how different nutrients (protein, carbs, fat, and alcohol) impact diseases or obesity. As an alternative, nutritional counseling can help avert conditions linked to nutrition, like the need to control weight. Nutritional counseling can be customized to treat patients with particular illnesses, help minimize side effects and/or complications, and enhance overall health. Active patient participation, as well as direction and support from the dietician or doctor, are necessary for prevention at all levels: primary (preventing disease), secondary (early diagnosis), and tertiary (preventing or slowing deterioration). Effective patient participation requires motivation, education, and counseling. Meal planning is frequently a part of dietary counseling in addition to patient education.

In addition to being crucial for patient safety, high-quality recordkeeping is also important for the provision and assessment of dietetic and nutrition care. All people have the fundamental human right to adequate nutrition. Nonetheless, among senior hospital patients in Western Europe, undernourishment is recognized as a common and significant health issue. Ensuring appropriate nutritional treatment and care is facilitated by nutritional documentation. The documentation of nutritional care by nurses in hospitals and in transitional care facilities has not been extensively studied. Currently available research indicates that documentation practices are inadequate. This chapter aims to investigate the ways in which nurses record the nutritional care and treatment provided to elderly patients in hospitals, as well as the ways in which nurses and student nurses exchange information regarding patients' nutritional status during the transfer of elderly patients between hospitals and nursing homes.

Norwegian laws pertaining to health care govern appropriate documentation and patient communication. Health care providers can use a patient's medical record as a working tool to deliver appropriate and safe patient care. To ensure the continuity of care and treatment, documented information needs to be organized and systematized. Health care providers also have a duty to record and share pertinent patient health status information amongst healthcare settings to follow up with patients. Furthermore, hospital medical staff members have a duty to counsel and direct the municipal health care services regarding the needs of their patients. Unfortunately, documentation of fundamental healthcare needs and communication of these needs amongst healthcare settings is inadequate. Furthermore, it was discovered that the documentation of nutritional care in the conducted studies was inadequate and primarily comprised data on various eating abilities or disabilities. Few studies have looked specifically at how nurses convey information about older patients' nutritional status between different healthcare settings. However, studies have indicated that there are obstacles pertaining to insufficient information transfer between different health care settings. Short hospital stays, resource demands, and differences in health professionals' nutritional knowledge and proficiency have all been identified as barriers..

Orientation and Directional Terms

Term	Definition	Illustration
Nutritional counseling	A process by which a health professional with special training in nutrition helps people make healthy food choices and form healthy eating habits.	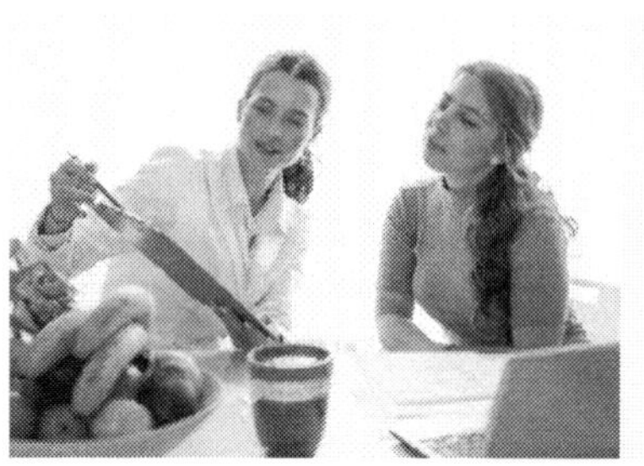
Food frequency questionnaire	Food frequency questionnaire is a questionnaire used to obtain frequency and, in some cases, portion size information about food and beverage consumption over a specified period of time, typically the past month or year.	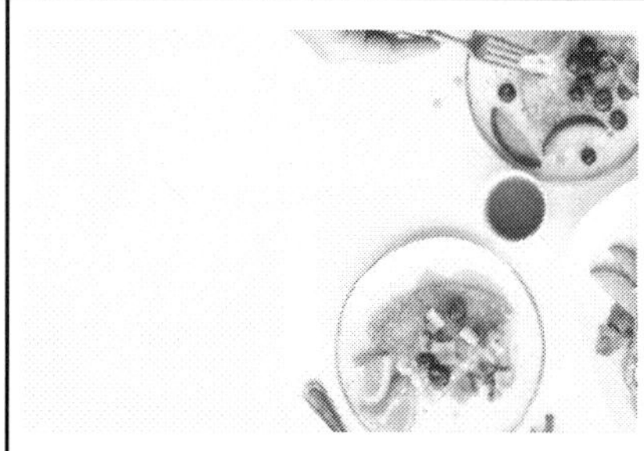
Nutrition education	Nutrition education is a set of learning experiences designed to assist in healthy eating choices and other nutrition-related behavior.	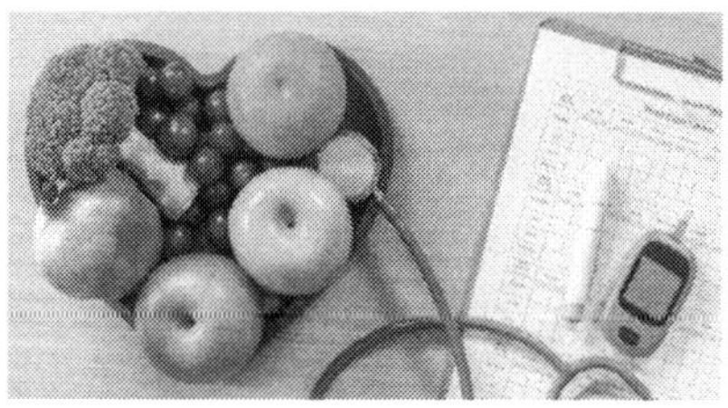
Nutrition informatics	Nutrition informatics is the management of the information dietetics professionals need to practice successfully while tailoring recommendations to meet each patient's specific needs.	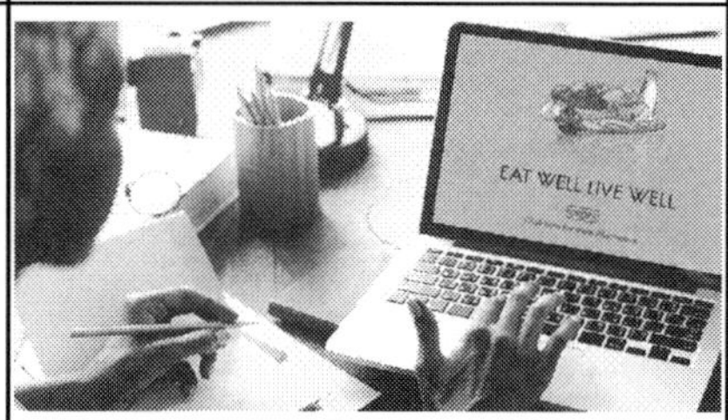
Obesity	Obesity is a chronic complex disease defined by excessive fat deposits that can impair health. Obesity can lead to increased risk of type 2 diabetes and heart disease, it can affect bone health and reproduction, it increases the risk of certain cancers.	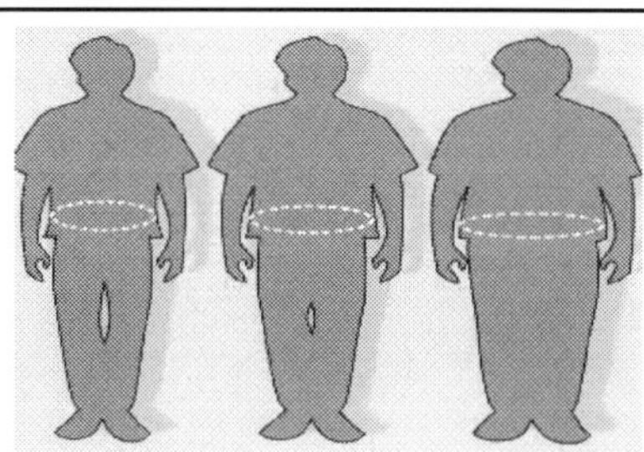

9.1. Nutrition Counseling Principles

To provide relevant information and assist the client in making healthy decisions at home, good counseling starts with asking questions about the client's symptoms and circumstances. Simply giving someone instructions does not guarantee that they will follow through, as knowledge alone cannot alter behavior. Counselors must be able to prioritize messages based on the needs of their clients and deliver them efficiently in a brief amount of time in addition to knowing what messages are appropriate. Experience and practice are needed for this. A variety of mnemonic devices have been created to aid the retention of counseling steps and provide guidance to counselors on sound technique. These can also be applied in supervision and mentorship visits, as well as during role-plays in training.

- **Ethical Principles for Counseling:** Upholding ethical standards is also essential for effective counseling.
    - **Provide Accurate Information:** Clients should be able to trust that counselors' words and actions are truthful and reliable.
    - **Keep Client Information Confidential:** Clients need to know that counselors will keep their information confidential except as needed for their treatment or recovery.
    - **Respect Autonomy of the Client:** Clients have the right to make their own decisions without coercion.
    - **Keep Interests of Clients in Mind:** Advise them based on professional assessment and offer alternatives if you cannot help them.
    - **Do No Harm:** Avoid any interventions that could harm or exploit clients emotionally, financially, or medically.
    - **Be Fair:** Treat all clients fairly and without discrimination. Respect clients' rights, dignity, and individual difference.

9.1.1. Effective Counselor-Client Relationship

The nutritional counseling process cannot be successful unless dietitians and clients interact effectively. Dietetics is the application of the health and disease sciences to the study of food composition and the different economic, social, psychological, and physiological factors that affect dietary behavior. Its main goal is to help clients translate abstract concepts and theoretical knowledge about a healthy lifestyle into actionable steps and useful behavioral skills. For the intervention to be successful, the patient's faith in the dietitian-patient relationship is also essential (Figure 9.2).

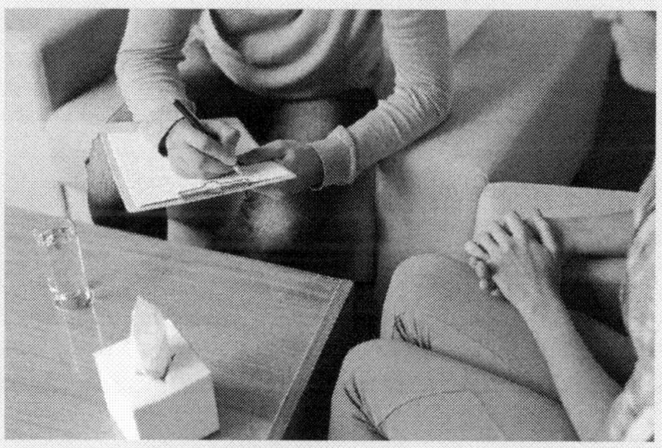

Figure 9.2. *Nutrition care process.*

Source: https://www.eatingdisorderhope.com/wp-content/uploads/2021/10/BPD-and-Therapy-2.jpg.

The primary objective of counseling is to assist those going through personal struggles in finding solutions and enhancing their emotional health. Building a transparent and reliable relationship with your patients is crucial to their success in therapy because it lays the groundwork for them to achieve their objectives in the most efficient manner.

Building genuine connections from a trusting counselor patient relationship is possible when these factors exist:

9.1.1.1. Empathetic People

Individuals who pursue careers in counseling are typically naturally sympathetic. It is commonly believed that the most important quality for a counselor to have is empathy. Throughout the counseling process, a wide range of delicate emotions will surface, and it is the counselor's responsibility to support their clients in feeling respected and understood. However, a healthy emotional balance is also necessary for a relationship to be successful. You should have empathy for your clients, but you should not pity them. You must show that you understand, but not to the extent that you condone unreasonable actions or ideas.

9.1.1.2. The Focus Is on the Patient

As therapy operates based on "they talk, you listen," counseling involves a great deal of listening. To obtain the necessary insight to make an accurate assessment and, eventually, create an appropriate treatment plan, it is your responsibility to maintain focus and provide each patient with the undivided attention they require.

9.1.1.3. Objectives Are Set

Establishing specific goals based on your client's needs and specific issues comes next, after you have carefully listened to them tell their story and taken thorough notes. You are giving your client hope that their problems can be resolved by outlining a clear set of goals with checkpoints along the way.

9.1.1.4. You Practice Unconditional Positive Regard in Your Therapy

This idea enables your patients to be forthcoming and honest about their emotions as well as actions that may have prompted them to seek counseling. The opposite will happen if your patient believes you are making a bad judgment about them based on what they have disclosed and discussed.

9.1.1.5. You Are Prepared

A competent counselor will review notes from past sessions to prepare for each one and create a plan based on evidence-based counseling practices and research for each patient's objectives.

Additionally, excellent counselors understand that research and ongoing education are critical to expanding their expertise, which is what sets exceptional counselors apart.

9.1.1.6. You Are Patient and Flexible

The client dictates how quickly they accept and use the counseling they are receiving. Flexibility and patience are needed for this. Although goals can be linked to a schedule, you may decide to alter a therapy session and change directions based on how slowly (or quickly) a client advances.

9.1.1.7. There Is No Coddling

It is your responsibility to assist your client in overcoming and managing their problems and anxieties; however, coddling them will only impede the process. Your client will make progress at a pace that suits them, and sometimes that progress will require some encouragement. Every session should conclude with a takeaway, or a "assignment" that your client can use to move one step closer to their objective in their daily lives.

9.1.1.8. Your Relationship Is Professional

Simply stated: you are the teacher and your patient is the student.

Effective counselors establish a clear boundary between being friendly in nature, and having a "friendship." Crossing that boundary can have serious implications on a effectiveness of the therapy, and in some cases can result in an ethics complaint against your license.

9.1.1.9. You Are Unbiased

Effective counselors are considerate of each client's lifestyle, culture, and religious preferences while remaining impartial in the face of their own personal preferences or beliefs.

If and when it makes sense, a competent counselor will seek to incorporate the belief of a client into a successful care plan.

9.1.1.10. You Seek Help Yourself

It is possible that you lack the experience necessary to manage every problem that a patient presents with.

Your patient is paying a hefty amount for counseling services, so you should treat them fairly and honestly. If you do not feel like you can help a patient with their problem, ask a colleague for advice or send the patient to a counselor who is more qualified to help them.

9.1.1.11. Proper Procedures Are Followed

Prior to starting any treatments or therapies, make sure you have the patient's informed consent.

In addition to being frequently mandated by law, it plays a critical role in assisting in the prevention of malpractice claims made against counselors.

9.1.1.12. Confidentiality Is Indisputable

A counselor never, ever compromises patient confidentiality—of any kind. While it is acceptable to use one client's case—possibly to demonstrate the efficacy of a recommended therapy—in another client's therapy, client names and specifics should never be disclosed. The recovery and progress of your patient will be the best indicators of the caliber of your counseling. Your relationship with your counselor and patient is also very important. Patients should become happier, perceive things differently, approach situations more optimistically, and be able to help themselves as sessions go on, rather than depending entirely on your advice to get them through difficult situations. They will be able to control their emotions, make wiser decisions, and maintain hope for the future.

9.1.2. Interviewing Skills: Non-Verbal Skills

Patient satisfaction is determined by the quality and effectiveness of communication between medical staff and patients throughout their hospital treatment. Complaints about healthcare services frequently center on communication problems. Since nutrition education is a key component of MNT, dietitians with strong communication skills can emotionally support their patients. When it comes to giving patients nutritional counseling, dietitians need to have the best possible communication skills. It is pointless to spend time interacting with a patient if they do not comprehend the information provided by the dietitian. It is crucial that healthcare professionals take dietitians' communication abilities into account and regularly assess their communication style. As a member of the healthcare team, a dietitian must not only have solid clinical knowledge and skills to provide patient nutrition care, but also excellent communication skills to help patients understand what you have to say. The most crucial quality that a dietitian should have is improved communication because they work closely with patients to help them make dietary changes.

Destiny is determined by attitude. When working with patients, a dietitian ought to have a cheerful disposition. Before the dietitian and the patient ever speak to each other verbally, nonverbal communication begins. Dietitians' body language and facial expressions convey a lot about them, and their level of intervention on any given day is entirely based on their mindset. It is easy to read body language, and the patient's acceptance of the treatment or counseling will depend on it. A smile bestowed upon the patient conveys the dietitian's upbeat demeanor and approachability. It is imperative that all dietitians in the healthcare industry have this ability and continue to improve it. Dietitian etiquette builds respectful relationships with patients and their families and goes beyond simple good manners. Gaining a patient's trust can be achieved in large part by showing kindness and empathy. When a dietitian treats a patient with civility and respect, it makes them feel more at ease and encourages them to communicate and engage with the dietitian more, which improves the patient's experience and yields better results.

Strategies for an effective non-verbal delivery:

- Posture;
- Movement;
- Gestures;
- Facial expression;
- Appearance.

Improving on body language:

- Keep an appropriate distance;
- Touch only when appropriate;
- Take care of your appearance;
- Maintain eye contact;
- Smile genuinely.

9.1.3. Listening Skills

Dietitians must be skilled in counseling to establish rapport and trust with their patients, which will help the patients adhere to nutrition therapies and change their eating habits. Effective communication involves both spoken and non-spoken elements in counseling. In verbal communication, one should actively listen to patients, speak clearly, and avoid using too much nutritional or medical jargon (e.g., monosaccharides or hepatitis), demonstrating empathy, understanding, and compassion, and having cross-cultural communication skills. Using facial expressions, body language, physical gestures, and eye contact are examples of non-verbal communication. Insufficient or nonexistent verbal and nonverbal communication can demotivate patients from adhering to nutrition therapies and altering their dietary habits.

Active listening to the patient is a crucial component of communication. Dietitians ought to urge clients to divulge any information they believe is essential for their appointment. It is not that patients listen to dietitians when they talk or explain about diets. Dietitians are crucial in providing patients with information about nutrition and stressing the importance of equipping patients with the skills necessary to control or reverse their medical condition through diet. Patients should feel reassured by dietitians' counseling.

9.1.4. Action Responses

The communication plans and strategies created during the preparation phase are expanded upon by response actions. The emergency's actuality, as well as how it has impacted the community and communication channels, should serve as the foundation for any response measures. The effectiveness of the overall humanitarian response should be supported by the design of communication response actions. Nutrition communication offers the framework to fulfill accountability responsibilities to impacted populations across nutrition programs through community engagement. The main goal of advocacy work should be to provide the necessary funding and favorable conditions to safeguard and enhance the nutritional status of impacted communities. Depending on the situation, it might be necessary to promote certain underfunded interventions. g. feeding practices for infants and young children in an emergency (IYCF-E), micronutrients, or particular underprivileged groups e.g., senior citizens.

9.1.4.1. Options for Communication in Nutrition Emergency Responses

Remember, emergency communication is most effective when high-quality, evidence-based messages are communicated through multiple channels or options.

- **Interpersonal:** Face-to-face, meetings, counseling, peer communication;
- **Participatory:** Street theatre, participatory video, dance;
- **Print Material:** Newspapers, posters, leaflets, flyers, newsletters; consider written or visual print depending on the literacy level of communities.
- **Radio:** Community, national and international, across all.

9.2. Counseling Process

Nutrition counseling is a continuous process wherein a health practitioner, typically a registered dietitian, collaborates with an individual to evaluate their typical dietary consumption and pinpoint areas that require modification. The nutrition counselor assists the client in making and maintaining the necessary dietary adjustments by offering information, educational resources, support, and follow-up. Supporting an individual in creating and sustaining dietary changes is the aim of nutrition counseling. A mental health patient may require dietary modifications to encourage better eating, to follow a therapeutic diet, or to prevent nutrient-drug interactions. A crucial component of treatment for people with eating disorders or chemical dependency is nutrition counseling. Individuals on certain medications, like monoamine oxidase inhibitors, which are used to treat anxiety and depression disorders, must adhere to a diet low in tyramine to prevent food interactions with their medication. Individuals taking medications for mental health issues may also benefit from nutrition counseling because many of these medications have the potential to cause weight gain or loss. Together, the person and the nutrition counselor evaluate the person's present eating habits and pinpoint areas in which adjustments are required. In addition to nurses, doctors, and health educators, registered dietitians are highly qualified to offer nutrition counseling because they have fulfilled specific educational and experience requirements.

9.2.1. Assessing Dietary Habits

Typically, nutrition counseling starts with an interview during which the counselor inquires about the client's usual food intake. Nutrition counselors evaluate typical food intake using various techniques. A list of all the foods and drinks a person has had in the last 24 hours is what is meant by the 24-hour recall method. A person may be asked by the nutrition counselor to recall what they consumed as their first meal or beverage the day before. Subsequently, the counselor notes the approximate quantities of all the meals and drinks the individual had throughout the remainder of the day. Energy and nutrient intake can be estimated using the 24-hour food recall. People frequently overindulge in or underestimate the amount of a given food, so a person's food intake on one particular day might not be representative of their daily food intake.

Occasionally, a food frequency questionnaire can give a more realistic impression of an individual's usual eating habits. The client may be questioned by the nutrition counselor about how frequently they eat particular food groups. For instance, the counselor might inquire about the number of servings that the client typically consumes of grains and cereals, dairy products, fruits, vegetables, meats, and fats in a given day, week, or month. Assessing food intake can also benefit from reviewing daily food records. A person maintains a written log of all the foods and drinks they have consumed in a specific time frame. Subsequently, the nutrition counselor can examine the real energy and nutrient intake using the food records. It is common practice to keep three-day food records spanning two weekdays and one weekend day.

9.2.2. Assessing Body Weight

Nutritionists can determine a person's body weight by comparing it to different weight-for-height tables. Generally speaking, a woman should aim for a body weight of 100 pounds (45 kg) for the first five feet (1.05 meters) of height plus an additional 5 pounds (2.03 kg) for each inch beyond that. For the first five feet (1.05 meters) of height, a man is permitted to weigh 106 pounds (48 kg), plus an additional 6 pounds (2.07 kg) for each inch beyond that. However, the frame size of an individual is not taken into consideration in this guide. BMI is one more metric for determining body weight. Weight in kg divided by height in meters squared yields the BMI. It is considered normal weight to have a BMI between 20 and 25, underweight to have a BMI <20, and overweight to have a BMI over 25.

9.2.3. Identifying Changes Needed

The foundation for identifying behaviors that require modification is established by the initial dietary assessment and interview. Sometimes, someone knows exactly what dietary adjustments are necessary, but they might need assistance in implementing the changes. At other times, the nutritionist can assist in enlightening a person about the implications of various food choices on their health. Together, the client and nutrition counselor identify what needs to change, decide what needs to change first, and Figure out how to make the changes. Dietary changes must be made gradually. A person may begin by making one or two simpler dietary adjustments in the initial weeks, then progressively add more or more challenging adjustments over the course of several weeks or months. For instance, a person might find it simple to go from 2% to skim milk or to make time in the morning for a quick granola bar or yogurt rather than skipping breakfast. Adding more servings of vegetables to your diet each day or learning to swap out high-fat meat options for leaner options may be more challenging adjustments. It is important to carefully consider each person's situation and background when making dietary changes. A person's worldview, religion, socioeconomic status, ethnic background, and group affiliation are some of the factors that influence their food choices.

9.2.4. Identifying Barriers to Change

The client and nutrition counselor discuss potential issues that might come up after determining the necessary adjustments. To alter eating habits, one could, for instance, plan ahead for social gatherings, buy new foods, involve others, or bring particular foods to work. Some common barriers to changing eating habits include:

- Inconvenience;
- Social gatherings;
- Food preferences;
- Lack of knowledge or time;
- Cost.

9.2.5. Setting Goals

Together, the client and the nutrition counselor establish behavior-based objectives. Instead of focusing on an absolute value, like reaching a specific body weight, goals should center on the behaviors required to make the intended dietary change. For example, a person whose goal is to avoid weight gain from taking certain medications may want to up their daily intake of fruits, vegetables, and whole grains. These adjustments would help stop weight gain while emphasizing necessary behaviors rather than weight itself.

9.2.6. Finding Support

It is recommended that family members participate in nutrition counseling sessions alongside the client, particularly if they are also responsible for the food preparation and selection. While making dietary changes and making food choices is ultimately up to the individual, success is more likely when family and friends are on board and understanding.

9.2.7. Maintaining Changes

The main challenge for the client includes making the initial dietary adjustments and keeping them up over time. The maintenance of dietary modifications can be facilitated by self-monitoring, reasonable expectations, and ongoing follow-up. Self-monitoring entails tracking eating behaviors and periodically comparing eating habits to desired goals. Maintaining a food journal on a regular or occasional basis gives the person a quick tool to assess eating habits and increases awareness of their eating behaviors. Occasionally, a condensed checklist may be utilized to ensure sufficient consumption of various food groups.

9.3. Tools for Nutrition Counseling

The field of nutrition counseling does not lack resources. A variety of sources, including government agencies, publishing houses, volunteer health and professional organizations, reviews published in scholarly journals, and professional networking sites, provide information on nutrition education materials. Additionally, organizations that support a particular food or food group and businesses that produce health products offer educational resources. The availability of educational materials is not the main issue, even though there might not be a teaching tool that fully fits a patient's learning profile. Dietitians are more frequently prevented from using a teaching tool customized to meet the individual needs of a client due to resources related to acquisition and storage.

9.3.1. Meal Planning Tools

Numerous clinical nutrition domains have used various nutrition education tool formats. These consist of exchange systems, menu strategies, counting techniques, and guidelines. Guidelines that offer fundamental knowledge to assist individuals in choosing healthful foods include the Food Guide Pyramid. They might provide some details about portion sizes and food preparation, but they won't have the same level of nutrient specificity as other sources. As a first-education tool, guidelines are useful when exact nutrient intake is not necessary. They might have enough information in them to help some people change their eating habits in a way that lowers their risk of illness and improves clinical indicators. Menus serve as a tool for providing customers with precise instructions on what to eat, including serving sizes, types of food, and preparation techniques. A few days' worth of menus that feature well-known foods and guarantee adequate nutrition can be prepared for survival education. The popularity of this approach is demonstrated by the number of patients who take great care to gather their tray menus during a hospital slay. The patient is typically consulted when using menu planning tools so that food preferences can be taken into account. In addition to being utilized at the practical and continuing education levels, menu planning can be integrated with other teaching modalities. Menu planning computer programs are now available; they take individual food preferences and nutrient prescriptions into consideration.

The use of counting techniques has grown in popularity recently. The conventional method of managing weight is calorie counting. Teaching materials for cancer prevention, weight management, and cholesterol reduction use fat gram counting. Although it was first thought to be a method for intensive insulin therapy, carb counting is now used for both initial and ongoing education in all forms of diabetes. Nutrition principles are taught through exchange approaches, which emphasize food groups over individual foods. The Exchange Lists for Meal Planning, which have been used for decades to educate diabetic patients, are a well-known example. A tool for instructing patients on how to choose a diet that satisfies a prescription for macronutrients is offered by the system. The exchange lists idea has been modified for use in weight management education and is occasionally used in conjunction with nutrient data found in prepared foods and recipe books.

In the Diabetes Atherosclerosis Intervention Study (DIAS), the plate model—a popular teaching aid in Europe—was found to be just as successful as the more quantitative exchange lists. The technique makes use of a visual aid that shows a plate split into three sections: two-quarters of the plate, one-half of the plate, and one-quarter of the plate. According to the guidelines, one-half plate should contain vegetables, such as salads; one-quarter section should contain starches; and the other quarter section should contain meat and substitutes. Fruits and dairy are served as side dishes. The Plate Model approach is a straightforward way to promote healthy eating choices and portion control. It has been modified for use in diabetes education. These tools come in a variety of versions to accommodate a wide range of unique learner characteristics. The most popular versions are those that have been translated into Spanish and simplified versions suitable for clients with low literacy or for initial education. Nutrition counselors can efficiently have a variety of teaching materials available to meet the needs of each individual client by investing in reproducible tools. Even more intriguing are arc computer software packages that offer resources for nutrition education. The provider can modify the content if it becomes outdated and customize materials based on patient characteristics, thanks to computer programs.

9.3.2. Skill Training

Nutrition education requires more than meal planning tools, even those that are carefully chosen and matched to specific learner characteristics. Individuals might pick up the necessary knowledge, but they might not have the practical skills to put it into practice. Learning how to read a nutrition label gives someone the skills needed to understand the information. It takes skill to apply that knowledge to choices made during meal preparation or at the point of purchase. If there are differences in the serving sizes of the two products, comparing their nutrition labels will require analytical skills. Further abilities are needed to incorporate the chosen food into the overall diet after using the nutrition label to choose a product. Tools for teaching clients a variety of nutrition skills are available in print, video, CD-ROM, and three-dimensional models.

However, some clients are unable to learn certain skills or decide not to. One good example is to plan your meals. Regardless of their level of education and training, some people find that organizing their meals makes it difficult to follow orders. "Just tell me what to cat" is their common complaint. Preprinted menus offer a solution in some cases. The American Diabetes Association introduced the first of their Month of Meals publications in 1989 and quickly added four more editions in response to the demand. Books offering low fat and/ or low-calorie menus are abundant, as well.

However, people who lack the interest or skills to prepare meals from menus are not served by menus. The challenge that many people face when incorporating complicated dietary recommendations into their meals was addressed by the Cardiovascular Risk Reduction Dietary Intervention Trial. The trial compared a prepared meal program that was nutritionally complete with two different approaches: (1) a diet that was prescribed to match the same nutrient levels as the prepared meals and (2) usual-care dietary therapy. When compared to the other two interventions, the prepared meals program produced noticeably higher weight loss, lower blood pressure, and improved lipid and glucose levels than usual-care therapy.

9.4. Nutrition Informatics

The administration of the data required by dietetics professionals to practice effectively and customize recommendations to unique needs of each patient is known as nutrition informatics. Furthermore, it guarantees adherence to electronic health record (EHR) regulations. Nutrition informatics experts work with a vast amount of health and nutrition-related data. They work with disease-related nutritional data, food allergies, weight loss recommendations, and more in addition to nutrition data, such as food analysis and nutrient analysis tables. The data that these specialists deal with is intended to make it easier for nutritionists to give recommendations that are specific to each patient's needs.

A wide range of healthcare practitioners use nutrition informatics data in practice in various ways. To assist physicians, nurses, and registered dietitian nutritionists in developing a customized dietary plan, critical data from a paticnt's EHR may be compared with information on nutrition, disease management, and other topics. These programs may help obese patients lose weight or help diabetic patients better control their blood sugar levels. In a hospital or other clinical setting, doctors, and nurses, for example, can use the data provided by nutrition informatics specialists to develop customized diet plans for their patients.

9.4.1. Need of Public Health in Nutrition Informatics

Most public health professionals are not familiar with the field of nutrition informatics. As a result, those in charge of making information science and technology decisions in the field of public health as well as other domains frequently lack a thorough understanding of the fundamental sciences and crucial experiences in this field. The public health community has only lately started to realize the importance of such awareness. This has influenced the creation of the current patchwork within all levels of public health agencies. The rapid development and widespread use of data management software, web-based resources, mobile applications, and nutrition information systems with a specific focus have all contributed to the increased awareness of the advantages of information and communication strategies that take a comprehensive approach in public health practices.

Nutrition informatics is not just limited to those who work in or have an interest in technology it impacts all areas of dietetics practice, for example:

- **Clinical:** EHRs, clinical decision support, telehealth.
- **Consumer-based:** Apps and wearables, m-health, social media.
- **Food and Nutrition Management:** Staffing and workload statistics, recipe analysis.
- **Public Health:** Disease surveillance, disease prevention, surveys.
- **Research:** Clinical trials, other data collection, and analysis.
- **Retail:** Consumer purchasing trends, sales history, inventory.
- **Public Policy:** Evidence-based policymaking, measuring policy outcomes

9.4.2. Informatics Specialist

An informatics specialist exhibits familiarity with user support, hardware, software, and standard technologies in addition to system design. Proficiency in the analysis, administration, and assessment of technology and applications, as well as knowledge of technology-related regulations, are examples of skills. Another is the capacity to act as a technological information resource for others.

9.4.3. Public Health Informatics Expert

Public health experts participate in research on nutrition informatics and collaborate with other healthcare providers to create innovative approaches and guidelines for the administration of data and information. Public health professionals may utilize nutrition informatics tools such as databases that hold the footprints of recognized pathogens, which enable prompt identification of the cause of outbreaks.

Global positioning systems provide precise coordinates for mapping, which aids in problem solving and decision making when determining the location of epidemics.

It is feasible to create algorithms that can be utilized to create best practices for the safe production of food by using clinical decision support. Social media can be used to quickly disseminate information to the public and field workers. These professionals serve as future nutrition informaticists' teachers.

9.5. Medical Record

The patient's history, clinical findings, diagnostic test results, pre- and postoperative care, progress, and medication are all explained in detail in their medical records. Everybody has a distinct record, some having significantly more data than others. Medical staff can have a significant influence on medical records since each doctor is unique and takes notes in a different way. Nonetheless, almost all comprehensive medical records share a few common elements.

- The medical record may include records maintained in an electronic medical / record system, e.g., an electronic system framework that integrates data from multiple sources, captures data at the point of care, and supports caregiver decision making.
- The medical record excludes health records that are not official business records of UC, such as personal health records managed by the patient (Figure 9.3).

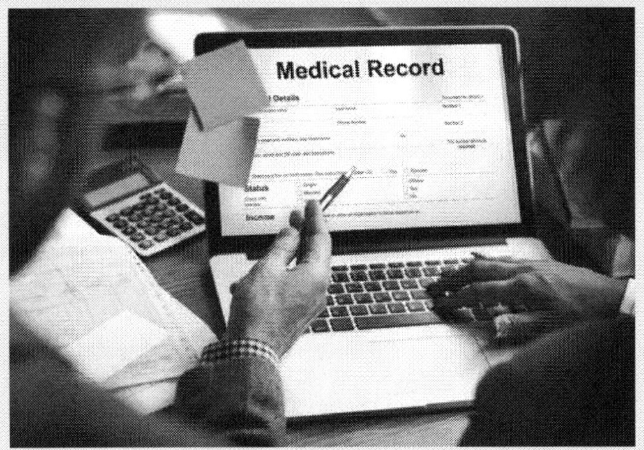

Figure 9.3. *A medical record.*

Source: https://us.123rf.com/450wm/rawpixel/rawpixel1609/rawpixel160968576/62855623-medical-report-record-form-history-patient-concept.jpg?ver=6.

Every medical record must have enough precise information to identify the patient, validate the diagnosis, explain the course of treatment, record the events and outcomes, and encourage continuity of care between medical professionals. Any source and any format, including but not limited to print media, audio/visual recordings, and/or electronic displays, may contain the information.

- **Designated Record Set ("DRS"):** A group of records that include protected health information (PHI) and that is maintained, collected, used, or disseminated by, or for, a covered entity (e.g. the UC Medical Center) for each individual that receives care from a covered individual or institution.

The DRS includes:

i. The medical records and billing records about individuals maintained by or for a covered health care provider (can be in a business associate's records);

ii. The enrollment, payment, claims adjudication, and case or medical management record systems maintained by or for a health plan; or

iii. The information used, in part or in whole, to make decisions about individuals.

9.5.1. Components of a Complete Medical Record

Almost everyone born in a hospital has some kind of medical history. A medical record contains all information of a patient's health and medical history. Medical records may differ based on the extent or necessity of a patient's care, but they will all share certain common details. Medical records are a vital piece of evidence that follows us around the world. In addition to being a legal document, they have some restrictions and rights that keep the information out of the wrong hands or from being shared illegally. In line with the U.S., only the individual or their personal representative may access these private records, according to the department of health and human services.

A medical record, to keep things simple, is a collection of data about the health and medical history of a patient. Patients will differ greatly in terms of the type, quantity, and level of information provided.

The amount of care a patient needs will largely dictate what documentation they need. Everybody has medical records, so it is important to know what information is in them and your rights when it comes to these important documents. It is equally important for industry professionals who might need to obtain medical records to familiarize themselves with these documents and comprehend their basic structure.

9.5.1.1. Identification Information

The first item on our list is vital identification information, which may not surprise anyone. Information linking a medical record to a patient is required. Simple examples of this include your name and birthdate, as well as any government-issued identification number, social security number, or state identification number.

9.5.1.2. The Medical History of a Patient

Everybody has a medical background. People with no medical history even have a history of not visiting a hospital or seeing a doctor. It appears that the absence of a medical history counts as a medical history. Nonetheless, most people living in the US do have a medical background of some kind.

This history could include:

- Past and present diagnosis;
- Medical care;
- Treatments;
- Allergies.

A patient's medical history includes even the times when they did not require medical attention. With regard to identifying which conditions or illnesses are acute, chronic, situational, or even seasonal, this information helps to paint a picture of the patient.

9.5.1.3. Medication History

A medical file also contains information about anything they eat or take in other ways that might have an impact on their health. This medication history may include herbal remedies, prescription or over-the-counter medications, and even illicit substances they have previously used. A portion of this data is obtained through patient testimonies, and some may be derived from previously written prescriptions that are already stored. The past use of medications by a patient can also provide insight into their current state of health and any potential complications. For example, certain drugs interact poorly with other drugs and may exacerbate existing symptoms or result in the development of new ones (Figure 9.4).

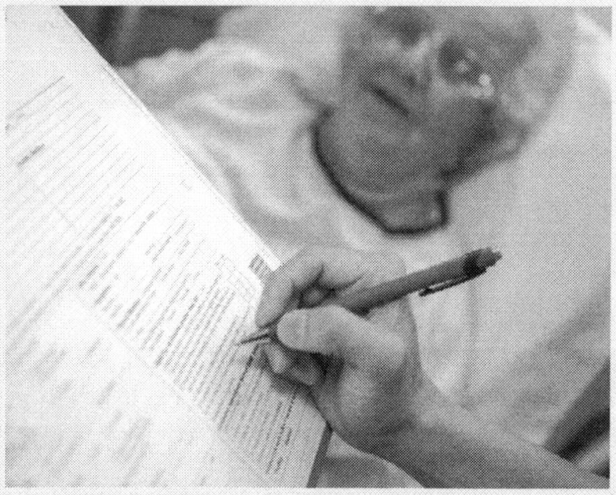

Figure 9.4. *Best possible medication history (BPMH).*

Source: https://geriatric-ed.com/bpmh-guide/.

9.5.1.4. Family Medical History

The medical history of a patient's family is extremely important to their health. Important additions are those that address health issues and concerns that are genetic in nature. Although the majority of family health issues are not cause for concern, certain cancers and other genetic illnesses can be inherited. Therefore, if available, a person's family medical history is frequently included in their medical records.

9.5.1.5. Treatment History and Medical Directives

Medical directives and the patient's treatment history are the last two essential pieces of information found in a medical record. Every treatment that has been administered, together with information about its effectiveness, should be included in a treatment history. Medical directives include things like a person's living will or DNR (do not resuscitate) orders. These are crucial records that specify a patient's desires and objections to certain treatments if they are unable to communicate.

9.5.1.6. What Are Medical Records Used For?

Though they are not the only pieces of information on these records, the previously discussed fundamental elements of medical records are the most typical. These records, along with any information that could enhance care, are crucial for helping present and future medical professionals understand the health and wellness of the patient. But there are other uses for medical records besides this. These are a few popular applications for medical records that are not related to healthcare.

Depending on the circumstances, medical records may be useful in legal proceedings. A well-known example of this is personal injury law, where records pertaining to a client's medical condition would undoubtedly be required in a court of law. Access to these records is subject to the consent of the individual. Finding medical records for legal purposes, however, can be a bit of a pain. Choosing the best medical document retrieval service can facilitate a quicker outcome.

Another area in which your medical records might be useful is insurance claims. When reviewing claims, insurance companies frequently ask for medical records to ensure that any associated medical expenses correspond with the claims. To view and review medical records, they will require a person to sign a release form. Medical research, Social Security disability, and even simple curiosity are other common uses for medical records. Yes, you can get your medical records—including your doctor's notes—if you would like to know more about what might be wrong with your health.

9.5.1.7. Understanding Health Insurance Portability and Accountability Act (HIPAA)

There are certain restrictions even though health information and medical records are private. The Health Insurance Portability and Accountability Act, or HIPAA, is a major player in the field of medical documentation.

This act was passed by congress in 1996 and continues to provide the following services for individuals around the country:

- Reduce any health care fraud or abuse.
- Creates and mandates the standard for health care information on electronic billing or any other processes.
- Protects and establishes confidentiality standards for protected health information, documentation, and records.

HIPAA covers a lot of various complexities involving medical documentation. You can visit the U.S. Department of Health and Human Services to learn more.

9.5.1.8. Medical Document Retrieval

It can be a bit of a hassle for businesses that need to access medical records. Retrieval can be costly in addition to taking a long time.

If you know how to do it correctly, this is not the case. The medical records must be obtained from the appropriate location. At American Retrieval, we recognize that HIPAA-compliant, secure, and quick document retrieval is essential for your business.

A dependable service for retrieving medical records is invaluable, whether you are attempting to win a case or settle a claim.

9.6. Standard Language and Medical Abbreviations

The language of medicine is crucial for advancing scientific knowledge and sharing clinical data. Connecting the worlds of the laboratory and medical practice through effective communication allows educators, researchers, and healthcare providers to stay up-to-date on advancements in practice, technology, and the sciences. However, a challenge arises due to the abundance of outdated terms, complexities, and conflicts in medical terminology, especially as research and clinical investigations expand rapidly. Medical terminologies are universal in the healthcare industry, providing a common language for all healthcare professionals to understand and communicate effectively. It is not limited to just doctors and nurses, but also essential for medical billers, coders, assistants, and other workers in the healthcare field. Those unfamiliar with medical terms risk being unable to perform their jobs effectively and may even jeopardize patient care. Accurate descriptions of the patient's condition and required treatments are provided by using medical terminology. In the event that healthcare personnel lack the necessary training and knowledge, there is a chance that patients won't receive the right care in the end. Communicating in a clear, succinct, and understandable manner is essential when working in a high-stakes, fast-paced industry like healthcare. Medical terminology guarantees that nothing is lost in translation and that medical and healthcare personnel speak a single, universal language.

- **How to Learn and Get More Familiar with Medical Terms?** Proper education about medical terms can bring the following benefits:

1. **Standardized Communication between Professionals:** Standard terms helps healthcare professionals understand patients' conditions and issues, help them decipher complex information to provide a more accurate diagnosis, and helps answer the following questions:
   - Why is the patient in the hospital?
   - What needs to be done to help the patient?
   - What treatment is recommended for the patient?
2. **Easy Documentation and Communication:** Medical jargon is filled with acronyms and easily transcribable terms, which are particularly helpful in a hectic work setting. Since medical terms are standard, abbreviations used by practitioners who deal with a large number of patients on a daily basis will still make sense to other practitioners in the field.
3. **Avoid Errors:** Not properly communicating or documenting medical records of a patient may get them in trouble and the patient might suffer larger health issues. Medical terms help describe the medical history of a patient through medical records and should the patient require additional care, these records help inform healthcare professionals details that can help them diagnose the patient more accurately and provide the appropriate treatments. Example: A doctor that learns that a patient is under certain medications or has been through certain medical procedures before, he would have a good idea on things like if there is medicine that should not be used.

9.6.1. Importance of Medical Terminology

Having a solid understanding of medical terminology is essential for anyone working in the healthcare industry, regardless of whether they see patients on a daily basis or never set foot in a clinic. When performing their daily tasks, employees in clinical and nonclinical roles in a healthcare system need to be able to comprehend written, spoken, and written medical terminology with ease. Medical terminology courses can help cut through the confusion that may surround words that seem like Latin nonsense to those who are not familiar with the field of medicine. Gaining knowledge of medical jargon can enhance your productivity at work or increase your appeal to employers seeking candidates for healthcare jobs.

Some of the top reasons to learn medical terminology include:

1. **Speaking the Standardized "Language of Medicine:"** All medical professionals can effectively communicate and understand one another thanks to medical terminology. Everyone can perform their jobs appropriately, such as delivering medication or billing for medication, when they all understand what a condition, medication, or procedure is. All staff members can fully comprehend staff communications and training—including infection control and HIPAA compliance training—if they are conversant in medical terminology. To establish a secure environment for both patients and staff, these trainings are essential.
2. **Improved Patient Safety:** Effective communication between all members of a healthcare team lowers error rates, which enhances patient safety. For example, it helps a doctor prescribe a safe, effective treatment for a patient if the doctor is aware of the patient's entire medical history, including surgeries or previous conditions. The care for a patient may significantly differ if terminology is misunderstood and the incorrect condition or procedure is entered into the chart. The course of treatment might be riskier or less effective.
3. **Improved Patient Experiences:** A team that includes members who are conversant in medical jargon can also assist the patient in understanding what those terms mean. Improved patient satisfaction results from patient education, which encourages patients to participate more actively in their care team. Understanding medical jargon can also help you avoid billing or coding errors that could require a patient to call you to fix, which would be extremely annoying for them.
4. **More Efficient Care:** Every day, medical personnel might see dozens of patients. Doctors and nurses may write quickly and scribble common abbreviations to provide care more efficiently. To deliver the best care, all members of the care team should be able to understand these terms and abbreviations.

Medical terminology frequently makes use of medical abbreviations. This can be attributed to the fact that most medical terms and phrases are rather lengthy. Sharing medical information with someone else is made quicker and frequently simpler with the help of these abbreviations. Until you study them and understand their meanings, the abbreviations may appear strange to you. You will soon be able to comprehend the meaning of the prescriptions you are on and the orders from other doctors. To differentiate an acronym from a similar one, remember that all abbreviations are case sensitive.

The following list contains some of the most common abbreviations found in medical records:

- AAD — "Average American" Diet
- AHS — Adventist Health Study
- Apo A-1 — Apoprotein A-1
- Apo B — Apoprotein B
- BD — Background Diet
- BMI — Body Mass Index
- BP — Blood Pressure
- BW — Body Weight
- CD — Conjugated Diene
- CHD — Coronary Heart Disease
- CHO — Carbohydrate
- CI — Confidence Interval
- CVD — Cardiovascular Disease
- DASH — Dietary Approaches to the Study of Hypertension
- DHA — Docosahexaenoic acid, 22:6n-3
- EPA — Eicosapentaenoic Acid, 20:5n-3
- EURAMIC — European Multicenter Case-control on Antioxidants, Myocardial Infarction and Breast Cancer
- F — Female
- FDA — Food and Drug Administration (U.S.)
- Fe — Iron
- FFQ — Food Frequency Questionnaire
- GISSI — Gruppo Italiano per lo Studio della Sopravivenza nell'Infarcto miocardico
- Hb — Hemoglobin
- Hcy — Homocysteine
- HD — Habitual Diet
- HDL_2-C — A Fraction of HDL-Cholesterol
- HDL-C — High-Density Lipoprotein Cholesterol
- IDL — Intermediate-Density Lipoprotein
- IHD — Ischemic Heart Disease
- IU — International Unit
- LDL_3–C — A Fraction of LDL-Cholesterol
- LDL — Low-Density Lipoprotein
- LDL-C — Low-Density Lipoprotein Cholesterol
- LF — Low Fat
- LFMR — Low-Fat, Monounsaturated Fatty Acid-Rich
- Lp (a) — Lipoprotein (a)
- LpL — Lipoprotein Lipid
- M — Male
- MBW — Mean Body Weight
- MI — Myocardial Infarct/Infarction

- MRFIT Multiple Risk Factor Intervention Trial
- M:S Ratio of Monounsaturated to Saturated Fat
- MUFA Monounsaturated Fatty Acid
- NHS Nurses' Health Study
- NO Nitric Oxide
- NOS Nitric Oxide Synthase
- P:S Ratio of Polyunsaturated to Saturated Fat
- UFA Polyunsaturated Fatty Acid
- RBC Red Blood Cell
- RD Reference Diet
- RDA Recommended Dietary Allowance
- RN Registered Nurse
- RR Relative Risk
- SD Standard Deviation
- SDA Seventh-day Adventist
- SF Saturated Fat
- SFA Saturated Fatty Acid
- TBARS Thiobarbituric Acid-Reactive-Substance
- TC Total Cholesterol
- TE Total Energy
- TF Total Fat
- UFA Unsaturated Fatty Acid
- USDA United States Department of Agriculture
- VLDL Very Low-Density Lipoprotein
- VLDL-C Very Low-Density Lipoprotein Cholesterol

9.7. Problem-Oriented Medical Record (POMR)

The problem-oriented medical record, known as the POMR, has been highly successful in helping doctors organize and review patient notes efficiently. This method, endorsed by the American Institute of Medicine, has been widely adopted by healthcare providers. However, as more doctors utilize computer systems to implement the POMR, limitations of this structure have become apparent. There is a clear opportunity to enhance the model to improve data quality and enhance its meaning. This chapter examines the shortcomings of the POMR and explores potential areas for expansion. The goal is to develop a more practical and user-friendly approach that can be easily implemented. Proposed extensions include incorporating encounters, episodes, subproblems, and a new perspective known as the Timeline. The chapter also clarifies the terminology used for these expansions and describes the mechanisms for implementing them. Suggestions are offered for automating the management of these extensions within healthcare systems. However, any enhancements to the POMR must be mindful of not disrupting the patient-doctor interaction and adhere to reporting requirements set by professional and governmental bodies. Additionally, practical considerations related to software and hardware limitations must be considered during implementation.

The comprehensive method of storing and retrieving patient medical data is known as the problem-oriented medical record, or POMR. The POMR was created in the 1960s by Lawrence Weed, MD, and is used to collect data from all members of the patient's care team to make a diagnosis and develop a treatment plan. A patient's history, a list of symptoms, test results, a treatment plan for each concern, progress notes, and a discharge summary with any necessary follow-up actions are usually included in the POMR. First described in 1968 by Dr. Lawrence Weed, MD, the medical record-keeping system dubbed "Problem Oriented Medical Records," or POMR, offers advantages to both provider and patients, not the least of which is a more patient-focused approach. However, many physicians object to its use as being too cumbersome, data synthesis restrictions, lengthy progress notes, etc. However, the proponents of this system insist that when used properly, POMR does just the opposite and results in concise, complete and accurate record keeping, especially with reporting and managing chronic care conditions.

The POMR arose from the recognized need for better management of chronic illness involving multiple encounters and interventions, increasing the need for tracking care over time while providing individualized medical solutions for each unique patient.

- **Problem Oriented Medical Records consists of the following components:**

1. A defined information data base
2. A complete problem list, further broken down into:

- Filter problems by status: current (either improving or worsening), dormant (no change) or resolved
- Grouped in chronological order, either by encounter date or entry date.
- As originally conceived, the system only allowed for one problem to be considered at a time. As many providers can attest, however, one visit can engender reporting of multiple problems.

3. A plan of action for every listed problem broken down into the following:
   - Basis;
   - Status;
   - Disability;
   - Goal;
   - Following the course;
   - Additional investigation;
   - Awareness of possible complications.
4. Notes on the progress documenting follow-up, feedback from patient and others and adjustments to the plan over time.

- **Limitations of the Problem Oriented Medical Records System:** Some possible limitations that cause POMR to be under-utilized include:
- The perception by providers is that the system, while usually quickly understood and learned in the first stages, is too complex overall to maintain once entries have begun.
- Multiple problems may be discussed by patients during a single visit ('encounter'). Some providers may feel overwhelmed by "data overload" as a result.
- Information may belong under multiple 'problem' headings such as blood pressure measurements showing under the headings of "ischemic heart disease" and "hypertension."
- There is often a need to link across entry boundaries, i.e.: when one 'problem' is caused by or closely linked to another, such as "pneumonia (secondary

problem) following prolonged bed confinement due to the operation for a broken hip (primary problem.)

- Working within the scope and limitations of the provider's own EHR system, including software and hardware reporting capabilities, as well as within governmental and other reporting constraints.
- **The Value of the Problem Oriented Medical Records:** The subjective/objective/assessment/plan, or SOAP note, is a type of documentation that enables clinicians to include notes in the patient record. In the context of today's EMR, the POMR is compared to this type of note. Along with the patient's medical history, test results, and other relevant data, the SOAP note in the POMR also includes the doctor's observations, a prioritized list of issues, and explanations for the problems' particular arrangement. Furthermore, it is divided into three distinct components for diagnostic, therapeutic, and patient-education plans. Medical solutions specialist, certified trainer, and HIT compliance officer at the Center for Computer Resources, the POMR was widely used from its inception through the 1980s. "The POMR was a functional way of documentation," she says. "Through to the '80s, a doctor could follow the format similar to that of the current SOAP note and be able to articulate his findings and recommendations by being focused on a problem—not just on the symptoms and facts around the problem."
- **Places for a Problem Oriented Medical Records:** Some settings are more conducive to POMR use than others.

Approach can create the following challenges:

- Failure to link conditions to underlying causes for accurate combination code assignments. "Congestive heart failure, for example, may be an entry in the problem-based record with the underlying cause (i.e., hypertension, valvar disease, ischemic cardiomyopathy) possibly entered as a separate problem and the conditions are not linked
- Listing a body system, sign, or symptom without associating a diagnosis. "For example, a physician may list the problem as renal rather than the associated diagnosis such as chronic kidney disease or acute kidney injury.

  Listing a differential diagnosis in a format that appears to be a definitive diagnosis: "You sometimes see a physician document UTI [urinary tract infection] without using uncertain terms such as 'possible' or 'likely,' then she or he stops treatment after negative cultures, but never says the UTI was ruled out.

9.8. Organization and Nutrition Document

A vital component of development and health is nutrition. Increased immunity, safer pregnancies and deliveries, a decreased risk of non-communicable diseases (like diabetes and cardiovascular disease), longer life spans, and better nutrition are all associated with better health outcomes for mothers, babies, and children. At baseline and 5 months into the project, medical records of residents in a nursing home ward were consulted to document the nutritional information. It was discovered that there was more documentation of specific nutritional treatment measures between the baseline and follow-up. There was a notable rise in the quantity of inhabitants who were under a nutritional care plan (NCP). Conversely, the research revealed a noteworthy decline in the percentage of inhabitants who had recorded their weight and nutritional condition.

9.8.1. Subjective Data, Objective Data Assessment Plan (SOAP) Documentation

A problem-oriented method called SOAP documentation is used by nurses to list and identify the health concerns of their patients. Primary health care settings frequently employ it.

Documentation is generally organized according to the following headings:

S = subjective data

Example: What is the patient experiencing or feeling, how long has this been an issue, what is the frequency, intensity, duration, what makes it worse or better, any past history, family history, home monitoring results (BP, weight, glucose monitoring), etc.

O = objective data

Example: Results of the physical exam, relevant vital signs, what the nurse observes, etc.

A = assessment

Example: What is the nursing diagnosis or medical diagnosis (for existing problems), identification of the problem, etc.

P = plan

Example: What interventions are done during the visit, what is the follow-up, what medications have been prescribed or changed, what further testing or investigations are required, when will the patient be seen again, etc.

9.8.1.1. A Sample Chart Note

S: In for refills and review of diabetes. Home glucose monitoring – taking BG readings three times/week in morning only (fasting). Average BG 7-8. Has been trying to avoid sugary snacks but has just quit smoking so is finding this difficult. Walking 5 times/week for 30 minutes.

O: Blood work – A1C 7.2 (was 7.3), LDL 1.9, Ratio 3. BP 118/70. HR 72 regular.

A: Diabetes (A1C not at target)

P: Provided with information on A1C, diabetes and targets. Provided with support and information related to nutrition and strategies to reduce sugary snacks. Reviewed blood glucose testing and will check postprandial sugars 2/week until next visit.

- Encouraged to book eye exam
- Due for foot exam next visit
- Increase metformin to 1000 mg bid
- Repeat BW in 3/12 (annual inc nephropathy screening) – encouraged to check glucometer with bloodwork
- RTC 3/12

9.8.2. The Problem, Etiology, Signs, and Symptoms (PES) Statement

A PES statement, also known as a nutrition diagnosis statement, is a structured sentence that identifies the particular nutrition issue that you, the dietitian, are in charge of managing and attempting to resolve, as well as the cause or causes of the issue and the supporting data. All nutrition assessments, with the exception of those that have "no nutrition diagnosis," require a PES statement. "

Three components make up the PES statement:

1. The Problem (P) – the Nutrition Diagnosis.
2. The Etiology (E) – the causes of the nutrition problem (Nutrition Diagnosis).
3. The Signs and Symptoms (S) – the evidence that the nutrition problem (Nutrition Diagnosis) exists.

The PES statement is a structured sentence, hence has a specific format to follow. Here is a sample of how to structure your statement:

- Nutrition diagnosis term (the nutrition problem) related to.
- The etiology (the causes of the problem or nutrition diagnosis) as evidenced by.
- The signs and symptoms (the evidence that the nutrition problem or nutrition diagnosis exists).

9.8.2.1. The Problem (P) – The Nutrition Diagnosis

The nutrition diagnosis pinpoints the particular nutrition issue that needs to be addressed and resolved by the dietitian. The nutrition diagnosis makes use of particular eNCP terminology. There are three classifications of the nutrition diagnosis: Intake, clinical, and behavioral.

- **Intake:** These relate to nutrition and intake related problems
- **Clinical:** These diagnosis include medical or physical conditions that have a nutritional impact.
- **Behavioral:** This category covers the nutritional problems associated with nutrition knowledge and belief (including attitude), physical activity and function (e.g. ability to self-care) and food access and safety).

The nutrition diagnosis should be specific to the role dietitian. The nutrition diagnosis is something that you as a dietitian can resolve (ideally) or improve.

9.8.3. The Etiology (E) – The Causes of the Nutrition Problem/ Nutrition Diagnosis

The PES Statement's initial letter "E" stands for etiology. "The cause, set of causes, or manner of causation of a disease or condition" is the definition of etiology.

The etiology pf the PES statement explains the reason behind the nutrition diagnosis. The goal of the nutrition intervention should be to address the etiology, or the root cause, of the nutrition issue.

Free text makes up the etiology statement. Etiologies are classified into groups based on the reason for the diagnosis.

There is no incorrect etiology statement, but it should include these general points:

1. The Etiology is the "root cause" of the Nutrition Diagnosis.
2. The Nutrition Intervention, should aim to resolve or at least attempt to improve the Etiology.
3. The Etiology is supported by the nutrition assessment data.

9.8.3.1. Signs and Symptoms (S) – Evidence That the Nutrition Diagnosis Exists

- Signs are objective data obtained through direct physical examination, observation, lab values and test results.

- Symptoms are subjective data reported by the client's or their families rather than actual results.

The PES Statement's signs and symptoms are free text, just like the etiology. The ability to recognize the Signs and Symptoms that indicate the existence of a nutrition diagnosis is crucial for dietitians. The diagnosis of nutrition should be supported by the signs and symptoms statement. To assess changes, it needs to be precise enough to be tracked and measured.

9.8.4. The Assessment, Nutrition Diagnosis, Monitoring/Evaluation (ADIME) Documentation

A: Assessment

D: Nutrition Diagnosis

- → Problem-high risk code assigned
- → Etiology-the cause of the problem or risk code
- → Signs/Symptoms-the evidence collected that trigger the high-risk code to be assigned

I: Intervention – Specific behavior change identified to address the Nutrition Diagnosis

M/E: Monitoring/Evaluation – next steps, follow-up information and referrals

- **ADIME Note Example 1:**

  A: Per mother, continues to offer formula in the bottle which she feels keeps infant fuller longer & sleeps better. Mother states infant eats well, likes mashed potatoes. Mother is surprised infant likes to self-feed. Offered three (oz) bottles of formula/day and 6oz apple juice/day.

  D: Limited adherence to nutrition related recommendations r/t infant feeding practices AEB mother offering cereal in the bottle with belief infant is fuller longer and sleeps better.

  I: Begin protein foods such as plain meat and beans. Recommended/encouraged to spoon feed cereal and avoid offering cereal in bottle.

  ME: No RD F/U unless requested by client. F/U on how introduction to protein foods went.

- **ADIME Note Example 2:**

  A: RD referral for Code 115. Mom feels child is growing perfectly, she agrees more with MD assessments that growth is WNL. Reports child digests 2% milk fine and MD has recommended Neocate three 8 oz bottles mixed to less than package directions. Tests indicated blood in stool and further tests are pending results, follow up in 1 month. Just moved to AZ from CA and MD's for child are in San Jose CA. Mom is hesitant to transfer care in middle of allergy testing. Brought Rx (not on WIC form) for 2% milk from MD in CA, approved for 1 more month, no duration listed. Mom is happy with the variety in his food groups except for grains, however, he eats corn and rice frequently.

D: Nutrition diagnosis of altered GI function r/t intolerance to high fat foods AEB blood in stool.

  I: Praised for offering a variety of foods and encouraged to continue. Discussed policies of AZ WIC for 2% milk and Neocate, RD will follow up with details of accepted out of state Rx's. Assured that corn and rice are grain foods. Discussed option to have WIC provide Neocate if prescribed by MD. Provided with 2 blank Rx forms for 2% milk and Neocate.

M/E: (1) Tell me about the results of the most recent testing. MD recommending to continuing Neocate?

(2) How do you feel about the amount of grains he eats.

9.8.4.1. Intervention, Evaluation, Revision (IER) Notes

IER is simplified version of SOAP.

- Intervention refers to what has been done for the patient and the patient's response to the treatment.
- Evaluation refers to the assessment part of SOAP, the diagnosis and evaluation based on the data gathered. It often includes a brief summary of the plan and an evaluation of the treatment's effectiveness.
- Revision of care refers to any changes recommended or ordered in the patient's treatment.

9.8.4.2. Problem, Intervention, and Evaluation (PIE) Notes

PIE (Problem, Intervention, and Evaluation) notes are also a blending of other types of charting.

- Problem identifies the specific nutrition problems for the client.
- Intervention refers to the nutrition treatments and steps designed to resolve the problems.
- Evaluation outlines the progress toward resolution of the nutrition problems.

9.8.5. Nutrition Charting Templates

Any nutrition practice has to maintain accurate health care charts. It's ideal to have a conversation that flows with your client, but it's also important to maintain an orderly and professional record. Using health care charting templates can help you save time, simplify record keeping, and make sure you're getting all the client data you need.

Here are a few reasons you may want to use health care charting templates:

1. **Better Direct Your Conversation with Your Clients:** You can use charting templates as a framework for your client conversations. You will be more familiar with the questions to ask and motivational interviewing prompts to use after assisting a few clients.
2. **Concisely Record the Information You Need to Know:** Nutrition chart templates save you from taking on the role of a transcriptionist. When your clients are talking, it could seem simpler to scribble everything down, but using a template makes it easier to get the important details.
3. **Maintain Better Records for Insurance, Physician Referrals, and Yourself:** Although thorough charting facilitates the process of submitting insurance claims, facilitating communication with referring providers, and helping you recall details if it has been a few weeks since you last saw your client, formal health care charts are not always required.
4. **Charting is Required for Insurance-based Nutrition Practices:** If you choose to accept insurance in your nutrition practice,

it is crucial to maintain accurate health care charts. In the event of an insurance audit, your chart notes will be examined. By using a charting template, you can ensure consistency in your documentation across all clients and guarantee that you are recording relevant client information. This practice will help protect both you and your business. Now that you recognize the significance of health care charting templates for your private practice, here are some key pieces of information that you may want to collect while taking notes.

5. **Charting for Initial Nutrition Consultations:** The charting for your initial nutrition consultation is probably going to be more thorough than the subsequent nutrition consultations. It is critical to obtain a comprehensive picture of your client's medical history and dietary habits.

We suggest including the following information in your initial nutrition charting templates:

- Reason for visit and nutrition goals;
- Diet history;
- Health history;
- Weight and recent weight changes;
- Current vitamins, supplements, and medications;
- Food allergies and restrictions;
- Current diet and lifestyle;
- Next steps or plan of care;
- Follow-up scheduled?

More simply:

- Nutrition history;
- Goals;
- Struggles;
- Next steps.

Having well-designed nutrition charts is crucial when explaining your treatment plan to other medical professionals. Charts used in healthcare are regarded as legal documents. It serves as evidence that you provided the best possible care for your client. Good charting techniques depend on capturing the data as soon as possible after it comes to mind.

A Closer Look

Meal Planning

Meal planning is a strategic approach to nutrition that involves thoughtful consideration of dietary needs, preferences, and goals to create balanced and nutritious meals. Taking a closer look at meal planning reveals its importance in promoting health, supporting dietary adherence, and facilitating efficient food preparation. The process typically begins with an assessment of individual dietary requirements, including energy needs, macronutrient goals, and any specific dietary restrictions or preferences. Based on this assessment, a variety of foods from different food groups, such as fruits, vegetables, whole grains, lean proteins, and healthy fats, are selected to ensure a diverse and nutrient-rich diet. Portion sizes and serving sizes are carefully considered to meet nutritional needs while promoting satiety and preventing overeating. Incorporating a variety of colors, flavors, and textures into meals not only enhances sensory appeal but also provides a wide range of essential nutrients, vitamins, and minerals. Meal planning also involves practical considerations such as budgeting, time constraints, and food availability, with an emphasis on finding convenient and affordable options that align with individual preferences and lifestyle. Additionally, meal planning can help individuals achieve specific health goals, such as weight management, blood sugar control, cholesterol reduction, or improving overall nutritional status, by incorporating foods that support these objectives. By taking a proactive approach to meal planning, individuals can make healthier food choices, reduce reliance on processed or convenience foods, and gain greater control over their dietary intake. Moreover, having a plan in place can alleviate stress and uncertainty around mealtime, making it easier to stick to nutritious eating habits and maintain dietary consistency over the long term. Overall, meal planning is a valuable tool for promoting healthful eating patterns, supporting dietary adherence, and fostering a positive relationship with food.

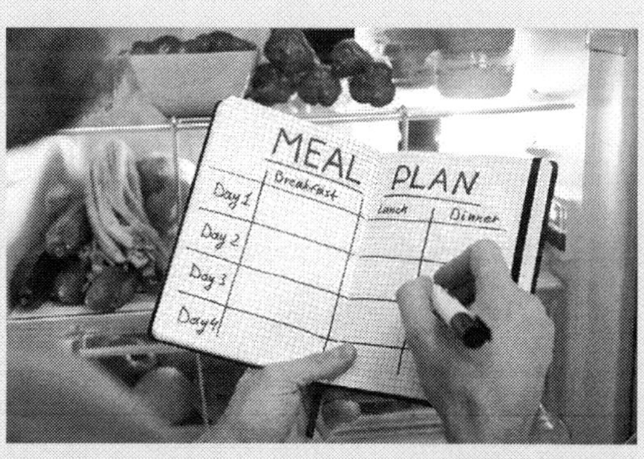

Source: *https://morningfresh.com.ng/wp-content/uploads/2020/04/meal-planning.jpg.*

Summary

- Nutrition counseling aims to help clients understand important information about their health and focuses on practical actions to address nutrition needs, as well as the benefits of behavior change.
- Dietary counseling provides individualized nutritional care for encouraging the modification of eating habits.
- The foundation of effective counseling is asking questions about the client's symptoms and situation to be able to give appropriate information and support the client to make healthy choices at home.
- The fundamental goal of counseling is to help individuals who are experiencing personal challenges be able to resolve them and improve their emotional well-being.
- Good and effective communication between the health professionals and the patients during their treatment journey in the hospital determines patient satisfaction.
- Good communication skills of dietitians provide emotional comfort to the patients as nutrition education is an important aspect of medical nutrition therapy.
- Counseling skills are a necessity for dietitians to build trust and rapport with their patients in order for the patients to comply with nutrition therapies and to improve their dietary behaviors.
- Nutrition counseling is an ongoing process in which a health professional, usually a registered dietitian, works with an individual to assess his or her usual dietary intake and identify areas where change is needed.
- Nutrition counseling usually begins with an interview in which the counselor asks questions about a person's typical food intake.
- Health care informatics was developed as an area of specialization within informatics devoted to management of health information.

References

1. Boaz, M., Rychani, L., Barami, K., Houri, Z., Yosef, R., Siag, A., Berlovitz, Y., & Leibovitz, E. (2013). Nurses and nutrition: A survey of knowledge and attitudes regarding nutrition assessment and care of hospitalized elderly patients. *Journal of Continuing Education in Nursing*, *44*, 357–364.
2. Duerksen, D. R., Keller, H. H., Vesnaver, E., Laporte, M., Jeejeebhoy, K., Payette, H., Gramlich, L., Bernier, P., & Allard, J. P. (2016). Nurses' perceptions regarding the prevalence, detection, and causes of malnutrition in Canadian hospitals: Results of a Canadian Malnutrition Task Force Survey. *JPEN. Journal of Parenteral and Enteral Nutrition*, *40*, 100–106.
3. Hall, A. M., Ferreira, P. H., Maher, C. G., Latimer, J., & Ferreira, M. L. (2010). The influence of the therapist-patient relationship on treatment outcome in physical rehabilitation: A systematic review. *Physical Therapy*, *90*, 1099–1110.
4. Hand, R., Abram, J., Brown, K., Ziegler, P., Scott Parrott, J., & Steiber, A. (2015). Development and validation of the Guide for Effective Nutrition Interventions and Education (GENIE): A

tool for assessing the quality of proposed nutrition education programs. *Journal of Nutrition Education and Behavior*, *47*, 308–316.

5. Holli, B. B., Calabrese, R. J., & Maillet, J. O. S. (2009). *Communication and education skills for dietetic professionals*. Philadelphia, PA, USA: Lippincott Williams and Wilkins.
6. Huebner, J., Marienfeld, S., Abbenhardt, C., Ulrich, C., Muenstedt, K., Micke, O., Muecke, R., & Loeser, C. (2014). Counseling patients on cancer diets: A review of the literature and recommendations for clinical practice. *Anticancer Research*, *34*, 39–48.
7. Johansen, N., Kondrup, J., Plum, L. M., Bak, L., Nørregaard, P., Bunch, E., Bærnthsen, H., Andersen, J. R., Larsen, I. H., Martinsen, A., & et al. (2004). Effect of nutritional support on clinical outcome in patients at nutritional risk. *Clinical Nutrition*, *23*, 539–550.
8. Lee, R., & Garvin, T. (2003). Moving from information transfer to information exchange in health and health care. *Social Science & Medicine*, *56*, 449–464.
9. Lu, A., & Dollahite, J. (2010). Assessment of dietitians' nutrition counselling self-efficacy and its positive relationship with reported skill usage. *Journal of Human Nutrition and Dietetics*, *23*, 144–153.
10. MacLellan, D., & Berenbaum, S. (2007). Canadian dietitians' understanding of the client-centered approach to nutrition counseling. *Journal of the American Dietetic Association*, *107*, 1414–1417.
11. MacLellan, D., & Berenbaum, S. (2003). Client-centered nutrition counseling: Do we know what it means? *Canadian Journal of Dietetic Practice and Research*, *64*, 12–15.
12. MacLellan, D., & Berenbaum, S. (2006). Dietitians' opinions and experiences of client-centered nutrition counseling. *Canadian Journal of Dietetic Practice and Research*, *67*, 119–124.
13. Mahan, K., & Raymond, J. (2017). *Krause's Food and Nutrition Care Process* (14th ed.). St. Louis, MO, USA: Elsevier.
14. McMahon, A.-T., Tay, P. C., Tapsell, L., & Williams, P. (2016). Building bridges in dietary counselling: An exploratory study examining the usefulness of wellness and wellbeing concepts. *Journal of Human Nutrition and Dietetics*, *29*, 75–85.
15. Murimi, M., Kanyi, M., Mupfudze, T., Amin, M., Mbogori, T., & Aldubayan, K. (2017). Factors influencing efficacy of nutrition education interventions: A systematic review. *Journal of Nutrition Education and Behavior*, *49*, 142–165.
16. Orell, H., Schwab, U., Saarilahti, K., Österlund, P., Ravasco, P., & Mäkitie, A. (2019). Nutritional counseling for head and neck cancer patients undergoing (chemo) radiotherapy—A prospective randomized trial. *Frontiers in Nutrition*, *6*, 1–12.
17. Patience, S. (2016). Advising patients on nutrition and healthy eating. *British Journal of Nursing*, *25*, 1182–1186.
18. Perry, L., Hamilton, S., Williams, J., & Jones, S. (2013). Nursing interventions for improving nutritional status and outcomes of stroke patients: Descriptive reviews of processes and outcomes. *Worldviews on Evidence-Based Nursing*, *10*, 17–40.
19. Ravasco, P., Monteiro-Grillo, I., & Camilo, M. (2012). Individualized nutrition intervention is of major benefit to colorectal cancer patients. *American Journal of Clinical Nutrition*, *96*, 1346–1353.

20. Ravasco, P., Monteiro-Grillo, I., Vidal, P. M., & Camilo, M. E. (2005). Dietary counseling improves patient outcomes: A prospective, randomized, controlled trial in colorectal cancer patients undergoing radiotherapy. *Journal of Clinical Oncology*, *23*, 1431–1438.

21. Rosal, M., Ebbeling, C., Lofgren, I., Ockene, J., Ockene, L., & Herbert, J. (2001). Facilitating dietary change: The patient centered counseling model. *Journal of the American Dietetic Association*, *101*, 332–341.

22. Ross, L. J., Mudge, A. M., Young, A. M., & Banks, M. (2011). Everyone's problem but nobody's job: Staff perceptions and explanations for poor nutritional intake in older medical patients. *Nutrition & Dietetics*, *68*, 41–46.

23. Rüfenacht, U., Rühlin, M., Wegmann, M., Imoberdorf, R., & Ballmer, P. E. (2010). Nutritional counseling improves quality of life and nutrient intake in hospitalized undernourished patients. *Nutrition*, *26*, 53–60.

24. Schofield, P., Diggens, J., Charleson, C., Mariglanie, R., & Jefford, M. (2010). Effectively discussing complementary and alternative medicine in a conventional oncology setting: Communication recommendations for clinicians. *Patient Education and Counseling*, *79*, 143–151.

25. Singh, S., Midha, S., Singh, N., Joshi, Y. K., & Garg, P. K. (2008). Dietary counseling versus dietary supplements for malnutrition in chronic pancreatitis: A randomized controlled trial. *Clinical Gastroenterology and Hepatology*, *6*, 353–359.

26. Sladdin, I., Ball, L., Bull, C., & Chaboyer, W. (2017). Patient-centred care to improve dietetic practice: An integrative review. *Journal of Human Nutrition and Dietetics*, *30*, 453–470.

27. Street, R. L., Jr., Makoul, G., Arora, N. K., & Epstein, R. M. (2009). How does communication heal? Pathways linking clinician-patient communication to health outcomes. *Patient Education and Counseling*, *74*, 295–301.

28. Tappenden, K. A., Quatrara, B., Parkhurst, M. L., Malone, A. M., Fanjiang, G., & Ziegler, T. R. (2013). Critical role of nutrition in improving quality of care. *Journal of Parenteral and Enteral Nutrition*, *37*, 482–497.

29. Volkert, D., Beck, A. M., Cederholm, T., Cruz-Jentoft, A., Goisser, S., Hooper, L., Kiesswetter, E., Maggio, M., Raynaud-Simon, A., Sieber, C. C., et al. (2019). ESPEN guideline on clinical nutrition and hydration in geriatrics. *Clinical Nutrition*, *38*, 10–47.

30. Xu, X., Parker, D., Ferguson, C., & Hickman, L. (2017). Where is the nurse in nutritional care? *Contemporary Nurse*, *53*, 267–270.

31. Barry, C. A., Stevenson, F. A., Britten, N., Barber, N., & Bradley, C. P. (2001). Giving voice to the lifeworld. More humane, more effective medical care? A qualitative study of doctor–patient communication in general practice. *Social Science & Medicine*, *53*(4), 487–505.

32. Bjorvell, C., Thorell-Ekstrand, I., & Wredling, R. (2000). Development of an audit instrument for nursing care plans in the patient record. *Quality Health Care*, *9*(1), 6–13.

33. Bjorvell, C., Wredling, R., & Thorell-Ekstrand, I. (2003). Experiences of using the VIPS-model for nursing documentation: A focus group study [corrected]. *Journal of Advanced Nursing*, *43*(4), 402–410.

34. Björnsdottir, K. (2001). Language, research and nursing practice. *Journal of Advanced Nursing*, *33*(2), 159–166.

35. Bueche, J., Charney, P., Pavlinac, J., Skipper, A., Thompson, E., & E., M. (2008a). Nutrition care process and model part I: The 2008 update. *Journal of the Academy of Nutrition and Dietetics, 108*(7), 1113–1117.

36. Bueche, J., Charney, P., Pavlinac, J., Skipper, A., Thompson, E., & E., M. (2008b). Nutrition care process part II: Using the International Dietetics and Nutrition Terminology to document the nutrition care process. *Journal of the Academy of Nutrition and Dietetics, 108*(8), 1287–1293.

37. Charney, P. (2012). Practice paper of the academy of nutrition and dietetics abstract: Nutrition informatics. *Journal of the Academy of Nutrition and Dietetics, 112*(11), 1859.

38. Chen, Y., Hsu, C.-Y., Liu, L., & Yang, S. (2012). Constructing a nutrition diagnosis expert system. *Expert Systems with Applications, 39*(2), 2132–2156.

39. Classen, D. C., Lloyd, R. C., Provost, L., Griffin, F. A., & Resar, R. (2008). Development and evaluation of the institute for healthcare improvement global trigger tool. *Journal of Patient Safety, 4*(3), 169–177.

40. Corado, L., & Pascual, R. (2008). Successes in implementing the nutrition care process and standardized language in clinical practice. *Journal of the American Dietetic Association, 108*(9), A42.

41. Ehrenberg, A., Ehnfors, M., & Ekman, I. (2004). Older patients with chronic heart failure within Swedish community health care: A record review of nursing assessments and interventions. *Journal of Clinical Nursing, 13*(1), 90–96.

42. Ehrenberg, A., Ehnfors, M., & Smedby, B. (2001). Auditing nursing content in patient records. *Scandinavian Journal of Caring Sciences, 15*(2), 133–141.

43. Enrione, E. B. (2008). Content validation of nutrition diagnoses. *Topics in Clinical Nutrition, 23*(4), 306.

44. Fesler-Birch, D. M. (2005). Critical thinking and patient outcomes: A review. *Nursing Outlook, 53*(2), 59–65.

45. Gearing, P., Olney, C. M., Davis, K., Lozano, D., Smith, L. B., & Friedman, B. (2005). Enhancing patient safety through electronic medical record documentation of vital signs. *Journal of Healthcare Information Management, 20*(4), 40–45.

46. Gingras, J., Asada, Y., Fox, A., Coveney, J., Berenbaum, S., & Aphramor, L. (2014). Critical dietetics: A discussion paper. *Journal of Critical Dietetics, 2*(1), 2–12.

47. Greenhalgh, T., Robb, N., & Scambler, G. (2006). Communicative and strategic action in interpreted consultations in primary health care: A Habermasian perspective. *Social Science & Medicine, 63*(5), 1170–1187.

48. Gunningberg, L., & Ehrenberg, A. (2004). Accuracy and quality in the nursing documentation of pressure ulcers: A comparison of record content and patient examination. *Journal of Wound, Ostomy and Continence Nursing, 31*(6), 328–335.

49. Gunningberg, L., Lindholm, C., Carlsson, M., & Sjoden, P. O. (2000). The development of pressure ulcers in patients with hip fractures: Inadequate nursing documentation is still a problem. *Journal of Advanced Nursing, 31*(5), 1155–1164.

50. Hakel-Smith, N., Lewis, N. M., & Eskridge, K. M. (2005). Orientation to nutrition care process standards improves nutrition care documentation by nutrition practitioners. *Journal of the Academy of Nutrition and Dietetics, 105*(10), 1582–1589.

51. Hammond, M. I., Myers, E. F., & Trostler, N. (2014). Nutrition care process and model: An academic and practice odyssey. *Journal of the Academy of Nutrition and Dietetics, 114*(12), 1879–1894.

52. Hellesø, R. (2006). Information handling in the nursing discharge note. *Journal of Clinical Nursing, 15*(1), 11–21.

53. Hughes, R., & Desbrow, B. (2005). Aspiring dietitians study: A pre-enrolment study of students' motivations, awareness, and expectations relating to careers in nutrition and dietetics. *Nutrition & Dietetics, 62*(2–3), 106–109.

INDEX

W

FSC
www.fsc.org
MIX
Papier | Fördert gute Waldnutzung
FSC® C083411

Kolibri 360 GmbH
Ferdinand-Jühlke-Straße 7
99095 Erfurt, Deutschland
produktsicherheit@kolibri360.de